Intensive Care

AN ILLUSTRATED COLOUR TEXT

D1581077

Commissioning Editor: Alison Taylor
Development Editor: Siân Jarman
Project Manager: Jess Thompson
Designer: Erik Bigland
Illustrator: Cactus
Illustration Manager: Merlyn Harvey

Intensive Care

AN ILLUSTRATED COLOUR TEXT

Michael Avidan MBBCh FCA
Associate Professor of Anesthesiology and Surgery
Division Chief, Cardiothoracic Anesthesiology & Cardiothoracic Intensive Care
Washington University School of Medicine
St Louis, MO, USA

Kara M. Barnett MD
Resident in Anesthesiology and Critical Care
The Hospital of the University of Pennsylvania
Philadelphia, PA, USA

Laureen L. Hill MD MBA
Vice Chairman, Department of Anesthesiology
and Associate Professor, Anesthesiology and Cardiothoracic Surgery
Washington University School of Medicine
St Louis, MO, USA

Lara Hopley MBBCh DA(SA) FCA(SA)
Senior Clinical Lecturer
Department of Anaesthesiology
Faculty of Medicine and Health Sciences
Senior Clinical Lecturer, University of Auckland
Department of Anaesthesiology and Department of Perioperative Medicine
and Anaesthesia, and Consultant Anaesthetist
Division of Anaesthesia and Perioperative Medicine
Auckland City Hospital, Auckland, New Zealand

Nicola Jones MD
Infectious Disease Physician
Nuffield Department of Clinical and Laboratory Sciences
Department of Microbiology
John Radcliffe Hospital
Oxford, UK

Johan Michael van Schalkwyk MBBCh FCP(SA) (Critical Care)
Perioperative Physician
Department of Perioperative Medicine and Anaesthesia
Auckland City Hospital, Auckland
New Zealand

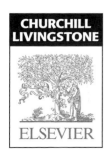

EDINBURGH   LONDON   NEW YORK   OXFORD   PHILADELPHIA   ST LOUIS   SYDNEY   TORONTO   2008

CHURCHILL
LIVINGSTONE
ELSEVIER

First published 2008

ISBN: 978-0-443-10060-4

British Library Cataloguing in Publication Data
A catalogue record for this book is available from the British Library

Library of Congress Cataloging in Publication Data
A catalog record for this book is available from the Library of Congress

Printed in China

Preface

Intensive Care Medicine is a new and rapidly evolving medical specialty. The intensive care unit (ICU) is the total body shop; it is where patients are admitted for an overhaul to recover from the most egregious insults, which in past times would have proved fatal. Patients on the ICU are generally the sickest in the hospital. They frequently have failure of multiple organ systems and present numerous diagnostic and management challenges. In order to increase the likelihood of a positive outcome, practitioners with diverse backgrounds and expertise contribute to the care of critically ill patients. Historically, anaesthetists, respiratory physicians and surgeons have run the majority of adult ICUs. As complexity of care evolves and as more sophisticated treatment modalities become available, there is increasing need for intensive care specialists and even sub-specialists. Advice on management in ICU is frequently sought from consultants from diverse specialties ranging from psychiatry to dermatology.

The global demand for intensive care is increasing apace. People are living longer and are expecting to live longer, even when they are stricken with severe illness. Frail, old people are undergoing complex surgery with an anticipation of returning to a healthy existence. Deadly infectious diseases, whose obituaries were written in the last few decades, are enjoying a sadly inevitable resurgence.

The chief authors and editors responsible for this book have global experience of working in ICUs on five continents: Europe, Australasia, North America, Africa and Asia. This eclectic experience coupled with their diverse backgrounds allows a broad and international perspective on intensive care medicine. The contributors to this book include intensivists, infectious disease physicians, respiratory physicians, anaesthestists (anesthesiologists in the USA), surgeons, ICU nurses, radiologists and ethicists. There is a rich collective medical knowledge base upon which this project is built.

This Illustrated Colour Text is intended to fill an important niche. It is designed as an entry-level textbook for practitioners who are plunged into the daunting ICU environment. Increasing numbers of hospital in-patients will be cared for in ICUs. The authors hope that this book will be accessible and will help medical students, student nurses and trainee doctors to overcome some of their trepidation about ICU. Like other books in this series, this book is designed to be informative, concise and clinically relevant. Each topic is covered in a double page spread. There are summary points and clinical case studies to provide context and to improve memory and understanding. While the book is by no means exhaustive, it provides a solid foundation and encourages readers to delve deeper into the varied and challenging areas of intensive care medicine. Relevant journal articles and further texts are suggested for most of the sections.

We hope that you enjoy reading this book as much as we have enjoyed writing it. We welcome your comments and feedback.

M. A., June 2007

Acknowledgements

It is hard to think that this thin book has taken so many people with such diverse expertise, ranging from medical to editorial, years to produce. It is challenging to write a crisp, creative and succinct illustrated textbook. The end product was the result of synergy, mutualism and, sometimes, disagreements. It was usually fun. It was always hard work. The staff members at Elsevier have consistently provided encouragement, creative input, editorial wisdom and constructive criticism. In the early phases, Joan Morrison kept prodding us and ensured that production never ground to a halt. Siân Jarman has been remarkable. Without her intervention, it is unlikely that we would have completed this book. She really engaged with this project and energized each and every author. The book would have faltered at the final hurdle without the input of Karin Skeet, our production editor. Like Siân, Karin has been far more involved with our book than could reasonably have been expected. Siân and Karin, we are truly indebted to you. The impact of this book owes much to the illustrations. We are grateful to Susan Tyler and Kate Nardoni for their insightful, funny and creative drawings. Michael Parkinson was the commissioning editor of this project. He has been consistently supportive of our efforts and we have enjoyed working with him. We look forward to building a constructive relationship with Alison Taylor, who has taken over the role as commissioning editor for this project.

We are also massively grateful to Maureen Arends who has an intimate knowledge of medical publishing. She has assisted with this project from its inception to its completion. It's not easy to coordinate authors who are dotted around the globe on three continents and to facilitate communication among them and the publishers in Edinburgh. Maureen also helped with editing and proofreading.

Apart from the authors listed on the cover of this book, many others – listed under contributors – have provided input to this book. We are deeply grateful to all of you for your magnificent offerings. Many of the contributors are world experts in their fields including medical ethics, echocardiography and trauma critical care. This book would have been much the poorer without the images provided by Doctors Humberto (Tito) Rosas, Tammie Benzinger and Christine Menias, all from the Mallinckrodt Department of Radiology at Washington University. Dr Li Ern Chen, a surgeon with a keen talent for photography, kindly helped with some of the photographs.

Finally, our thanks go to the many patients around the world who agreed to their photographs being published in this book. Their message was consistently, 'it is our pleasure if young doctors and nurses will benefit'.

Contributors

The following is a list of the clinicians who contributed to this book and sections that they co-authored:

Dr Ryan Fields	Fibreoptic bronchoscopy in the ICU
	Chest radiographs
Dr Kenneth Cummings	Oxygen delivery
	Endocrine emergencies
Dr Steven Schwulst	Carbon dioxide
Dr Scott Marrus	Electrolyte abnormalities
	Fluid therapy on the ICU
Dr Aaron Scifres	Neurological assessment
	Central nervous system injury
	Seizures
	Cholecystitis and pancreatitis
	Burns
	Trauma
Dr Stephen Streat	Organ donation
	Ethics: limiting and withdrawing treatment
Dr Frank Rosemeier	Ischaemic heart disease
Dr Charl De Wet	Heart failure in the ICU
Brian Torres	Arrhythmias
	Pacing
Dr Troy Wildes	Respiratory failure
	Toxicity: poisonings and overdoses
Dr David Fessler	Asthma
	Chronic obstructive pulmonary disease
Dr Marcus Tan	Gastrointestinal motility disorders
Dr Gordon Collins	Bleeding in the ICU
Dr May Hua	Inflammation

Contents

Introduction 1

The history of intensive care 2

What is intensive care? 4

Safety and quality in the ICU 7

Evidence-based intensive care 8

Critical care transport 10

Drug interactions 12

Evaluation of the ICU patient 15

Clinical excellence 16

Monitoring in the ICU 18

ICU procedures 21

The airway in ICU 22

Vascular access in the ICU 24

Fibreoptic bronchoscopy in the ICU 26

Cerebrospinal fluid, lumbar puncture and lumbar drain 28

Organ support 31

Mechanical ventilation 32

Renal replacement therapy 34

Mechanical circulatory support 36

Homeostasis 39

Circulation 40

Oxygen delivery 42

ICU acid–basics 44

Carbon dioxide 46

Thermal disorders 48

Food, salt and fluids 51

Feeding and starving in ICU 52

Electrolyte abnormalities 54

Fluid therapy in the ICU 58

Blood and blood components 60

Central nervous system 63

Neurological assessment 64

Central nervous system injury 66

Weakness in the ICU 68

Seizures 70

Altered mental states 72

Analgesia in the ICU 74

ICU sedation 76

Organ donation 78

Cardiovascular system 81

Monitoring the cardiovascular system 82

Ischaemic heart disease 84

Heart failure in the ICU 86

Arrhythmias 88

Pacing 90

Cardiac surgery 92

Pulmonary hypertension 94

Valvular and congenital heart disease 96

Respiratory system 99

Respiratory failure 100

Asthma 102

Chronic obstructive pulmonary disease 104

The ICU chest radiograph 106

Gastrointestinal/renal system 109

Renal failure 110
Gastrointestinal bleeding 112
Gastrointestinal motility disorders 114

Cholecystitis and pancreatitis 116
Liver failure 118

Endocrine system 121

Endocrine function in the ICU 122
Diabetes mellitus in the ICU 124

Endocrine emergencies 126

Haematological system 129

Clotting and bleeding: a delicate balance 130
Bleeding in the ICU 132

Thrombosis in the ICU 134

Infection 137

Prevention and treatment of infections 138
Sepsis and septic shock 140
Central nervous system infection 144
Pneumonia 146

Infections associated with prosthetic material in the ICU 148
The immunocompromised patient in critical care 150
Tropical medicine 152
Clever bugs and defunct drugs 154

Special topics 157

Inflammation 158
Burns 160
Obstetric critical care 162
Toxicity: poisonings and overdoses 164

Deliberate attacks: chemicals, radiation and bioterrorism 166
Advanced cardiac life support 168
Ethics: limiting and withdrawing treatment 170
Trauma 172

Appendix 1: Reference material 174

Appendix 2: Clinical case answers 184

Index 193

Introduction

The history of intensive care

The first intensive care unit (ICU)

Intensive care represents the coming together of many disciplines and many aspects of care. Because of this synergy, it is difficult to pinpoint where and when ICUs started, but many would choose Copenhagen on 27 August 1952. A poliomyelitis epidemic was raging and, after an initial, horrendous mortality of 87% (27 of the first 31 cases), interdisciplinary cooperation emerged, leading to a specific ventilatory 'ICU' unit.

Henry Lassen, a physician, reluctantly sought the help of Björn Ibsen, an anaesthetist. Ibsen pointed out that patients were dying from the inability to ventilate their lungs, with accumulation of carbon dioxide. Ibsen proposed hand ventilation using cuffed endotracheal tubes inserted via tracheostomy (Fig. 1). On 27 August, Ibsen graphically demonstrated the merits of this approach on 12-year-old Vivi Ebert, dying of polio. Physicians, anaesthetists and surgeons then cooperated in setting up a ventilatory facility, allowing up to 70 patients at a time to be hand ventilated by nurses and medical and dental students working in 6-h shifts. The mortality rate dropped to 25% or less.

In addition to tracheostomy, tracheal intubation, suctioning of secretions and manual ventilation, many other components of critical care came to the fore soon afterwards. Engström's positive pressure ventilator was shown to work well. Astrup's innovation was to determine pH in blood and then repeat the measurement at a *known* partial pressure of CO_2 – which allowed the original P_{CO_2} to be determined.

There have been counterclaims about 'intensive care' preceding the Danish effort at Blegdamshospitalet and the subsequent establishment of a unit by Ibsen at the Kommunehospitalet in 1953. For example, Johns Hopkins University in Baltimore asserts that a postoperative neurosurgical unit established in 1928 by Walter Dandy was the first ICU, a burns 'ICU' was created at the Massachusetts General Hospital in 1942 after the tragic Coconut Grove fire, and many hospitals temporarily established facilities to manage victims of poliomyelitis epidemics in the 1940s and 1950s.

Technical components of intensive care – a few highlights

Cardiovascular monitoring and support

In the 1960s, interest proliferated in the monitoring of heart rhythm after myocardial infarction, and resuscitation from ventricular fibrillation. 'Coronary care' units were established worldwide. These developments were incited by the work of Zoll, who showed that *external* direct current (DC) countershock can terminate ventricular fibrillation and, to some extent, by the work of Safar and colleagues on mouth-to-mouth resuscitation, and Jude's demonstration of closed-chest cardiac massage.

There were numerous other important developments between 1950 and 1970. The first cardiac pacemaker was created by Hopps, Bigelow and Callaghan in 1950. The first successful open heart surgery was performed by John Gibbon on 6 May 1953, and the Starr–Edwards valve was used successfully in the early 1960s. In 1970, Swan and Ganz developed their controversial catheter, over 50 years after Forssmann performed the first cardiac catheterisation. Swan apparently had the idea watching a yacht in the bay, on one of his rare days off from the ICU! Refinements and new ideas followed thick and fast.

Ventilatory monitoring

Although pH electrodes had been constructed in 1909 by Haber and Klemensiewicz, and blood pH was measured by Kerridge in 1925, commercial measurement of blood pH only became available in the 1950s. Using blood pH, and blood carbon dioxide content measured by the Van Slyke method, it became possible to work out the partial pressure of carbon dioxide in blood. This approach was first utilised on a large scale in 1952 in the Copenhagen polio epidemic. The first O_2 electrode was created by Clark in 1952, and Stow devised a CO_2 electrode in 1957. The pulse oximeter was created in 1972 by Takuo Aoyagi, after he had brilliantly worked out its principles of operation.

Renal replacement therapy

Thomas Graham first described the *process* of dialysis (and invented the term) in 1861, but an artificial kidney was not developed until 1913 by Abel, Rowntree and Turner. They tested it on rabbits, using the crushed heads of leeches (hirudin) for anticoagulation. A 15-min human dialysis was performed by Haas in 1924, but it took nearly 20 more years before Kolff created a practical machine based on cellulose acetate sausage skin (1943), working in the Netherlands during the Nazi occupation. He was motivated to do so after helplessly watching the slow uraemic death of a 22-year-old man he was caring for. The first life saved by dialysis was that of a 67-year-old woman dialysed by Kolff in 1945. Refinements and acceptance took years. In 1962, Scribner invented both the shunt named after him and the bioethics committee.

Other vital components – a few highlights

Adrenaline (epinephrine) was discovered by Cybulski in 1895, and rediscovered several times after this (by Abel, Takamine and von Furth). Takamine purified and patented it, and injection of adrenaline of varying purity was introduced shortly thereafter. Inhalation of adrenaline for its beta-agonist effect was only introduced by Graeser and Rowe in 1935. Takamine's original adrenaline isolate was contaminated by noradrenaline (norepinephrine), which was identified in sympathetic neurones in 1946.

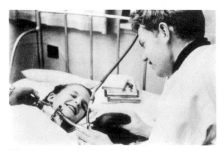

Fig. 1 **Manual ventilation of a poliomyelitis patient in 1952.** From Severinghaus JW, Astrup P, Murray JF (1998) *Am J Respir Crit Care Med* 157(4): S114–S122, with permission.

Feeding in ICU has often been desultory. When enteral feeding failed for a prolonged time, this was a death sentence until the 1960s, when Dudrick and Roads introduced total parenteral nutrition. In addition to amino acids (Robert Elman had shown in the 1930s that protein lysates could safely be given intravenously) and glucose, stable intravenous fat solutions were now available (Intralipid), and made all the difference.

Blood transfusion was described several centuries ago, but the history of the procedure is chequered with deplorable incidents often involving the death of the recipient and, it is said, sometimes even of the donors! Landsteiner made the necessary advance when he described the ABO system in 1901, and Ottenberg performed the first typed, cross-matched transfusion in 1907. Transfusion of stored, cooled blood was first used in England in 1916. Kolff may have been the first person to start a transfusion service in continental Europe.

Infection control long antedates antibiotic therapy, and preceded intensive care by 100 years. In 1847, Semmelweiss demonstrated that handwashing dramatically lowers death rates from puerperal sepsis (Fig. 2).

The antimicrobial era started in 1932 with the discovery and *use* of sulphonamides by Domagk. He gave the red dye prontosil, which was metabolised within the body to the active agent sulphanilamide. Although penicillin was discovered by Fleming in 1928, its use as a life-saving antibiotic was delayed until March 1942, because purification in sufficient quantities was immensely difficult. Purification was finally achieved by Heatley, Florey and Chain. (All except Heatley received the Nobel prize.) Penicillin achieved prominence when it was used after the Coconut Grove fire in November 1942, and was then used willy-nilly so that, by the end of the decade, many strains of *Staphylococcus aureus* were already resistant to penicillin. This pattern has been repeated again and again with every antibiotic coming into use.

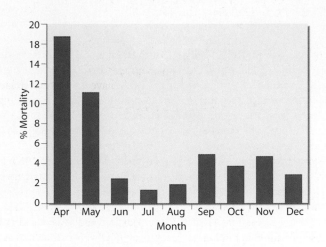

Fig. 2 **Death rates from puerperal sepsis** in patients cared for by doctors at the Vienna lying-in hospital, 1847. Handwashing was introduced in May. Adapted from Noskin GA, Peterson LR (2001) *Emerg Infect Dis* 7(2): 354–357.

care is more about identifying seriously ill patients, and segregating them from less ill patients in an area where dedicated staff can look after them, then intensive care may go back further than many realise. For example, in 1854, Florence Nightingale defined the concept of keeping patients recovering from surgery in a separate part of the hospital. During the Second World War, injured soldiers were segregated in 'shock wards'.

Significant dates in ICU

- 1895: Adrenaline discovered.
- 1907: First typed, cross-matched blood transfusion
- 1932: Start of the antimicrobial era.
- 1942: Therapeutic use of penicillin.
- 1943: First practical dialysis.
- 1950: First pacemaker.
- 1952: First ICU; blood pH and P_{CO_2} determination.
- 1953: First successful open heart surgery.
- 1960: Coronary care units, total parenteral nutrition.
- 1970: Swan–Ganz catheter.
- 1972: Pulse oximeter.
- 2000+: 'Human factor' engineering.

'history'. There are many possible scenarios but, whatever happens, it is highly likely that ICU will remain an expensive and constrained resource. Advances will come largely through encouraging a culture of safety and communication, with a well-balanced utilisation of modern technology to 'first do no harm' (see p. 16).

As at the start, we need a vital synergy between all the experts the world has to offer. This includes all the traditional 'medical and paramedical' personnel, as well as human factor, communication and engineering experts, to name only a few.

ICU as organisation

The previous sections have concentrated on the 'therapy' component of ICU. If we take the alternative, entirely reasonable perspective that intensive

ICU – back to the future

As with taking a history from a patient, we must not only dwell in the past: we should also look to the future and include what *will* happen in the

Summary points

- Major technical and pharmacological advances currently allow us to monitor and support nearly every organ system within our patients.
- The intensive care of patients has been a synergistic melding of every different speciality, all with their own exceptional contributions, since the beginning of 'modern medicine'.
- Untold lives have been saved by the combination of sheer genius and unmitigated hard work, and yet we still have much to learn.

What is intensive care?

Intensive care is commonly seen as synonymous with 'having a patient on a ventilator'. Although such a perception correctly emphasises the importance of support for a failing system, here the respiratory system, it falls far short of a good definition of an intensive care unit (ICU) for three reasons. The first is that critically ill patients may require support of a variety of other organ systems, and may well *not* be on a ventilator. Keen anticipation of and fending off problems may well prevent the need for ventilatory support! The second limitation is that it neglects the most important component of ICU: the *staff!* The third limitation is that it ignores the process of patient care (Box 1), which is a complex interaction of competing and complementary systems.

As the name 'intensive care' suggests, a key component of an ICU is having adequate levels of 'care'. Again, there are many different views of what constitutes such care, but emphasis is often placed on staffing ratios, the number of nurses per patient. A critically ill patient will usually require a dedicated nurse to observe and manage them, but patients on complex support (for example, ventilatory support combined with the use of an intra-aortic balloon pump and multiple complex infusions) may require two or three nurses in attendance. As important as having sufficient provision of staff is having a sufficient level of competence within the staff.

What ICU is *not!*

Some place great emphasis on the ICU environment and equipment available (Box 2), but such an approach is fallacious, as it again de-emphasises the critical role of good staff (particularly good nursing staff) in the delivery of intensive care. Good staff can deliver intensive care even in a locale that is far from ideal (although this is not advisable), but no amount of fancy equipment can compensate for inadequate staff numbers, training or commitment.

The ICU as part of the hospital

An ICU cannot exist divorced from the hospital(s) it services, so a vital, but often neglected component of an ICU is its interface with the 'rest of the hospital'. As intensive care resources become constrained, such an interface becomes ever more valuable.

Intensive care is often seen as the 'last resort' for placement of seriously ill patients, but the role of the unit should be different and greater. If there is sufficient resource, then intensive care specialists can provide valuable input on patients outside ICU, changing their trajectory and forestalling deterioration and ICU admission.

In addition, a fully functional ICU can derive great benefit from input by a variety of external experts within the hospital, including nutrition experts, infectious disease specialists, pulmonologists, cardiologists, renal physicians and many others.

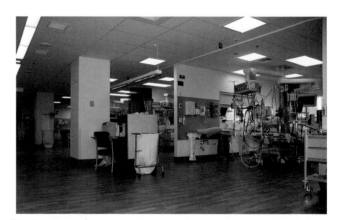

Fig. 1 **A modern ICU is well laid out, functional and well lit.** Reproduced with permission.

Box 1. *Intensive care as a process – the interplay between the various systems is intricate*

- *Patients* who are seriously ill, often with multiple organ systems that are compromised or where compromise is anticipated.
- *Staff members* who are suitably trained and present in sufficient numbers to care for the patients. This includes not only nurses and doctors, but also dieticians, physiotherapists, pharmacists, laboratory staff and health care assistants.
- *Equipment* and staff for sterilisation, maintenance and calibration of equipment are vital components of safety structures (see Box 2 for equipment).
- *Safety considerations* including guidelines and protocols, physical factors, patient and other alarms and responses to such alarms (including fire alarms).
- The *ICU's physical environment*, which has a size, position and other ergonomic characteristics (such as natural lighting) that make it conducive to patient care and staff comfort (Fig. 1).
- A *management structure* that ensures a flow of information, assessment of outcomes and feedback of information to interested parties and continually strives to improve the quality and cost-effectiveness of care.

Box 2. *Commonly encountered facilities in the ICU*

- Appropriate beds, scales and blankets (including forced air warming);
- Numerous monitoring devices (p. 18);
- Equipment for airway manipulation and ventilatory support (pp. 22 and 32);
- Emergency resuscitative equipment and suction (p. 10);
- Equipment for fluid management and haemodynamic support (pp. 24, 36, 40, 58 and 87);
- Temporary pacing devices (p. 90);
- Dialysis and ultrafiltration (p. 110);
- Intracranial pressure monitoring (p. 28);
- Continuous electroencephalogram monitoring capability (p. 70);
- Positive and negative pressure isolation rooms;
- Immediate access to information including medical records, poison databases, contact numbers of crucial personnel.

Open and closed units

There are two possible strategies for managing admissions to and discharges from ICU:

- The 'closed' unit, where admissions and discharges are regulated by senior ICU staff, usually under the governance of an ICU director.
- The 'open' unit, where such admissions (and often discharges) are controlled in full or in part by the primary physician (or others) who does not work primarily in intensive care. The management of the patient is predominantly that of the primary physician with input from the critical care specialist.

There is now evidence that ICUs under the control of an ICU director have better outcomes than those operating in other situations, so it seems reasonable to recommend this as the preferred strategy (Fig. 2).

ICU functioning

An advantage of seeing the ICU as a process is that one is then inclined to ask questions about the process, particularly:

1 What is the input into the process?
2 What is happening during the process?
3 How might functioning be improved?
4 What comes out?

Commonly, emphasis is correctly placed on patient outcomes. We must however remember that monitoring of staff outcomes is as important, particularly if the ICU is to continue functioning viably. There is no point in having a superb ICU where patients have optimal outcomes if permanent staff members all 'burn out' after 5 years, and junior staff hate the experience and leave vowing never to return. Some studies show higher levels of burnout in ICU than in other nursing settings, but others show the converse – a lot seems to depend on the particular unit, and perceptions by the nurses and doctors that they control their destiny!

Another neglected effect of the ICU is that on family members of patients in ICU. Staff who work there every day often rapidly become 'acclimatised', but family members may find even brief attendance stressful and intimidating.

A human factor and safety culture approach to improving functioning within the ICU is starting to highlight the competing systems involved within the process. These can now be used to allow the systems to support and facilitate each other (see p. 16).

Summary points

- Intensive care is more than just an isolated time period of patient care, and it is not simply 'the place where organ support is achieved'.
- Intensive care is the process of caring for the patients within the hospitals that an ICU serves. This involves pre-empting patients' deterioration and supporting their continued improvement after discharge.
- 'Closed' units may function more safely and efficiently than 'open' ones.
- The systems approach to patient safety and staff well-being is starting to change the structure and function of modern intensive care.

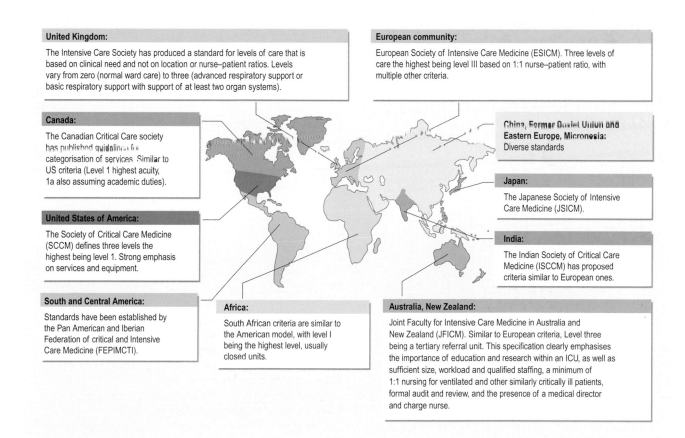

United Kingdom:

The Intensive Care Society has produced a standard for levels of care that is based on clinical need and not on location or nurse–patient ratios. Levels vary from zero (normal ward care) to three (advanced respiratory support or basic respiratory support with support of at least two organ systems).

European community:

European Society of Intensive Care Medicine (ESICM). Three levels of care the highest being level III based on 1:1 nurse–patient ratio, with multiple other criteria.

Canada:

The Canadian Critical Care society has published guidelines for categorisation of services. Similar to US criteria (Level 1 highest acuity, 1a also assuming academic duties).

China, Former Soviet Union and Eastern Europe, Micronesia: Diverse standards

Japan:

The Japanese Society of Intensive Care Medicine (JSICM).

United States of America:

The Society of Critical Care Medicine (SCCM) defines three levels the highest being level 1. Strong emphasis on services and equipment.

India:

The Indian Society of Critical Care Medicine (ISCCM) has proposed criteria similar to European ones.

South and Central America:

Standards have been established by the Pan American and Iberian Federation of critical and Intensive Care Medicine (FEPIMCTI).

Africa:

South African criteria are similar to the American model, with level I being the highest level, usually closed units.

Australia, New Zealand:

Joint Faculty for Intensive Care Medicine in Australia and New Zealand (JFICM). Similar to European criteria, Level three being a tertiary referral unit. This specification clearly emphasises the importance of education and research within an ICU, as well as sufficient size, workload and qualified staffing, a minimum of 1:1 nursing for ventilated and other similarly critically ill patients, formal audit and review, and the presence of a medical director and charge nurse.

Fig. 2 **ICU around the world.**

Safety and quality in the ICU

Evidenced-based intensive care

Medicine is a science, albeit an imprecise science. One of the major criticisms levelled at intensive care medicine is the paucity of evidence driving practice in the intensive care unit (ICU). This is valid, and it is important that health professionals in the ICU conduct well-designed clinical research to attempt to answer some of the many uncertainties with which we are faced. It is also necessary to keep an open mind and a balanced perspective. There are those who promote evidence-based medicine with religious fervour. Doubtless there is some merit to their missionary zeal; doctors have traditionally been reluctant to embrace the scientific method, preaching that medicine is an art. But, in science especially, there is room for uncertainty. If physicists can accept doubt in quantum mechanics, health professionals should accede that evidence cannot be applied uniformly to human beings who are diverse in their genetic makeup and whose individual responses to therapies may be unpredictable (Fig. 1).

When the Prowess study was published in the *New England Journal of Medicine* in 2000, many of us were lobbying our hospitals to free up activated protein C because it would decrease the mortality in sepsis by a staggering 8%. We did not stop to consider the cost of applying this expensive therapy across the board. Nor did we go into some of the controversies surrounding the conduct of the study. We did not consider the bleeding risks associated with the intervention. And we were not aware that, if there is benefit, it may accrue only in certain subgroups.

Ambiguous evidence

Even studies that have been impeccably conducted have uncertain clinical implications. For example, the ARDSNet study showed that people with acute respiratory distress syndrome (ARDS) have better outcomes when the tidal volume is set at 6 mL/kg rather than 12 mL/kg. But what about values between these? There was a multicentre Canadian study that suggested that mortality is lower when the transfusion trigger for red blood cells is a haemoglobin value of 7 g/dL rather than 10 g/dL. But this study was conducted before routine leucocyte reduction of packed red blood cells.

Conflicts of interest

These illustrations are not intended to suggest that we should ignore the evidence and follow our own instincts. They are intended only to heighten awareness and to promote rigour. People with conflicts of interest may seek to slant the evidence and may undermine our patients' best interests. Clinicians may wish to do procedures, such as pulmonary artery catheter insertions, because these are lucrative. Drug companies exert subtle pressure on doctors to prescribe their medicines. This may lead to antibiotic resistance, inappropriate use of medicines and frittering away of scarce health care resources. Perhaps most pertinent for practising clinicians, when we have been adhering to a particular practice for many years, we are reluctant to admit that we may have been mistaken and that we may have been subjecting our patients to potential harm.

The evidence base

Despite gaps in knowledge and questionable evidence, medicine is not all voodoo practice. Without antibiotics, many patients with infections would succumb; without ventilators, acute respiratory failure would herald death; without dialysis, renal failure would be fatal. Certainly there have been important recent additions to the ICU evidence base, which, if applied, improve our patients' prognoses (Table 1).

As regards ICU staffing, the Leapfrog Initiative and several other studies have demonstrated that mortality is reduced when fully trained ICU physicians run the ICU and are available 24 h a day. This is partly because such practitioners

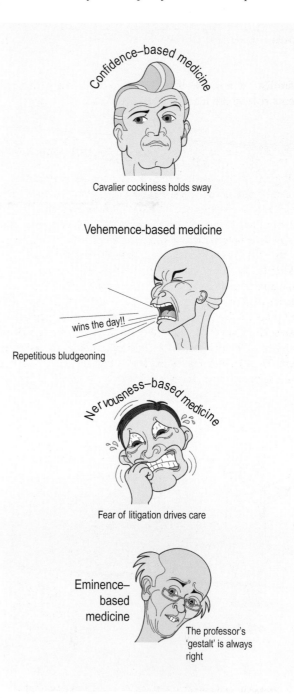

Confidence-based medicine

Cavalier cockiness holds sway

Vehemence-based medicine

wins the day!!

Repetitious bludgeoning

Nervousness-based medicine

Fear of litigation drives care

Eminence-based medicine

The professor's 'gestalt' is always right

Fig. 1 **Alternatives to evidence-based medicine.** How poor decisions may be made on the ICU.

Table 1 Recent additions to the ICU evidence base

Field	Intervention	Outcome	Reference
Neurology	Hypothermia	Decreases death following cardiac arrest	*N Engl J Med* 346(8): 549–556
	Daily waking	Decreases ICU length of stay	*N Engl J Med* 342(20): 1471–1477
Cardiovascular	Continuous positive airway pressure (CPAP)	Decreases need for intubation with cardiogenic pulmonary oedema	*N Engl J Med* 325(26): 1825–1830
Respiratory	Low tidal volumes	Improves outcome in ARDS	*N Engl J Med* 342(18): 1301–1308
Haematology	Low haemoglobin transfusion threshold	Decreases mortality with no ischaemic heart disease	*N Engl J Med* 340(6): 409–417
Metabolic	Tight glucose control with insulin	Decreases mortality especially after heart surgery	*N Engl J Med* 345(19): 1359–1367
Infection	Activated protein C	Decreases mortality in severe sepsis	*N Engl J Med* 344(10): 699–709
	Decreased antibiotic course	Eight days as good as 15 for most pneumonias	*JAMA* 290(19): 2588–2598
GIT	Ulcer prophylaxis	There is less GI bleeding with ranitidine than sucralfate	*N Engl J Med* 338(12): 791–797
Renal	Low-dose dopamine	Does not decrease renal dysfunction	*Lancet* 356(9248): 2139–2143
Endocrine	Low-dose hydrocortisone + fludrocortisone	Decreases mortality in sepsis with adrenal insufficiency	*JAMA* 288(7): 862–871
	Growth hormone	Increases ICU mortality	*N Engl J Med* 341(11): 785–792
Nutrition	Enteral feeding	Decreases GI bleeding in ventilated patients	*Crit Care Med* 27(12): 2846–2847
Resuscitation	Early goal-directed therapy	Decreases mortality with sepsis	*N Engl J Med* 345(19): 1368–1377
Monitoring	PA catheter	No improvement in high-risk surgical patients	*N Engl J Med* 348(1): 5–14
ICU staffing	Pharmacist on ICU rounds	Decreases prescribing errors	*JAMA* 283(10):1293
	High intensity ICU physician staffing	Decreases mortality and ICU stay	*JAMA* 288(17): 2151–2162

ARDS, acute respiratory distress syndrome; GIT, gastrointestinal tract; ICU, intensive care unit; PA, pulmonary artery.

are familiar with the pertinent evidence and ensure that ICU patients receive the highest standard of care.

Evidence-based protocols and guidelines

It is important that we try to draft evidence-based protocols that can be tailored to the specific needs of individual ICUs. Ventilator weaning protocols decrease intubation and mechanical ventilation times. Sedation and analgesia protocols facilitate adequate analgesia and decrease the likelihood that patients are too heavily sedated. Many doctors and nurses work on ICUs. Not all have extensive ICU experience. Having simple and unambiguous protocols provides important guidance to staff working on the ICU and facilitates evidence-based practice. The experienced intensivist should help to devise such protocols and should also intervene when strict adherence to the protocol is not appropriate for the individual patient (Fig. 2). Guidelines should also be evidence based, but are not as prescriptive as protocols.

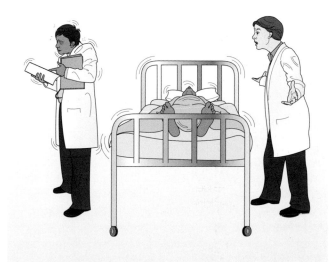

Fig. 2 **Protocols and guidelines.** "Dr Patel, what are you doing? The patient's dying and you're leafing through pamphlets!" Dr Patel: "I'm worried that if I institute the wrong protocol the consultant will be ticked off."

Myth debunked

A meta-analysis published in 1999 in the *British Medical Journal* suggested that albumin administration might be associated with increased mortality. In an inflammatory editorial, a comment was made that, if a clinician administered albumin to one of the author's family members, he would consider legal proceedings. In 2004, a well-designed, randomised, double-blinded, multicentre study – the SAFE study, published in the *New England Journal of Medicine* – found that albumin is no more hazardous than normal saline.

Clinical case

A randomised, double-blinded, prospective study titled 'High dose dexamethasone is safe and decreases contrast medium nephropathy' was reported in the *Journal of Medically Unwarranted Stupid Hypotheses* (MUSH). Forty ICU patients with suspected pulmonary emboli were sent for computerised tomography (CT) scans with intravenous contrast agent. Twenty patients received 200 mg of dexamethasone in 1000 mL of normal saline prior to the scan. The 20 patients in the control group received no intervention. There was a statistically significant increase ($P < 0.05$) in the creatinine in the control group compared with the intervention group. There was a non-significant increase in pneumonia in the intervention group ($P = 0.07$). The authors concluded that high-dose dexamethasone decreases the incidence of renal dysfunction without increasing the risk of infection in this setting. What are the glaring errors apparent in this study?

Summary points

- Evidence does not constitute scientific fact; it merely suggests likely superior clinical practice.
- Conflicts of interest may obscure the evidence.
- The Leapfrog Initiative suggested that ICUs should be run by dedicated ICU staff, including specialist intensivists.
- Protocols are useful for guiding staff and implementing evidence-based practice in the ICU.

Critical care transport

Transportation of critically ill patients within the hospital or between facilities is potentially hazardous. Significant adverse events, including death, have occurred in association with patient transport. Critical incident reporting has allowed investigators to analyse specific causes of breakdown in the transport process. Contributing factors identified are related to patient condition/stability, personnel, equipment, monitoring and communication. There are important considerations and methods for improving patient transport safety.

Is patient transport necessary?

The decision to transport a critically ill patient must be based on a careful assessment of the potential benefits of transport weighed against the potential risks. Generally, *intra*hospital transport is done to facilitate additional diagnostic testing or procedural intervention that cannot be performed in the intensive care unit (ICU). Common destinations include diagnostic radiology or the operating theatre. When patients are deemed unstable or unfit for transport, alternative bedside techniques may be considered.

Increasing regionalisation and specialisation of care may necessitate *inter*hospital transport of patients. Data support the validity of transfer of critically ill patients to tertiary centres for specialised care, demonstrating improved outcomes in multiple trauma, head injury, coronary care, adult and paediatric critical illness.

Interfacility transport

A number of factors must be considered in deciding to transport critically ill patients to another facility. The referring physician must first determine that a patient requires a level of care that exceeds available resources. Once an appropriate facility and accepting physician have been identified, the mode of transport must be determined. Options for transport may include ground ambulance, helicopter or fixed-wing aircraft. Factors that will influence the mode of transport include patient stability, distance of travel, weather, geography and available personnel or resources. Ground ambulance is usually the most readily available and least expensive method of transport, while fixed-wing aircraft are preferable for long-distance travel if a patient's condition can tolerate the effects of altitude.

Improving patient transport safety

The transport process must be well organised and efficient to minimise potential harm. Research and experience have led to the publication of numerous guidelines and recommendations regarding patient transport. Five primary areas of focus have been identified to improve transport safety, which will be discussed briefly: (1) pretransport planning and communication; (2) transport personnel; (3) equipment/medications; (4) monitoring; and (5) patient preparation.

Pretransport planning and communication

When a new team will be assuming responsibility for patient care, continuity of safe patient care requires physician-to-physician and nurse-to-nurse communication to review important information regarding the patient's condition and ongoing treatment plan. This holds true whether the patient is moving to another care area within the hospital or to another facility. All preparations should take place prior to transport to ensure that all necessary personnel, supplies and equipment are available, including coordination with support personnel such as hospital security, lift teams, etc. When patients are transferred to another facility, additional preparatory efforts are required to coordinate the timing of the transport and to provide copies of all relevant medical records, diagnostic studies and care summaries for the receiving health care team.

Transport personnel

There is continued debate about the composition of the transport team, but it is generally agreed that a minimum of two persons, in addition to vehicle operators, should accompany a critically ill patient. Generally, one member of the transport team is a registered nurse with special training in critical care. Other members of the transport team may include other nurses, respiratory therapists, critical care technicians, paramedics or physicians, depending on available resources, local regulations and the level of care required. Ideally, a dedicated team composed of members familiar with the transport of critically ill patients and skilled in airway management and critical care would provide for all transportation of critically ill patients within and between hospitals. Several studies have sought to determine whether physicians should be present on all interhospital transports and, indeed, some prospective studies have demonstrated improved outcomes with direct physician attendance. Some professional societies now advocate the presence of a physician with training in airway management, advanced life support and critical care training or equivalent for the transport of unstable patients.

Equipment/supplies

Careful preparation of equipment and supplies prior to transport is essential (see Figs 1 and 2). Critically ill patients may require assisted ventilation or continuous intravenous infusions, and all patients will require ongoing monitoring of various physiological parameters. Portable equipment necessary to provide these functions must be available and checked to ensure proper functioning prior to transport. Adequate battery charge and/or additional battery capabilities must be confirmed to prevent important equipment failures that may lead to harm. Transport vehicles must have the room to transport any necessary equipment with backup battery and oxygen supplies in the event of vehicle breakdown.

Ventilation problems may occur as a result of loss of a secure airway, endotracheal tube malpositioning, inadequate oxygen supply, ventilator failure or improper ventilator settings. Haemodynamic instability may result from infusion pump failure or an inadequate supply of intravenous medications or fluids. Such critical events must be anticipated, and efforts aimed at preventing or minimising their occurrence must be undertaken. Many advocate the

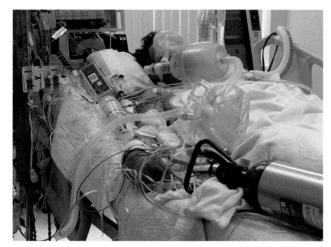

Fig. 1 **Never transport with a tangled mess.**

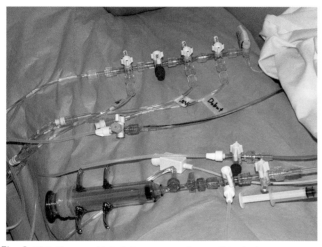

Fig. 2 **Tidy lines and labels improve patient safety during transport.**

development and implementation of a pretransport checklist, similar to that used by flight crews prior to takeoff. Studies have demonstrated that the use of such equipment and patient checks have prevented or limited harm.

Monitoring

Minimum requirements for monitoring in the critically ill patient should include:

- continuous electrocardiography
- oxygen saturation
- regular measurement of blood pressure
- end-tidal carbon dioxide detection in ventilated patients.

Selected patients may warrant additional monitoring, including:

- intra-arterial blood pressure
- intracranial pressure
- central venous or pulmonary artery pressure.

Patient preparation

Lastly, patients must be stabilised and prepared for transport when at all possible. Avoid the 'scoop and run' mentality.

- Patients must have a safe airway; intubation may be necessary prior to transport.
- Proper endotracheal tube position should be verified and secured.
- Oxygenation/ventilation status should be confirmed and optimised.
- Adequate intravenous access must be established.
- Haemodynamic stability should be attempted with fluids and medications as necessary.
- Ensure a sufficient supply of fluids and medications for the duration of transport.
- Spinal immobilisation should be maintained for patients without adequate evaluation to rule out spinal injury risk.
- Additional devices such as a Foley catheter or nasogastric tube may be indicated in selected patients.
- Thoracostomy tube will be necessary for even a small pneumothorax in patients requiring flight. Provide suction, water seal or one-way valve. DO NOT CLAMP!
- Restraints or the use of sedative and analgesic medications may be necessary to prevent agitated or combative patients from harming themselves or crew members.
- Patients and equipment should be secured to prevent mishaps during movement.
- Tidy lines and cables. Tangles increase hazard and promote errors (Figs 1 and 2).

Clinical case

You are caring for a 55-year-old woman with a history of rheumatic heart disease and atrial fibrillation with prior mitral valve replacement. She requires head magnetic resonance imaging (MRI) following surgery for cerebral aneurysm clipping. She is currently sedated and mechanically ventilated, and is receiving esmolol and sodium nitroprusside for blood pressure management. How will you prepare for her transport?

Summary points

- Always confirm the presence of a safe and secure airway prior to transport.
- A laryngeal mask airway is not an acceptable option.
- Always travel with a self-inflating bag in the event that you lose your oxygen source.
- Simplify and minimise your intravascular lines to avoid mishaps and tangles.
- The patient and any necessary equipment must be secured to prevent falls or accidents.
- Obstetric patients should be transported with left lateral displacement to prevent aortocaval compression.

Drug interactions

The magnitude of the problem

Critically ill patients usually enter the intensive care unit (ICU) on several drugs, and more drugs are often added daily. As is shown in Fig. 1, with each added drug, the risk of interaction with drugs already present is thought to increase exponentially.

Many drug interactions are mild but, in a precariously poised patient, even a small insult may tip the balance. It has been estimated that medical error kills up to 98 000 people each year in the USA alone. This is the equivalent of a 747 passenger jet crashing on a daily basis. Many such errors will be drug errors. We have *no idea* how many people end up in intensive care because of drug interactions, or how many develop a serious interaction while in the ICU.

How drugs interact

Important concepts

Key concepts are:

- Pharmacokinetics – how a drug is absorbed, distributed and eliminated.
- Pharmacodynamics – the action of a drug at the (receptor) site where it has its effect.

Drugs can interact in many ways. Mechanisms are listed in Box 1.

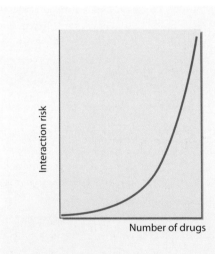

Fig. 1 **The exponential increase in drug interactions with increasing drug number.**

Box 1. *Ways drugs interact*

Interference with absorption
Alterations in distribution
Changed elimination
Pharmacological interactions at a receptor level
Physiological interactions on the same system, with altered physiology increasing the likelihood and severity of interactions.

Types of interaction

By far the most important drug interactions are related to metabolism, and we will consider such interactions in detail. Occasionally, drugs may interfere in other ways, for example with the absorption of other drugs (e.g. sucralfate interferes with quinolone absorption when the drugs are given together). Further potentially lethal non-metabolic interactions are considered in Box 2.

Finally, we should never forget the *pharmacological interaction* of drugs. It makes little sense to continue giving a beta-blocker together with an inotrope that has beta-agonist activity! Even more silly is to give 'small' doses of dopamine together with an antihypertensive! A life-threatening 'serotonergic crisis' may occur when drugs with monoamine oxidase inhibitory activity (e.g. moclobemide or linezolid) are combined with agents that raise serotonin levels (e.g. fluoxetine, tricyclic antidepressants, tramadol or fentanyl).

The cycle of therapy

The common occurrence and potential lethality of drug interactions suggests that the 'cycle of therapy' shown in Fig. 2 may be appropriate.

Once we have made an initial decision that a drug is required (and noted dosing, formulation and route), we need to examine *all* current drugs, and weigh up the benefit and risk. Only if the potential benefit exceeds the risk should we give the drug.

Cytochrome P450 – a brief note

In Table 1, we list CYP interactions for several fairly commonly used drugs. Probably over half the drugs we use in clinical medicine are metabolised by cytochrome P450,

Box 2. *In vitro interactions and a myth debunked*

There is another group of common interactions – in vitro interactions (from the Latin for *in glass*!). These interactions occur when incompatible drugs are mixed. In the past, intensivists have often succumbed to the temptation to, say, mix the dopamine into the total parenteral nutrition (TPN)! Even allowing drugs to meet by infusing them through the same line may cause harm.

There is a common (but wrong) belief that simply looking at a mix is an adequate test of compatibility!

Never allow two drugs to meet unless you are *certain* that they are compatible.

Practice point

In ICU patients, vascular access may be difficult, and multiple infusions are often running simultaneously. It is certainly possible that two incompatible drugs might be infused through the same port or may be mixing on exiting two closely situated ports.

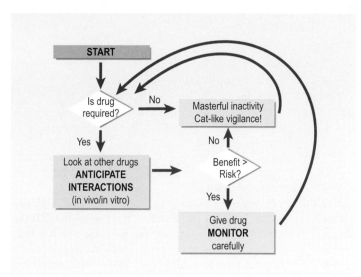

Fig. 2 **The cycle of therapy.** Once we have made an initial decision that a drug is required (and noted dosing, formulation and route), we need to examine *all* current drugs, and weigh up the benefit and risk. Only if the potential benefit exceeds the risk should we give the drug.

Table 1 **Important CYP interactions**		
Inhibitors (blue) and inducers (green)	**CYP isoenzyme**	**Substrates**
Azole antifungals,		
Cimetidine	3A4	Macrolide antibiotics
HIV protease inhibitors		Midazolam, other benzodiazepines
Calcium channel blockers		Ciclosporin and tacrolimus
Macrolide antibiotics		HIV protease inhibitors
SSRIs		Haloperidol
Amiodarone		Diltiazem, verapamil
Ciprofloxacin		Statins
		Cisapride
Rifampicin		Methadone
Carbamazepine		Quinidine
Phenytoin		
SSRIs	2D6	SSRIs, tricyclic antidepressants
Quinidine		Haloperidol
		Propafenone, mexiletine
		Codeine, tramadol, oxycodone, venlafaxine
Azole antifungals		Warfarin
Sulphonamides	2C9	Phenytoin
Amiodarone		Glipizide
Isoniazid		Non-steroidal anti-inflammatories (some)
Rifampicin		Losartan, irbesartan
Omeprazole		Diazepam
Ticlopidine	2C19	Omeprazole, some other PPIs
Azole antifungals		Phenytoin, phenobarbitone
Fluoxetine		
Disulfiram		Paracetamol
Chronic ethanol use,	2E1	Volatile anaesthetic agents
Isoniazid (INH)		Ethanol
Cimetidine, quinolones		Theophylline
	1A2	Tricyclic antidepressants
Rifampicin, phenytoin, phenobarbitone		Clozapine

HIV, human immunodeficiency virus; PPIs, proton pump inhibitor; SSRIs, selective serotonin reuptake inhibitor.

otherwise known as 'CYP'. CYP uses iron to metabolise drugs, usually to more water-soluble metabolites. An old-fashioned term for the action of CYP is 'phase I metabolism', phase II being the subsequent conjugation of the metabolites to, for example, glucuronide to make them even more water soluble. The liver is the main CYP organ, although substantial amounts are also present in the kidney.

There are about 50 *isoforms* (different types) of CYP in man, but only a handful are very important in drug metabolism. Of particular importance are CYP 3A4, 2D6, 2C9 and 2C19, but 2E1 and 1A2 are also worth a mention. (Don't worry too much about the combination of numbers and letters but, for those who are interested, the first number refers to a CYP *family* of similar genes, the

letter tells us the *subfamily*, and the final number refers to a *specific gene*. Members of families have at least 40% sequence homology, and members of subfamilies are more closely related still, with 55% homology.)

Clinical case

A reformed drug addict in his 50s has been on a stable methadone dose of 110 mg/day for the past 12 years. He has hepatitis C, but no evidence of cirrhosis, and a cardiomyopathy of moderate severity, managed on small doses of furosemide, combined with an angiotensin-converting enzyme (ACE) inhibitor. He is admitted in cardiac failure, which improves with furosemide diuresis, but then develops recurrent episodes of ventricular tachycardia which respond to amiodarone therapy, which is continued.

Several days later he is found obtunded and bradypnoeic with pinpoint pupils. How would you manage him, and how might you explain his condition? What would your comments be if you were told that he had also recently received a course of oral itraconazole for his refractory onychomycosis?

A myth exposed!

Traditionally, pharmacologists have emphasised the importance of drugs displacing other drugs from binding sites on albumin. Although such sites exist and bind drugs such as warfarin and phenytoin, as well as benzodiazepines and ibuprofen, the clinical relevance of competition for binding sites (if any) remains to be demonstrated.

Summary points

- Drug interactions are common.
- Avoid mixing drugs.
- Most interactions are CYP based. Anticipate interactions between drugs that are metabolised by CYP. Know the drugs you use!
- The more drugs you give, the more interactions you will encounter. Minimise drug therapy and justify the use of each drug.
- Watch for interactions. They are there and can kill!

Evaluation of the ICU patient

Clinical excellence

The need for clinical medicine

Intensive care is expensive and causes iatrogenic harm (harm due to investigation or treatment). With the complexity of intensive care unit (ICU) patient management goes enormous potential for errors. The guard against error in ICU is clinical medicine – the synthesis of all aspects of patient care into a unified whole. *Only* a good clinician can be a good intensivist.

Error checking in clinical medicine

Clinical medicine is dynamic and imprecise. We should and can never be certain – we will make mistakes; and aggressive, undirected investigation can mislead us and worsen our error! The corollary is that there is a lot of room to improve the quality of clinical medicine. How might we do so? Clearly, we need to identify, manage and even forestall errors.

The nature of error

There are several ways in which we can err. These include problems of diagnosis and treatment, as shown in Box 1.

Why we err

Why do we make diagnostic errors? There are many reasons, including the following:

- Undirected 'routine' testing might focus our attention on 'problems' that aren't really there (Box 2)
- Blind acceptance of test results (Box 3)
- It is quite common (and very human) to concentrate on one component of a disorder to the exclusion of other important information (fixation error)
- We tend to remember recent cases we have seen, and focus on features present in those cases, even if the current problem is not the same
- We may gloss over areas where we are ignorant, rather than looking things up.

Therapy: cause or association?

When it comes to therapy, timing is everything, and it is common to over- and undertreat. In the ICU, once we have decided that a patient's problems have a particular *cause*, we institute therapy that we believe will *cause* an improvement. Ideas of causality hold together the science of diagnosis and treatment (Practice point 2).

We come close to 'proving' causation using prospective randomised controlled trials but, even here, we can only *assume* (within certain statistical boundaries) that the apparent benefit of a particular intervention is related to the treatment given to that group. We then assume that similar treatment will benefit our patient, particularly if our patients

---

Box 2. *Misleading numbers*

Information can mislead us. We all tend to believe laboratory results, perhaps even more than our senses. To see why such belief may sometimes be inappropriate, let us look at sampling of blood levels of an arbitrary substance (let us call it 'Chemical X'):

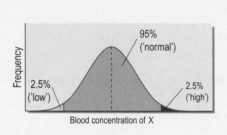

Fig. 1 **A normal curve, with confidence limits.** As is commonly done in laboratory medicine, we have set 95% confidence limits. Blood levels of X are considered 'abnormal' if they are below the lower limit (we might call this 'hypoXaemia') or above the upper limit (hyperXaemia).

If we take blood samples from many individuals in a population, we will find that 5% of those individuals have X values outside the 'reference range'. In the artificial situation in which we have many such tests, each used to diagnose a particular disease, we are forced to the reluctant conclusion that *each 'disease' occurs with the same frequency – 2.5%*. Clearly this is absurd, but worse is to follow. For if we take an individual, and perform many tests (say 20 tests) on that individual, statistically we are almost certain to come up with an 'abnormal' result – a 'disease'! The 'noise level' in the system is increased by such testing.

Box 1. *Areas of potential error*

1 Miss a substantial problem
2 See a problem that isn't there
3 Misdiagnose a problem
4 Delay therapy or withdraw it too soon
5 Continue therapy too long
6 Tinker officiously and create a substantial problem
7 Contribute to system errors.

Box 3. *Potential errors with studies involving single diagnostic tests*

1 Measurement errors (random errors of 'precision'; or systematic errors – test bias)
2 Failure of studies to adequately sample both normal and diseased populations
3 Failure to identify the effect of co-morbidity on a test
4 'Verification bias' (workup bias) – a positive test makes the clinician pursue a diagnosis more enthusiastically, so he *does* find the disease more often!
5 'Diagnostic review bias' (and 'incorporation bias') – the result of the test contributes to (affects) *making* the final diagnosis
6 'Test review bias' – knowledge of the diagnosis influences interpretation of the test
7 Failure to take into account 'uninterpretable' tests.

resemble the patients in the trial. This process of extrapolating from one group to another – creating a general theory from specific observations – is called 'scientific induction'. Our assumption of benefit of a particular therapy is strengthened if we have a powerful underlying *model* of how that therapy is working.

The personal approach to error trapping

A personal commitment to preventing and trapping errors goes a long way to improving patient care. Box 4 lists important strategies.

A systems approach to error

We must be aware of our potential for error, but individual awareness isn't enough. In the complex ICU environment, we need to *engineer* the system so that errors are picked up and corrected. Important points are:

1 Minimise complexity. A necessary minimum of tests and interventions provides less substrate for error (see pp. 12 and 18)
2 Multiple levels of checking within a team culture
3 Checklists, guidelines and *ongoing training* all help
4 Shouting at people doesn't usually help.

Most important of all may be a team culture of error awareness, openness and avoidance of blame. Learn from the airline and rail industries how to engineer low-error systems and create a culture of good 'crew resource management'. Where errors are likely (particularly drug errors), two people should check therapy. A well-engineered computer system is a useful adjunct, but deskilling human participants will probably result in harm when the computer fails.

Clinical medicine – actively pursuing the problem

In clinical medicine, we have three major advantages over undirected testing:

1 We usually have at least one initial *problem* that needs addressing
2 We direct our initial acquisition of information based on a *model* of the problem at hand
3 We can often use *multimodal* sensory inputs to cross-check our information.

As an example, consider the patient in the clinical case. What is your *model* of the problem? How certain are you of your model? How does this model govern further investigation and management of the patient? Where do you 'draw the line' in terms of further investigation?

Clinical case

A comatose patient is admitted to the ICU. We hear from the person accompanying the patient that he is diabetic, has recently been unwell and has not been taking his insulin. We have corroborative clinical notes from past admissions. We feel the patient's thready pulse and cold hands. We smell the ketones on his breath, and see his laboured 'Kussmaul' breathing.

Practice point 1: VOMIT

Undirected 'routine' testing may falsely identify 'disease'. The term VOMIT has even been coined to describe the results of such practice (an acronym for 'victim of medical investigative technology')!

Practice point 2

Modern scientists realise that all our statements of 'fact' are theory laden, and no theory in science is ever 'proven beyond doubt'. Good theories in science (and medicine) are susceptible to disproof!

Practice point 3

Despite uncertainty, we can still help patients, but we must be cautious:
1 We need a good model of what is happening
2 We need to check our model against perceived reality repeatedly
3 If the model fails, we must reformulate it.

Practice point 4

A vital component of good clinical medicine is synergy between all the participants in patient care. A competent nurse at the bedside is of more value than a million dollars worth of fancy equipment, but only if the intensivist who decides on therapy is attentive to the nurse's concerns about the patient!

Box 4. Important personal strategies for reducing error

1 Don't order tests unless you have *reasonable* justification and an idea of how you will react to the information
2 Be aware of your limitations, and *look it up* if you don't know
3 Continuously compare your model of a problem against reality
4 Admit error!
5 Seek help from experts
6 Check what you're doing with others (especially giving medication)
7 Communicate effectively with staff, family members and, where possible, the patient.

Summary points

- Avoid undirected testing.
- No diagnosis is ever 'proved' – there is always doubt.
- Repeatedly check your model of the patient's problems against your perception of reality.
- Listen to the nurse at the bedside.
- Both individual and system errors are common in the ICU.

Monitoring in the ICU

The need for monitoring

Monitoring in the intensive care unit (ICU) is complex (Fig. 1). But is it all necessary? Monitoring in the ICU has become fairly 'standardised' without good evidence that monitors actually contribute to patient safety or help with management. Box 1 lists several ways in which 'routine' monitoring may adversely affect the patient.

Conversely, monitoring may play a valuable role in alerting us to problems, and even anticipating problems before they occur. Fig. 2 shows a rational approach to the process of monitoring.

Monitor precision and accuracy

Precision versus accuracy
Fig. 3 demonstrates the difference between precision and accuracy using a picture of targets.

Trusting the monitor
A monitor is useless if you cannot trust the results – it needs to be checked against a reference standard. For example, if the blood pressure reading is 220/140, action almost certainly needs to be taken, *unless* the true blood pressure is, say, 150/70, and the reading is high

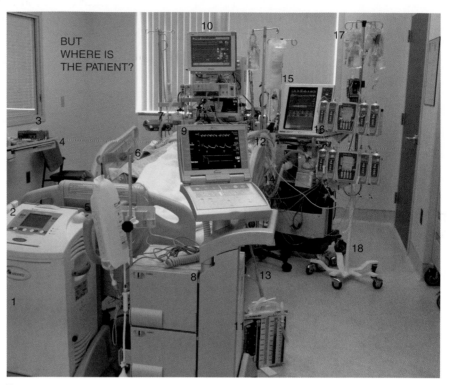

Fig. 1 **ICU bedspace**, with numerous monitors in situ. 1, Heart assist device; 2, blood flow display; 3, gloves; 4, calf compression device; 5, pressure bag; 6, arterial line; 7, breathing tube; 8, another heart assist device; 9, heart and blood pressure monitor; 10, monitor with lots of information – numbers are flashing and alarms are beeping; 11, blood drainage monitor; 12, tubing; 13, tubing for urine catheter; 14, cables; 15, breathing machine; 16, electronic pumps – medicines for pain, sedation, to help the heart, to control blood sugar, to increase blood pressure; 17, intravenous fluids; 18, drip stands.

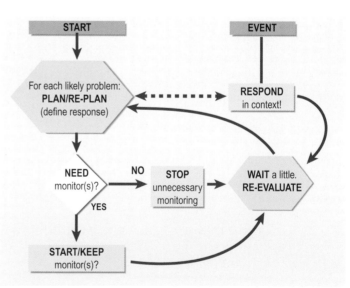

Fig. 2 **Monitoring flowchart.** We start with a plan and respond to events in the context of that plan. We regularly re-evaluate the need for monitoring and the plan. In the context of this flowchart, monitoring without an action plan is pointless.

Box 1. Potential adverse effects of monitoring

- *Overtreatment*, especially where responses to events are *generic*, that is not tailored to the patient, e.g. overtreatment of benign cardiac arrhythmias detected on electrocardiogram (ECG) monitoring
- Repeated *false alarms* may cause slowed responses to real events, e.g. failure to respond to hypotension/ asystole in the belief that the 'pulse oximeter is playing up again'
- *Information overload* may hide real abnormalities in a wealth of trivia
- 'Normal numbers' may *falsely reassure*
- *Injury* may occur due to the monitoring process, e.g. loss of a hand due to iatrogenic harm from an arterial line.

because the monitor has not been *zeroed* (see Fig. 4).

Ultimately, all clinical measurements need to be referred back to an international reference standard. The 'chain of command' from the reference standard to the bedside is called *traceable calibration*. At each step along the way, the amount of error should be known, so that we can say how confident we are in the final bedside reading. For example, an anaeroid

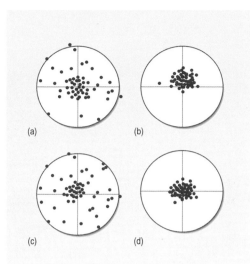

Fig. 3 **Precision and accuracy.** On target a, the bullet holes are loosely grouped around the centre; the shooting is accurate but not very precise. On target b, the bullet holes are precisely grouped but offset from the centre (inaccurate). On target c, shooting is both inaccurate and imprecise. On target d, the holes are both accurate *and* precise.

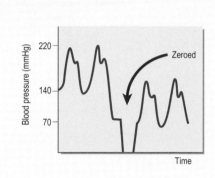

Fig. 4 **Zeroing an arterial blood pressure trace.** The tracing on the left shows apparent hypertension. The tracing on the right is the 'true' one, once the pressure has been 'zeroed' against the reference point of atmospheric pressure. Similar (but less dramatic) errors can be caused by lowering the pressure transducer below the reference point level with the patient's right atrium.

sphygmomanometer is useless unless it has recently been checked against a local reference standard, which in turn has been checked against a regional reference standard, and so on up the chain! ICUs should work closely with their Hospital Department of Clinical Engineering to ensure the chain is not broken.

Several modes of monitoring, combined with clinical acumen (see p. 16) will go a long way to alerting ICU practitioners to monitoring errors.

False alarms

The cardiac monitor that is continually 'going off' is not only a source of irritation, but it desensitises staff members to real emergencies. Here again, clinical insight is important – does the patient look as ill as the monitor says she is?

It is often valuable to look at trends rather than isolated numbers, and to relate the monitor information to your internal model of the patient's disease. It is enormously helpful to know what is normal for *that patient*! For example, a patient may have a 'baseline' blood pressure of 170/110 on admission to the ICU, but the patient may normally be normotensive, and the high pressures may be a response to pain.

Conversely, a blood pressure of 110/70 may represent substantial hypotension in somebody whose baseline blood pressure is 170/110. Many similar examples exist – see the clinical case.

Monitoring – the human factor

It has often been shown that computerised monitors outperform most humans in detecting abnormalities. Detecting every last abnormality may, however, not benefit the patient, or may even result in harm. Sophisticated computer algorithms are currently unable to integrate the totality of clinical information into a reliable management plan for the critically ill patient.

The attentive, dedicated nurse at the bedside of the critically ill patient remains our best monitor. Other monitoring modalities should be used intelligently as an adjunct to this monitoring.

> *Clinical case*
>
> A cyclist who competes internationally presents to the emergency department (ED) of your local hospital following a road traffic crash (car versus cyclist). Consider these two scenarios:
>
> *Scenario A.* The ED staff are concerned because of the bradycardia of 36/min. The patient is unconcerned. Blood pressure 90/60.
>
> *Scenario B.* The pulse rate is 80. The patient is feeling unwell. Blood pressure 90/60.
>
> What is your response to each scenario?

> *Summary points*
>
> - Trust your monitors, if they are trustworthy.
> - Unnecessary monitoring can cause harm – continually re-evaluate the need for each monitor.
> - Monitors must be used in the context of a response plan for likely events.
> - Multiple monitors give security.
> - 'Trust nobody, believe nothing, give oxygen' (an old anaesthetic adage)!

ICU
procedures

The airway in ICU

Early on during the development of the embryo in the womb, the trachea and lungs originate as an outpouching of the primitive digestive tract. This unfortunate association has enormous consequences in the critically ill. Owing to the anatomy of the mouth and pharynx, the larynx is relatively inaccessible (Fig. 1) but, even worse, the nearby oesophagus predisposes to aspiration – soiling of the lungs with stomach contents is common and life threatening if the airway is not protected.

In intensive care, we often further compromise the airway, of necessity. We sedate and even paralyse patients, rendering them incompetent to protect their own airway. We transgress their gastro-oesophageal junction with a nasogastric tube, predisposing to regurgitation of stomach contents into the oesophagus. When we lie patients flat, fluid in the oesophagus trickles towards the poorly protected larynx. Even cuffed endotracheal tubes do not provide unequivocal protection of the airway, as folds in the cuff commonly allow fluid to leak past it.

Anticipating airway problems

The most important concept in airway management in the intensive care unit (ICU) is *anticipating problems*. Important points are:

1 Have 'airway algorithm' available and practise it often in a proper simulated environment.
2 Do not intubate or perform any kind of airway manipulation alone. These actions should be done electively during daylight with the presence of senior, experienced staff to minimise the risk of failure.
3 Always call for expert help early on.
4 Failure of oxygenation kills patients. Failure of intubation does not.
5 Monitor and maintain oxygenation with a face mask or a laryngeal mask airway (e.g. Classic LMA or ProSeal® LMA) until the appropriate equipment and expertise arrives to help secure the airway.

There are certain recipes for airway catastrophes in ICU (Box 1).

Assessing the airway

Unlike an anaesthetist, who can often take time to assess the airway of an elective surgical patient, the intensivist is often reliant on information provided by others. This does not excuse intensive care staff from diligently examining the airway to the best of their ability (Box 2).

The airway in crisis

The following situations represent life-threatening crises and should be managed as shown in Box 3.

1 Where a non-intubated patient deteriorates and 'requires emergency intubation'
2 Where the orotracheal tube becomes dislodged unexpectedly
3 Where a blocked orotracheal tube needs to be exchanged
4 Where a tracheostomy tube becomes displaced or blocked.

The dislodged tracheostomy can be particularly problematic (Box 4), as it is all too easy to create a false tract by trying to reinsert the tube blindly. Such attempts can be lethal! Most tracheostomies in current ICUs are performed percutaneously, so intensive care practitioners are less familiar with surgical tracheostomies and the use of stay sutures.

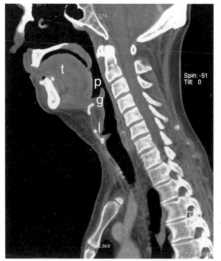

Fig. 1 **Magnetic resonance imaging of the airway,** showing how the tongue impedes access to the glottis, as well as the intimate relationship between the pharynx and larynx. g, glottis; l, larynx; p, pharynx; t, tongue.

Box 4. The dislodged tracheostomy

1 Oral intubation is best (see Box 3), even if jaw wires have to be cut

2 Do not blindly reinsert a dislodged surgical tracheostomy

3 Surgical tracheostomies should always have *stay sutures* in place (see Fig. 2). Use these sutures to pull the trachea up towards the skin and separate the tracheal hole

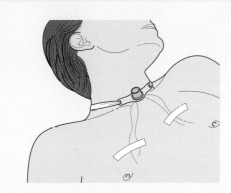

Fig. 2 **Tracheostomy with stay sutures.**

4 Intubate the trachea under vision (fibreoptic scope if you have one)

5 With recent extensive neck dissection, lay the wound open and visualise the trachea directly!

6 *Confirm tube placement* using in-line capnography.

Box 5. Note on rapid-sequence induction (RSI)

1 Failure of oxygenation kills patients. Failure of intubation does NOT

2 Monitor and maintain oxygenation until the appropriate equipment and expertise arrives to secure the airway

3 RSI is intubation in an expedient and organised fashion by an experienced team with the goal of providing a definitive airway safely, minimising the physiological or complications

4 It is often easier to insert a laryngeal mask airway (LMA) device (e.g. Classic LMA or Proseal LMA) than a tracheal tube. An LMA will relieve upper airway obstruction and will provide oxygenation and ventilation until appropriate expertise arrives

5 Emergency tracheostomy or jet ventilation via a percutaneous needle can be disastrous in the hands of the non-expert. Maintain oxygenation (see myth debunked)

6 Have a *designated leader* who oversees the entire crisis, not just the intubation. Many hands will help

7 All good anaesthetic texts have excellent descriptions of how to do a RSI. If you have not done one, call for help from someone who has

8 Do not ignore the circulatory system in the rush to intubate – predict a precipitous drop in blood pressure immediately after intubation. Have the appropriate intravenous fluids and adrenaline or noradrenaline infusion ready and connected.

Clinical case

A patient is sent to ICU with an 'armoured' orotracheal tube (spiral embedded tube, flexometallic tube) following head and neck surgery. You are experiencing difficulty ventilating the patient, with high pressures. What is your approach?

Myth debunked ($2 \times 7 = 14$)

Needle cricothyroidotomy with a 14 gauge cannula connected to a 2/3-mL syringe with a ETT connector pushed into the back of it connects to a self-inflating back BUT you CANNOT *ventilate* through this device. It will provide *oxygenation* with the self inflating bag limiting the oxygen pressure but don't squeeze the bag! (Fig. 3)

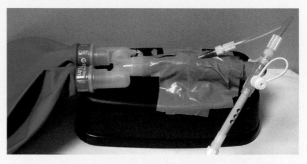

Fig. 3 The simple skill simulator showing how easy it is to deliver *oxygenation* via a 14 gauge cannula connected to an oxygen flow device. Note the holes in the oxygen tubing to allow free egress of oxygen to prevent wall pressure causing a high-pressure complication, e.g. pneumothorax or pneumomediastinum.

Clinical pearl

There is no substitute for hands-on practice – especially repeated practice in a *simulated* crisis situation.

Summary points

- *Anticipation* of airway problems is half the battle won.
- Have a management plan for airway crises.
- Practise airway management repeatedly.
- Get competent help early on during a crisis.
- Failure of oxygenation kills, failure of intubation doesn't (what I tell you three times is true!).

Vascular access in the ICU

The need for access

All patients in the intensive care unit (ICU) will have one or more catheters placed within their vessels. Such access comes at a price, and both the process of gaining access and the presence of a line or lead within a vessel can result in catastrophic complications. Vascular access is often life saving as it allows us both to monitor and to treat, but we cannot be blasé about such access. Each intravascular catheter should be sited for a clear reason, and left in no longer than is necessary.

Reasons to breach the patient's skin and place an intravascular foreign body are shown in Box 1.

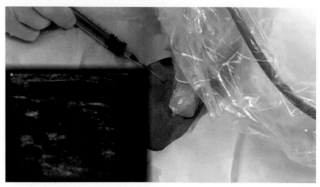

Fig. 1 **Insertion of a vascular line.**

Recent technical advances – ultrasound guidance

By far the most important recent advance in the placement of vascular catheters is the use of ultrasound imaging. Technical innovation has made ultrasound devices that provide two-dimensional imaging fairly affordable, and improved their quality immensely. The anatomy of central veins is variable, so it is difficult to justify performing blind cannulation (with a significant complication rate) now that cannulation under vision is readily available. As with all procedures, there is a learning curve, and ignorant use may result in substantial complications.

Ultrasound (US) should be used to guide needle placement in real time, rather than simply for delineating anatomy. Gel is placed on the probe, which is then covered in a sterile sheath and used to image the needle tip as it indents and enters the vein (see Fig. 1).

Key points regarding ultrasound-guided needle placement are listed in Box 2.

It can be tricky to distinguish between an artery and vein, even on ultrasound. Important points are:

1 The vein is usually readily compressible with *minimal* pressure
2 Venous distension varies with respiration
3 The arterial wall is thicker and more conspicuous
4 Arterial pulsation is usually prominent.

Once the intensivist has learned how to use ultrasound to image the jugular, femoral and axillary veins, he/she will

---

Box 1. Indications for vascular access

1 Infusion of fluid and drugs into the veins of the patient
2 Large, rapid fluid infusions through a large, short peripheral catheter
3 Small-volume but irritant fluid infusions through long, central catheters
4 Large-bore cannulae inserted for purposes of dialysis or extracorporeal circulation
5 Monitoring of beat-to-beat alterations in arterial pressure
6 A desire to monitor central vascular pressures or acquire mixed venous or arterial blood
7 Placement of a pacing lead, usually within the right ventricle.

Box 2. Requirements for ultrasound-guided needle placement

1 The operator must be trained or supervised and experienced in the use of the device.
2 Select probe and settings.
  1 Small footprint curvilinear (C11 – Sonosite) for long-axis imaging (LAX);
  2 Linear array (L38 – Sonosite) for short-axis imaging (SAX);
  3 Use highest resolution setting 7–14 MHz;
  4 Select depth – usually start at 3-cm depth.
3 Position US by ipsilateral chest and stand on contralateral side of patient (to ensure needle follows a path from needle to lateral).
4 Prepare sterile field and place US probe in sterile sheath. Use sterile US gel.
5 Place probe at cricoid level. Scan laterally to identify thyroid, carotid artery and jugular vein.
6 Scan cranially then caudally to assess the course of the jugular vein. Find a position where the vein is most lateral to the artery.
7 Select site of puncture to minimise the risk of arterial puncture. Position the neck and probe such that the artery is NEVER in the line of the needle.
8 Vessels should be confidently identified as venous or arterial (see text) *before* application of Doppler (if this modality is present on the machine, it is not an essential component) – use of Doppler adds little to help in distinguishing between the two.
9 Perform puncture of vein. Try to image the needle tip at all times – for SAX imaging, use an angle of 60°; for LAX, a needle angle of 30–45° is best.
10 Confirm puncture by aspiration and presence of needle/wire in vein (see the white spot in the insert of Fig. 1).
11 Complete cannulation as usual.

Practice point

It is usually *not* appropriate to use central venous lines for the purposes of resuscitation. A high resistance makes rapid infusion of large volumes difficult. Use a large-bore peripheral venous cannula.

appreciate the utility of this approach. The user quickly becomes aware of how, with spontaneous inspiration or minimal pressure, it is easy to obliterate (and therefore miss) the vein, as well as how remarkably the anatomy of the lateral subclavian and neck regions varies.

Access at various sites

Cannulation of vessels often involves introduction of a guidewire through a needle, subsequently feeding a cannula over the wire (the Seldinger technique). Complications of vascular puncture are listed in Box 3.

Deep vein cannulation

Deep venous cannulation is usually performed on the jugular, subclavian or femoral vein. The subclavian vein is not accessible to ultrasound location but, moving laterally, the axillary vein is. During jugular or axillary cannulation, the patient must be placed in a head-down position, both to distend the veins and to prevent air embolism.

Although less frequently performed than in the past, some patients may still warrant placement of a pulmonary artery catheter (PAC). This device, first described by Swan and Ganz in 1970 (p. 2) has a small, inflatable balloon at the end of a long catheter. The catheter is inserted via a sheath, and the balloon is then inflated, allowing blood flow to direct the catheter tip through the right heart into the pulmonary artery. The indications for and use of pulmonary artery catheterisation are covered on p. 82.

Arterial lines

Arterial cannulation is commonly performed on the radial artery of the patient's non-dominant hand (Fig. 2). Current perception is that performing Allen's test (checking for adequate collateral flow in the ulnar artery before cannulating the radial artery in that hand) is neither necessary nor useful. Many believe that cannulation of the brachial artery should be avoided if possible, because there is no convenient bony area against which the artery can be pressed to stop bleeding.

An arterial line may potentially damage or occlude the artery, although this complication is uncommon. Inadvertent

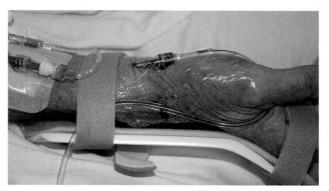
Fig. 2 **An arterial line in the radial artery.**

introduction of air or drugs into the arterial line has the potential to cause crippling ischaemic damage to the hand.

Pacemaker leads

In haemodynamically unstable patients with high degrees of heart block unresponsive to pharmacological intervention (usually following myocardial infarction), it may be necessary to insert a *temporary pacing lead*. The lead is introduced via a sheath, usually one placed in the right internal jugular vein using the Seldinger technique. Except in very unusual circumstances, placement of the pacing lead should always be performed under X-ray screening, with the ability to view the lead within the right ventricle, both anteroposteriorly and from the side. Viewing the lead from the side is particularly important as this will confirm the necessary placement of the tip of the pacing lead in the apex of the right ventricle.

Complications of vascular puncture

There are many possible complications of vascular puncture. Some are listed in Box 3.

Clinical case
After placement of a line in the right internal jugular vein, the follow-up radiograph demonstrates that the guidewire has been left in and is now sitting in the superior vena cava, with the tip in the right atrium. How can the guidewire be removed?

Box 3. Complications

1 Accidental injury to adjacent structures: arteries, nerves or the lung. Perforation of heart chambers has been reported on rare occasions
2 Blood loss
3 Air embolism. Entrainment of as little as 20 mL of air can cause cardiovascular collapse. If the patient has congenital heart disease with a right-to-left shunt, a few bubbles will be enough to cause a stroke
4 Infection, either local or systemic
5 Local venous thrombosis is common
6 Injection of drugs into the wrong site (e.g. an arterial line)
7 Major complications of PAC placement occur in at least 1% of cases (where carefully looked for) and include all of the above, as well as uncommon complications such as pulmonary infarction, rupture of a pulmonary artery branch (which is usually fatal) and knotting of the catheter.

Summary points

- Ultrasound guidance combats the common problem of variable vascular anatomy.
- The decision to place a cannula should be based on an assessment of risks and benefits.
- Arterial cannulation is commonly performed on the radial artery of the patient's non-dominant hand.
- Placement of a temporary pacing lead should always be performed under X-ray screening.
- During jugular or axillary cannulation, the patient must be placed in a head-down position.

Fibreoptic bronchoscopy in the ICU

A fibreoptic bronchoscope (FOB) is like a periscope that allows clinicians to inspect from within the trachea and the bronchial tree. Bronchoscopy has increased our ability to diagnose and treat several disease states and problems that affect intensive care unit (ICU) patients. Bronchoscopy is inexpensive, readily available and carries a low side-effect profile. The FOB is an essential tool for any ICU clinician.

Indications

Bronchoscopy may yield useful and rapid information when there is a change in a patient's pulmonary status. It takes minutes to perform a bedside bronchoscopy, which is much quicker than obtaining and interpreting a chest radiograph. Bronchoscopy may have high yield in situations where there are sudden unexplained changes, such as increasing peak airway pressures or decreasing oxygen saturation. Indications for bronchoscopy can be divided into diagnostic and therapeutic (see Table 1).

Bronchoscopy allows the clinician to visualise the bronchial tree directly to inspect for irregularities. This can be especially helpful in such situations as inhalational injuries, foreign body ingestion or a fresh bronchial or tracheal anastomosis.

For diagnostic purposes, bronchoscopy and bronchoalveolar lavage (BAL) are more specific for microbiological cultures for diagnosis of pneumonia than tracheal aspirates, which may be contaminated with upper respiratory flora and may not represent the bacterial population of the distal airways.

Bronchoscopy is useful to aid tracheal intubation, especially when there is a known or suspected airway abnormality making visualisation of the vocal cords with a laryngoscope challenging. Patients who are intubated may have copious secretions that are not amenable to clearance via tracheal suctioning. Bronchoscopy with irrigation and suctioning is a suitable way to clear the airway of thick or copious secretions or mucus plugs. Some patients who do not have a tracheal tube in place may be unable to cough and clear their own secretions. Irrigation with a FOB inserted through the nose may be sufficient to clear the airway secretions and stave off placement of a tracheal tube; tracheal intubation may be a safer option in such situations.

Bronchial anatomy

Fig. 1 shows the bronchial anatomy. The trachea branches into the right and left mainstem bronchi. The right mainstem bronchus then has three divisions: the right upper lobe (RUL), the right middle lobe (RML) and the right lower lobe (RLL). The left mainstem bronchus has two divisions: the left upper lobe (LUL) and the left lower lobe (LLL). Each of these divisions is accessible with a FOB.

Technique

A FOB is shown in Fig. 2. It consists of a set of optics for viewing (A), a light source cord (B), two-dimensional range-of-

Table 1 **Indications for bronchoscopy**	
Diagnostic	**Therapeutic**
Bronchoalveolar lavage (BAL)	Fibreoptic intubation
Biopsy	Suctioning of secretions/mucus plugs
Evaluate bronchial tree	Foreign body removal
Evaluate anastomosis postoperatively	

motion control (C), injection/instrument port (D), suction port (E) and the bronchoscope (F). The clinician should always have a bite block, suction, saline for irrigation and a specimen container available. Damage to the FOB can be minimised by using a bite block when the scope is introduced via an orotracheal tube.

The nostril is prepared with lidocaine jelly, and the posterior pharynx is sprayed with an aerosolised lidocaine solution. This prevents much discomfort. A vasoconstrictor such as phenylephrine in the nostril decreases the likelihood of bleeding. Small amounts of midazolam or propofol decrease discomfort. High oxygen concentration should be delivered via a face mask with a side port cut out. The FOB is advanced through the side port into the nostril and then into the posterior pharynx. When the vocal cords are seen, lidocaine spray onto the cords may prevent spasm and may ease passage of the FOB into the trachea. Further sprays of lidocaine may prevent coughing as the FOB is advanced.

Tracheal and tracheostomy tubes are convenient conduits for a FOB. Increase the F_iO_2 to 100% prior to bronchoscopy and ensure that the pitch of the pulse oximeter is audible. Fig. 3 demonstrates landmarks encountered during bronchoscopy. Once the FOB is in the trachea, the operator should orientate the bronchoscope. The tracheal rings are c-shaped with the non-cartilaginous part (the membranous trachea) orientated posteriorly (Fig. 3). Once the rings are identified, anterior, posterior, left and right can be appreciated. The membranous trachea has parallel fibres that run down the posterior tracheal wall.

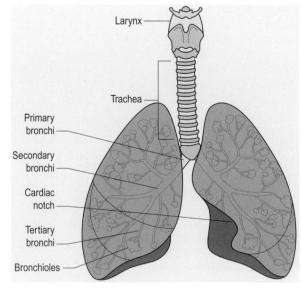

Fig. 1 **Bronchial anatomy.**

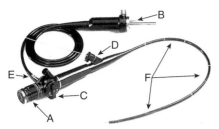

Fig. 2 **A fibreoptic bronchoscope.**

The tip of the FOB is controlled by an up–down lever on the handpiece. When the lever is pushed away from the operator, the tip flexes in the direction of a notch, which is visible at the periphery at the FOB's circular field. Rotation of the FOB accomplishes clockwise and anticlockwise movement of the flexed tip. Combining manipulation of the FOB's lever with a twisting action allows guided navigation of the FOB through the bronchial tree. When the FOB is in the trachea, the carina should be identified, ideally with the FOB's notch at 12 o'clock underlying the anterior portion of the tracheal rings. In order to navigate into the right mainstem bronchus, the tip is flexed towards the notch at 12 o'clock and the FOB is twisted clockwise. The takeoff of the RUL is seen superiorly close to the carina in the right mainstem and takes an acute angle at its origin. This is the most difficult lobe to access and is often missed.

When bronchoscopy is used is for BAL, the chest radiograph may suggest where there is suspicion of pneumonia, and the FOB may be directed to that area. The FOB should be advanced to the area of interest with minimal or no suctioning. If suctioning is necessary for navigation, 50 mL of saline should be flushed through the injection port and suctioned before collecting any specimen. The FOB should be advanced as deeply as possible into the lobe of interest. A specimen trap should be connected to the suction line. Saline (50 mL) is infused via the injection port. This is then suctioned into the specimen trap, which is sent to the microbiology laboratory. The priority is to identify infecting organisms so that antimicrobial therapy may be appropriately targeted and unnecessary therapy may be prevented.

Complications

In the awake patient, FOB can induce emesis and aspiration. Passage of the bronchoscope into the posterior pharynx can cause injury and bleeding. Insertion of the FOB through a nostril may precipitate severe epistaxis. A FOB should be used cautiously in patients with facial fractures or severe coagulopathy. The FOB may be passed into the oesophagus and perforation may occur. If the operator is not vigilant, when patients require assisted ventilation, prolonged bronchoscopy may be associated with oxygen desaturation. The clinician should always be aware of the patient's oxygen saturation. Bronchoscopy may lead to a loss of positive end-expiratory pressure (PEEP), which may further decrease oxygen saturation. Direct irritation by the FOB of the vocal cords and the airways may precipitate laryngospasm or bronchospasm. Those with asthma should receive a beta-agonist prior to bronchoscopy. The FOB may spread infection in several ways: there may be intrapulmonary seeding within the same patient, pathogen transmission from one patient to another and spread of infection from the patient to participating medical personnel. Gram-negative bacilli, particularly *Pseudomonas aeruginosa*, may be introduced into the lungs of those undergoing bronchoscopy. Standard protective precautions are recommended for all present for all bronchoscopies, including gloves, masks and eye protection. When there is suspicion of highly contagious and dangerous agents a power air-purifying respirator hood should be considered. For these patients, bronchoscopy should be performed in a negative pressure-ventilated room. The diagnosis should be made by techniques other than bronchoscopy if possible.

Clinical case

A 52-year-old man is brought to the ICU after a major abdominal operation. The anaesthetist reports no difficulty with ventilation during the surgery. The endotracheal tube is a size 8.0 tube secured at 25 cm at the lip. You are called to the bedside owing to concern about a persistent air leak around the tube despite repeated inflations of the tracheal tube pilot balloon. On chest radiograph, the tracheal tube is not visualised. A FOB is introduced. What are the most likely findings?

Summary points

- Bronchoscopy has diagnostic and therapeutic indications.
- Increase the inspired oxygen and ensure the pulse oximeter signal is audible prior to bronchoscopy.
- Specimens may be obtained for culture or pathology.
- The airway may be cleared of secretions and debris.
- Complications include spread of infection both to the patient and from the patient.

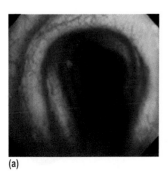

(a)

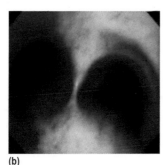

(b)

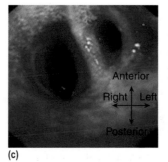

Anterior

Right | Left

Posterior

(c)

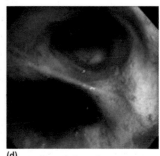

(d)

Fig. 3 **Landmarks encountered during bronchoscopy.** (a) Trachea; (b) Carina; (c) Lobar division on right; (d) Lobar division on left.

Cerebrospinal fluid, lumbar puncture and lumbar drain

Normal anatomy

The normal brain floats on a cushion of cerebrospinal fluid (CSF), which also acts as a metabolic sink for brain waste products. Encased within the rigid skull and weighing in at about 1.4 kg, the brain occupies about 80% of the intracranial volume. The remaining 20% is equally divided between the cerebrospinal fluid and blood. The rigid encasing skull is the basis of the Monro–Kellie doctrine (Box 1), which can be paraphrased as 'Something's gotta give'! As the brain swells, the compensatory reserves of the other components become exhausted, at which point tiny increments in volume will result in enormous increases in pressure.

Normal CSF pressure is about 5–18 cm of water, that is up to about 13 mmHg. As mean arterial pressure is usually about 90 mmHg, there is usually a generous *cerebral perfusion pressure* (CPP) of over 70 mmHg (the difference between mean arterial pressure and intracranial pressure). When the brain is injured, it is believed that a reduction in CPP much below 70 mmHg often results in serious and often irreversible brain injury, because of impaired flow of blood to the brain. Clearly, both raised intracranial pressure (ICP) and lowered arterial pressure can be harmful in these circumstances.

Traditionally it is taught that CSF is absorbed by the arachnoid villi, microscopic interfaces between the arachnoid and surrounding veins (Fig. 1). Recent evidence suggests that, even in man, lymphatic channels contribute, particularly nasal lymphatics near the cribriform plate.

Raised intracranial pressure

Sudden, sustained increases in ICP pose a serious threat to the brain. Common causes of raised ICP include substantial head trauma, intracranial space-occupying lesions (such as haematomas and tumours) metabolic causes of brain oedema such as liver failure, and obstruction to the flow of CSF (hydrocephalus). Obstruction to the flow of CSF (hydrocephalus) is another important cause.

Clinically, it is difficult to discern that ICP is high until overt brain injury has occurred so, in those at risk, invasive ICP monitoring is the gold standard. Features of massively raised ICP include impaired consciousness, raised blood pressure, irregular respiration and, terminally, slowing of the pulse. Papilloedema is often seen (Fig. 2), but may be absent in some individuals, even in the presence of grossly elevated ICP.

A lot of information can be derived from ICP monitoring. The mean pressure is important, but the pressure *waveform* also provides useful information. Marked variation in pressure with arterial pulsation suggests that further small increases in pressure will result in catastrophe. Sustained increases in pressure lasting more than a few minutes are termed 'Lundberg A waves' (Fig. 3) and are dangerous; less

Box 1. The Monro–Kellie doctrine

As volume is added to one component of the cranial contents, one of the other components must decrease in volume.

Clinical pearl

By visualising the subtle pulsation of the veins in the fundus of the eye that normally occurs with breathing, it is possible to *exclude* raised ICP.

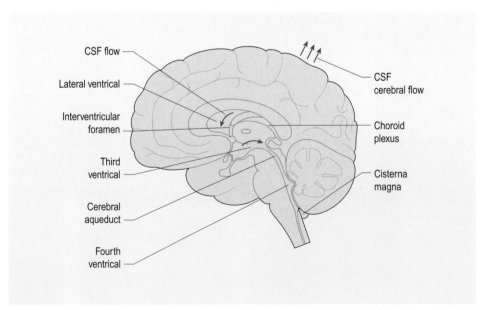

Fig. 1 **Ventricles and CSF flow.** Every day, about 0.5 L of CSF is produced by the choroid plexuses, vascular 'cauliflower-like' structures in the lateral ventricles (also present in the third and fourth ventricles). Fluid flows from the lateral ventricles through the cerebral aqueduct, ultimately exiting through holes in the roof of the fourth ventricle, to gain access to the subarachnoid space, which contains most of the CSF. The ventricles contain about 20 mL of CSF and the spinal region about 30 mL. The choroid plexuses have complex autonomic innervation!

Labels in figure: CSF flow · Lateral ventrical · Interventricular foramen · Third ventrical · Cerebral aqueduct · Fourth ventrical · CSF cerebral flow · Choroid plexus · Cisterna magna

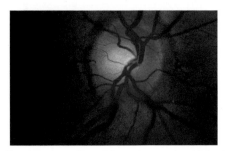

Fig. 2 **Papilloedema** – swelling of the optic nerve head following raised ICP (courtesy of Dr AD Woods, Nova Southeastern University, Fl, USA).

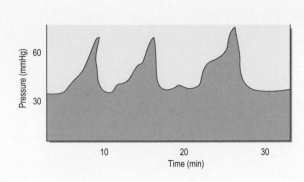

Fig. 3 **Lundberg 'A' waves** on ICP monitoring.

ominous are briefer, lower amplitude B waves of 5–20 mmHg, lasting 1–5 min.

ICP monitors

The main methods of monitoring are (Fig. 4):

1 Intraventricular catheters – the gold standard. The usual pressure reference point used is the level of the external auditory meatus. Such catheters can also be used to drain off CSF and lower pressure. Their major disadvantage is infection, which is more common if the catheter is left in for more than 5 days.
2 Intraparenchymal transducers. These (either wire or fibreoptic) are stable for about 4 days after initial calibration, and cause less infection than intraventricular catheters, but are slightly less reliable.
3 In the past, bolts have been placed through the skull, the tip entering the subarachnoid space, but these are more prone to error than the above methods. Epidural transducers (which do not enter the subarachnoid space) are also inaccurate.

Low intracranial pressure

Lowered ICP is often disregarded as a problem in the intensive care unit (ICU), but consequences can be substantial. Ongoing CSF leaks can result in not only infection, but also refractory headache (often relieved on lying down), cranial nerve palsies and even subdural haemorrhage.

Lumbar puncture

Provided ICP is not raised, and sterile techniques are used, it is usually safe to insert a fine-bore needle between the lumbar vertebrae (below L3) and into the spinal fluid. This procedure causes a significant incidence of post-lumbar puncture headache (1% even with a 27-gauge needle, and about 20% with a 21-gauge needle), but may provide valuable information including:

1 Pressure (provided the needle is immediately connected to a fluid manometer)
2 CSF biochemistry
3 Evidence of infection (CSF leucocytosis and isolation of infecting organisms or their antigens)
4 Presence of altered blood (xanthochromia) indicating subarachnoid haemorrhage.

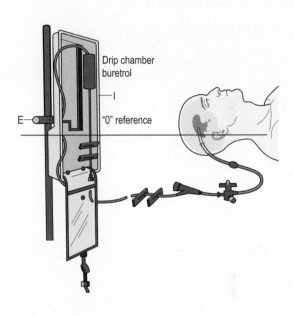

Fig. 4 **ICP monitoring.**

Clinical case

A 34-year-old nurse who trained in Africa presents with a week's history of headache and photophobia. Mild confusion is present and she has marked neck stiffness. Lumbar puncture shows an opening pressure of 37 cmH$_2$O, glucose 2.1 mmol/L (blood glucose taken at the same time was 5.3 mmol/L), protein 1.7 g/L, neutrophils 600/mm^3, mononuclear cells 100/mm^3, chloride 117 mmol/L. What are your concerns?

Summary points

- As the brain swells, so other components lose volume.
- Normal cerebral perfusion pressure is about 70 mmHg; as this pressure is lowered, so the risk of brain harm increases.
- Intraventricular catheters are the gold standard for ICP monitoring.
- Post-lumbar puncture headache is common.

Organ support

Mechanical ventilation

The respiratory muscles form an elegant pump which pulls air into the lungs. After a pause, air exits passively. Failure of this pump results in hypercarbia, hypoxia and eventual death.

In patients in whom recovery to a reasonable level of function is anticipated, it makes sense to support the failing respiratory pump using a mechanical ventilator (see p. 2).

Numerical values (especially blood partial pressures of oxygen and/or carbon dioxide) are often cited as criteria for 'respiratory failure' and a requirement to ventilate. Absolute numbers are unreliable, as baseline values differ in different individuals, especially in those with chronic lung disease, and blood gas values may not accurately mirror respiratory muscle function or anticipate its decline!

The decision to ventilate depends on an overall assessment of the patient's problems (see p. 16). Conditions other than failure of the respiratory muscle pump may necessitate intubation and ventilatory support, e.g. impaired level of consciousness and septic shock.

Ventilation basics (and terminology)

Ventilator terminology is confusing. Fig. 1 shows a common mode of ventilation called 'synchronised intermittent mandatory ventilation with pressure support' (SIMV + PS). Important points are:

- Pressure decreases to baseline in between breaths
- Positive end-expiratory pressure (PEEP) means that, during mechanical ventilation, we artificially splint the airway by introducing a positive pressure offset from baseline
- Continuous positive airway pressure (CPAP) refers to PEEP with the patient breathing *entirely spontaneously*
- *Pressure control ventilation* is superficially similar to pressure support, but (a) will be initiated by either patient or ventilator and (b) is *time* cycled, not flow cycled.

Other modes of ventilation include: pressure-regulated volume control, 'volume support', various forms of 'BiPAP' (bi-level positive airways pressure) and exotic methods such as

high-frequency oscillatory ventilation (HFOV), high-frequency jet ventilation (HFJV) and airway pressure release ventilation. These modes have not been shown to have a convincing advantage over conventional ones.

Ventilator problems

There are three major, non-technical problems with current approaches to ventilation:

1 Infection
2 Attempts to achieve normality rather than function
3 Lung harm caused by inappropriate ventilatory strategies.

Two major mechanisms are overdistension and lung collapse. Normal lung volumes depend largely on stature, gender and race, and not on body weight.

Overdistension ('barotrauma' or 'volutrauma')

The term 'barotrauma' has traditionally been used to describe pressure-induced lung injury. There is a well-characterised relationship between the pressure across the wall of an air space and the volume of that air space (Fig. 2).

Measurement of pressure at the mouth end of an endotracheal tube is inconstantly related to transalveolar

pressure because, in this dynamic system, pressure depends on flow and the resistance of the endotracheal tube. A large, variable pressure component is used to overcome chest wall resistance to filling (impedance). Incorporating a measure of intrapleural pressure would be more reliable, but is difficult to achieve. Some have used intraoesophageal pressure as a proxy for intrapleural pressure.

The ARDSNet trial demonstrated that small *volume* ventilation (6 mL/kg) at faster rates is preferable to large volumes (12 mL/kg) at slow rates, but we do not know where the optimal value is between (or even below) these extremes. It is often stated that ventilator *plateau pressures* should be kept under 30 cmH$_2$O and, in most cases, barotrauma is then unlikely. However, in some patients with a large thoracic wall impedance (e.g. those with rigid chest walls or massive obesity), slavish adherence to such a pressure rule may result in inadequate ventilation.

Lung collapse

Every patient who is exposed to very high concentrations of oxygen under general anaesthesia, especially 100% oxygen, will within minutes develop collapse of the dependent portions of their lungs ('atelectasis'). This has been well demonstrated even in normal

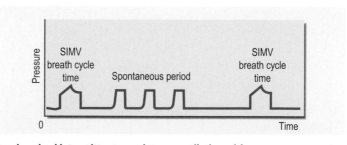

Fig. 1 **Synchronised intermittent mandatory ventilation with pressure support** (SIMV + PS).

SIMV: patient initiates a breath	**Pressure support:** Subsequent (in this case smaller) breaths in the 'spontaneous period' are initiated by the patient	If the patient doesn't initiate a breath for some time, then the machine takes over
The ventilator delivers a preset *volume*	When inspiratory *flow* drops sufficiently, expiration occurs – the breath is 'flow cycled'	The ventilator delivers a *mandatory* 'volume-controlled' breath
The *pressure* is determined by the characteristics of the patient and the inspiratory flow required to deliver that volume	*Supported* by the ventilator up to a certain pressure	

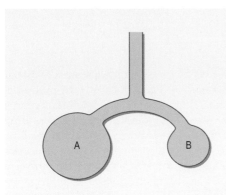

Fig. 2 **Laplace's law.** Transalveolar pressure depends on surface tension, and is inversely related to radius. Delta P is often called the 'recoil pressure'. According to Laplace's law, the transalveolar pressure in B forces air into A. Fortunately, in the lung, *surfactant* normally lowers the surface tension in B more than in A, thus maintaining balance.

individuals, and can be a catastrophic insult in the critically ill. Such collapse *cannot* be prevented by provision of moderate amounts of PEEP, e.g. 5 cmH$_2$O, but can be prevented by larger amounts (e.g. 12 cmH$_2$O), which may unfortunately result in some haemodynamic compromise, usually in the volume-depleted patient.

Once basal pulmonary collapse has occurred, there is extreme confusion about which patients have severe atelectasis, and which have 'acute respiratory distress syndrome'. A variety of approaches have been used to 'recruit' collapsed air spaces in the lung (see Box 1).

Infection

An endotracheal tube transgresses the normal laryngeal defence mechanisms and removes the patient's ability to cough. Lying the patient flat then strongly predisposes to lung infection. A major complication of conventional mechanical ventilation is thus 'ventilator-associated pneumonia' (see p. 146).

Striving for normality

In the critically ill, it is a great sin to aim for normality over function. There is no evidence that moderate degrees of hypercarbia or respiratory acidosis are harmful overall, and the same goes for moderate degrees of hypoxia. For example, in the ARDSNet trial, arterial oxygen saturation often ran at 88% in those patients who fared better. Great harm can be induced by ventilatory attempts to produce normocarbia and normoxia, commonly related to pressure/volume-related trauma. There is good evidence that, in asthmatics, adopting a strategy of 'permissive hypercapnia' is conducive to good outcomes, and the same probably holds for other states.

Box 1. A strategy for 'recruitment' of collapsed air spaces

The following approach should be considered experimental, although the results of a successful recruitment manoeuvre are dramatic and satisfying.

1 Select an appropriate patient
2 Ensure muscle relaxation
3 Monitor the patient fully
4 Administer 40 cmH$_2$O of PEEP for 90 s
5 Prevent 'derecruitment' (12–15 cmH$_2$O PEEP)
6 Wait and recheck the arterial blood gas

Liberation from ventilation

Traditionally, we talk about 'weaning' from ventilation. There is no evidence that gradual withdrawal of ventilation has any advantage over immediate removal of an endotracheal tube (ETT) that is not required any more, as ventilation is invasive and can be harmful. The decision to remove the ventilator (and/or the ETT) can be difficult, but tentative attempts may be even more harmful.

As with intubation, poorly prepared extubation may be dangerous or even fatal. Extubation should always be done by an expert, with the equipment, the time, the help and the correct frame of mind to reintubate as necessary (see p. 22). The commonest cause of failed attempts at extubation is failure to realise that substantial coexisting *non-respiratory* disorders contraindicate extubation (see Box 2).

Box 2. Important contraindications to extubation

1 Unstable haemodynamics
2 Heart failure
3 A spiking temperature
4 Marked abdominal distension
5 Gross electrolyte disturbance
6 A large pH derangement
7 Substantial central nervous system dysfunction.

Clinical case

A 'tight' asthmatic has a P_aO_2 of 180 mmHg, P_aCO_2 of 90 mmHg, pH 7.11 (use information given above to convert from mmHg to kPa). On SIMV with no PEEP, short inspiratory times and prolonged expiration at a rate of 10 breaths/min, tidal volume is 80 mL and plateau pressure is 54 cmH$_2$O. The blood pressure is declining and the patient is about to die. What is the problem and what should you do?

Summary points

With severe lung disease, there is no single approach – diseases differ, and so must management – get expert help.

■ Tidal volumes of ~6 mL/kg ideal body weight should probably be the standard of care.
■ *Volumes* are likely to be a better indicator of potential lung injury than pressures.
■ PEEP should be tailored to the case.
■ Permissive hypercapnia is an acceptable manoeuvre, but the role of pH correction is not resolved.
■ One should not aim for a 'normal' P_aO_2 – a haemoglobin saturation of ~90% is probably more than adequate, if achieving a higher saturation is likely to compromise the patient in other ways.
■ Respiratory rate is probably of little importance in the pathogenesis of lung injury.
■ Appropriate recruitment manoeuvres *may* be life saving, but all the necessary caveats must be adhered to.
■ Contrary to the outmoded practice of 'flattening' every ventilated patient, one should aim for an awake, cooperative and comfortable patient.

Renal replacement therapy

Prior to modern techniques of renal replacement therapy (RRT), mortality for acute renal failure (ARF) approached 100%. Today, there are machines that can replicate the essential functions of the kidneys to improve outcome in the intensive care unit (ICU). The goals of RRT include the removal of nitrogenous waste products while maintaining the normal acid–base, electrolyte and fluid balance of the body. There are two main methods by which RRT works. Dialysis or diffusion involves movement owing to an electrochemical gradient. Rate depends on the molecular weight of a particular substance. Convection or ultrafiltration is the dragging of solutes across a membrane's pores with water driven by a hydrostatic or osmotic force. Rate does not depend on the molecular weight.

Indications

RRT should be initiated before the complications of ARF occur and become an emergency (Table 1).

Types of renal replacement therapy

Intermittent haemodialysis (IHD) consists of 3- to 4-h sessions every day or every other day, with a high dialysate flow rate. It is less labour intensive with a lower cost and a decreased risk of infection than continuous therapy. There is rapid removal of poisons and electrolytes, and limited anticoagulation is needed. IHD is contraindicated in hypotensive patients because the rapid flow rate may promote haemodynamic instability.

Continuous renal replacement therapy (CRRT) is continuous dialysis with a low dialysate flow rate. It is labour intensive and requires a dedicated machine. There is no proven survival advantage over IHD, but it is used more frequently in the ICU. Theoretical advantages include haemodynamic stability and more reliable correction of hypervolaemia because it is continuous rather than episodic. With CRRT, the fluid and electrolyte shifts are more gradual. The prognosis for recovery of renal function may be better for those receiving CRRT compared with IHD if there are fewer hypotensive episodes. CRRT may be advantageous in terms of correction of metabolic acidosis as well as cytokine and solute removal. High calorie-containing fluids may be used for undernourished patients. Disadvantages of CRRT include the continuous need for anticoagulation, constant patient immobilisation and higher cost. Specific concerns include infection, bleeding and thromboses.

Continuous veno-venous haemodialysis (CVVHD) is the most used subtype of CRRT in the ICU. A pump drives blood through a filter with a permeable membrane from the patient's vein. A slow countercurrent dialysate flows through the filtrate compartment of the filter so that the fluid is not replaced, and clearance occurs through diffusion and convection. The blood is then returned to the patient's vein.

High-volume haemofiltration (HVHF) is a high ultrafiltrate rate with convection. It is considered to be a powerful immunomodulatory treatment with sepsis but, thus far, the data about outcome are conflicting. HVHF may decrease the sepsis-related inflammatory response, and proponents advocate that it should be started early in the treatment of sepsis, even without ARF. This is unwarranted in view of the current evidence.

Slow low-efficiency daily dialysis (SLEDD) is a new method of RRT, combining CRRT and IHD. It is classic IHD with a low dialysate and blood flow rate. There is a longer dialysis time (6–12 h/day) with improved tolerance. Advantages over IHD include more haemodynamic stability, better correction of hypervolaemia and more adequate solute removal. Advantages over CRRT are that it is cheaper because of the use of IHD equipment and patients are free to move around during much of the day.

Peritoneal dialysis (PD) is continuous dialysis with the movement of substances across the peritoneum. Dialysate solution is intermittently introduced and removed from the peritoneal cavity. PD does not require anticoagulation and can be used in a patient who is hypotensive or has poor vascular access. It is less efficient in metabolic clearance than other modalities and does not optimally control uraemic manifestations. Rapid glucose absorption may cause extreme hyperglycaemia. PD cannot be used for patients who have had abdominal surgery and has a high failure rate for those with a paralytic ileus. The fluid in the peritoneal cavity may impede diaphragmatic movement and compromise pulmonary function. There is a high rate of peritoneal infection.

Anticoagulation

Anticoagulation may be indicated to avoid clotting of the RRT machine or vascular access. It is one of the major problems of RRT, especially CRRT. Methods of anticoagulation include low-dose heparin, low-molecular-weight heparin, citrate, intravenous prostacyclin and direct thrombin inhibitors, such as bivalirudin and argatroban. The advantages of heparin are familiarity, cost, ability to monitor therapeutic effect, reversal if required with protamine and ease of use. The target partial thromboplastin time for heparin anticoagulation is typically between 50 and 80 seconds, and is checked about three times per day. Specific concerns relating to heparin are that prolonged use frequently results in heparin resistance and heparin-induced thrombocytopenia with life-threatening thrombosis.

Table 1 **Indications for renal replacement therapy**
Acidaemia (pH is < 7.2 or serum bicarbonate is < 15 mmol/L)
Electrolyte abnormalities (toxic levels of K^+, Ca^{2+}, Mg^{2+} or PO_4^{2-})
Intoxications (e.g. lithium, aspirin, ethylene glycol, methanol)
Volume overload (pulmonary oedema, anasarca)
Uraemia (pericarditis, encephalopathy, platelet dysfunction)

Complications

The major causes of death for those requiring RRT are infection and cardiopulmonary complications (Fig. 1). Poor prognostic indicators include the need for mechanical ventilation and the use of inotropes or pressors.

Clinical case

A 72-year-old male is on the ICU with ARF following exposure to contrast agent for cardiac catheterisation. Owing to haemodynamic instability following a myocardial infarction, CVVHD has been prescribed. The arterial blood gases have been followed, and a trend of worsening acidaemia has been noted. Bicarbonate infusion and the CVVHD flow rate are increased. The patient becomes confused and complains of nausea and headache. Apart from delirium, myoclonus is noted. The potassium is found to be 2.5 mmol/L 2 h after the adjustments to the CVVHD. The potassium 2 h previously had been 4.3 mmol/L. What is the probable explanation for the hypokalaemia and the change in mental status?

Discontinuation

There are three main reasons for stopping RRT: (1) the kidney function is improving; (2) the patient's prognosis is dismal; or (3) the patient (or their advocate) does not wish to continue with RRT. A trial of stopping RRT may be warranted when the patient is passing urine and there are no specific indications for RRT as described previously. For the survivors of ARF, 90% recover renal function and do not need lifelong dialysis. Full recovery may take several months, although most forms of ARF reverse within 8 weeks.

Summary points

- Mortality for patients with acute renal failure on the ICU has decreased but remains high.
- Indications for RRT include severe acidaemia, electrolyte abnormalities, intoxications, fluid overload and signs of uraemia.
- Continuous RRT is indicated when patients are haemodynamically unstable.
- Complications of RRT include bleeding, infection, fluid derangement, electrolyte abnormalities and acid–base disorders.

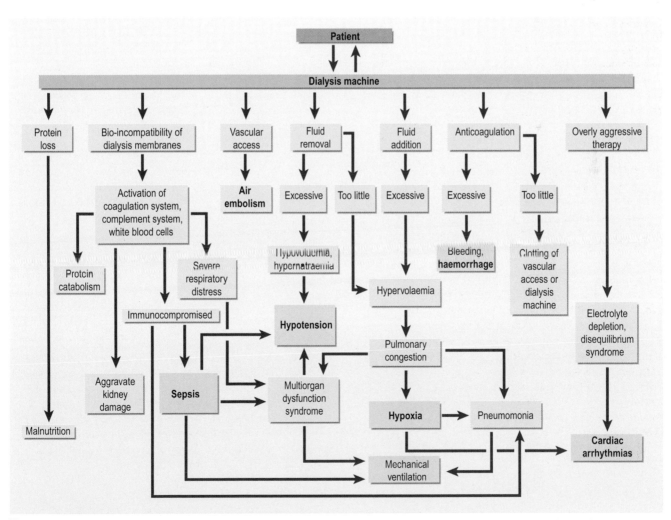

Fig. 1 **Complications associated with RRT***. Biocompatibility is the interaction between blood and the artificial membrane (synthetic polymers are more biocompatible then cellulose).

Mechanical circulatory support

Mechanical support may also be required for days (to allow time for recovery), for months (as 'bridging therapy' while a donor heart is found) or even years [as final (*destination*) therapy].

Devices for mechanical circulatory support (Box 1)

A vast amount of effort and emotion has been invested in replacing the human heart with a mechanical prosthesis. The first artificial heart was used as bridging therapy by Cooley in 1969. This was the Liotta heart, an air-driven biventricular pump. The number and variety of current mechanical devices for circulatory support is evidence that no one device is spectacularly effective (Table 1).

For short-term support, the older commonly available Medtronic Biomedicus pump may work as well as far more expensive centrifugal rotary devices. There are still numerous problems with mechanical circulatory support (Box 2).

Clinical pearl
When a patient with a left ventricular assist device (LVAD) is 'failing to thrive', consider preload optimisation (packed red cells), lowering afterload and treatment of right heart failure and pulmonary hypertension (e.g. inhaled prostacyclin).

Clinical case
A previously fit and well 10-year-old girl presents after 2 weeks of 'lethargy and fatigue' with gross cardiomegaly and cardiac failure. Despite optimal medical management, she had a progressive decline over the next 2 weeks and developed multiorgan failure and inotrope dependence. How will you manage her now?

Table 1 **Some devices for 'mechanical' circulatory support**

Device	Date (approx)	Make	Mechanism	Site/tcet	Output	Term/notes
IABP	1980	Various	Pneumatic	Aorta	30–40 mL	Short
ECMO	1979	Various	Roller pump	V/A		Short
BVS 5000 AB 5000	1988	Abiomed	Pneumatic, passive fill	Extracorporeal	6 L/min	Short FDA 1992
VAD, IVAD	1976	Thoratec	Pulsatile, LV ± RV	External/ implantable (IVAD)	7 L/min	Short/bridging FDA 1995
Novacor LVAS	1998	World Heart	Pulsatile, linear driver	Implantable	10 L/min	Bridging FDA 1998
Lionheart LVAS	1999	Arrow	Pulsatile	Abdomen, tcet	4.7 L/min	Destination
CardioWest	1985	Syncardia	Pneumatic	Orthotopic	6–8 L/min	Bridging FDA 2004
Heartmate IP	1986	Thoratec	Pneumatic	Abdomen	11.5 L/min	Bridging FDA 1994
Heartmate XVE	1990	Similar to IP, but 12-V DC motor controls pusher plate; REMATCH trial is of note. Textured surfaces				Destination FDA 2003
Impella Recover	2000	Abiomed	Impeller pump	Across aortic valve	2.5 L/min 33 000 rpm	7 days
Jarvik 2000	2000	Jarvik	Axial	Implantable, *intraventricular*	8 L/min, 8–12 000 rpm	Bridging, long term
INCOR	2002	Berlin Heart	Axial, maglev	Implantable (200 g)	7 L/min 10 000 rpm	Bridging, ?long term
Micromed DeBakey VAD	2004	Micromed	Axial	Implantable, small (110 g)	10 L/min 10 000 rpm	Bridging FDA (child)
Heartmate II	2003	Thoratec	Axial	Implantable (375 g)	10 L/min,6–15 000 rpm	Bridging
AbioCor	2001	Abiomed	Axial	Implant, tcet (500 g)	8 L/min, 3–10 000 rpm	Destination
CentriMag	2003	Levitronix	Centrifugal, maglev	Attach to CPB	9.9 L/min 5000 rpm	14 days Phase I 2003
TandemHeart pVAD	2002 Phase II	Cardiac assist	Centrifugal, LA to arterial!	Minimally invasive	4 L/min 3– 7500 rpm	Short Phase II 2002
Heartmate III	Awaited	Thoratec	Centrifugal maglev	Implantable textured, tcet	2–12 L/min 3–5000+ rpm	?Long term
VentrAssist	2005	Ventracor	Centrifugal maglev	298 g, fully implantable	2–3000 rpm 1–5+ L/min	Long term
C-Pulse	2005	Sunshine	Pneumatic	Around aorta	30% SV	Experimental

tcet, transcutaneous energy transfer; SV, stroke volume; LV, left ventricle; LA, left atrium; maglev, magnetically levitated; V/A, ventricular/atrial; CPB, cardiopulmonary bypass; FDA, FDA approval granted in some circumstances. Note: RELIANT trial is comparing Novacor LVAS and Heartmate XVE.

Box 1. *Devices for mechanical circulatory support*

Intra-aortic balloon pump (Fig. 1)
Pulsatile blood pump (Fig. 2)

Spiral impeller (Fig. 3)
Centrifugal rotary pump (total ventricular assist device; Fig. 4)

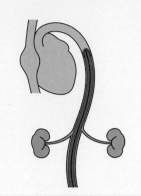

Fig. 1 **Intra-aortic balloon pump.**

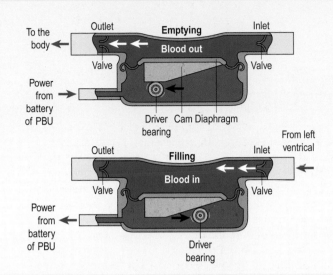

Fig. 2 **Pulsatile blood pump.**

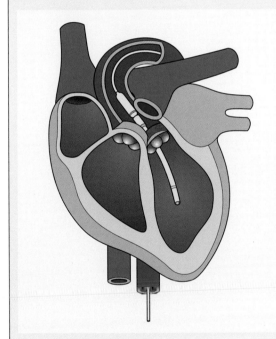

Fig. 3 **Spiral impeller.**

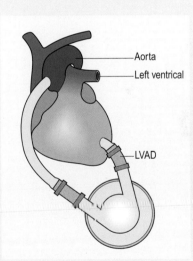

Fig. 4 **Centrifugal rotary pump.**

Box 2. *Common problems with long-term mechanical circulatory support*

- Haemorrhage: haemolysis with rotary devices depends on flow dynamics and speed – the slower the rotation the better
- Thrombosis and embolism: decreased with biocompatible coatings including diamond-like carbon and MPC
- Infection (28% in 3 months)*
- Device failure (35% in 2 years)*
- Organ dysfunction (renal and respiratory)
- Tied to a machine!

Percentages in parenthesis indicate incidence in the REMATCH study.

Summary points

- Uninterrupted, effective mechanical chest compression is the most important form of mechanical circulatory support.
- Many complex techniques have been used for mechanical circulatory support; most are still essentially experimental.
- Complications are common (notably infection and thrombosis), even in the best hands.
- The intra-aortic balloon pump is a temporising measure, with a high complication rate.
- Pneumatic pulsatile pumps have been extensively trialled.
- Centrifugal pumps have favourable flow characteristics.
- Despite their fast rotation speeds, axial pumps do not usually cause much haemolysis.

Homeostasis

Circulation

In 1628, the English physician William Harvey announced a revolutionary theory stating that blood circulates repeatedly throughout the body, with the heart acting as its driving force. This flew in the face of Galen's sacred hypothesis – widely accepted for over 1000 years – that the liver converts food into blood, which serves as direct nutrition for the various organs.

Many critically ill patients have circulatory failure or shock. One of the main challenges in managing such patients is discovering and redressing the causes of shock. In some settings, it is relatively straightforward to determine the origin of shock. A young man who has been stabbed in the femoral artery is suffering from hypovolaemic shock. An old man who has had a large heart attack is suffering from cardiogenic shock. But in the intensive care unit (ICU), where patients have complex diagnoses, there are frequently several factors contributing to shock.

Physiology

The circulation consists of a pump, the pulmonary circulation and the systemic circulation. The systemic arteries are resistance vessels, and the veins and pulmonary vessels are capacitance vessels, which act as a reservoir for intravascular volume.

The relationship between flow on the one hand and pressure and resistance on the other is shown in Fig. 1.

There are two important concepts that bear emphasising:

1 It is generally appreciated that, when the mean arterial pressure (MAP) decreases, there is a concomitant decrease in flow or cardiac output. What is not always considered is that flow is dependent on pressure gradient. This applies to flow in general. For example, with right heart failure and elevated central venous pressure, 'normal' MAP may not be adequate to maintain flow to vital organs. This principle also applies to regional flow or flow to organ systems. When there is elevated left ventricular end-diastolic pressure, increased diastolic blood pressure may be required to maintain coronary perfusion. When there is elevated hepatic or renal venous pressure, increased MAP may be required to maintain flow to these vital organs. Another important example relates to increased intracranial pressure. In such instances, maintaining a higher than 'normal' blood pressure may be critical to the maintenance of cerebral perfusion. It may therefore be more useful to think of perfusion pressure, rather than blood pressure in isolation.

2 Vital organ systems autoregulate their flow. This means that, largely through the release of local vasoactive mediators such as endothelins and nitric oxide, flow to these organs is maintained constant over a wide range of perfusion pressures. Patients on ICUs frequently have impaired autoregulation (Fig. 2). This occurs when organ systems are dysfunctional. Importantly, sedative agents such as propofol may obtund the ability of vital organs to regulate their flow. Another important consideration is that many patients on the ICU have coexisting diseases, including poorly controlled hypertension. This results in autoregulation of flow occurring at higher than 'normal' MAP. In such instances, an acute reduction in blood pressure to an apparently normal MAP of 90 mmHg may result in inadequate perfusion to vital organs, such as the kidneys.

Cardiac output (CO) or flow is defined by the following relationship:

$$CO \text{ (flow)} = \text{stroke volume} \times \text{heart rate}$$
$$\text{Stroke volume} \propto \text{preload} \times \text{contractility/afterload}$$

Preload is end-diastolic myocardial fibre length, which increases with increased intravascular volume. Stroke volume increases with increased preload as described by the Frank–Starling curve.

Afterload is the tension the heart muscle must develop just prior to the onset of contraction. Increase in afterload is associated with a decrease in stroke volume. It is intuitively understood that increased resistance to cardiac contraction, such as occurs with systolic hypertension, increased systemic vascular resistance and aortic stenosis, increases afterload. Less appreciated is that the geometry and radius of the heart and thickness of the heart muscle also determine afterload. When the heart's geometry is altered, such as by an aneurysm or a dyskinetic muscle segment, cardiac contraction loses efficiency. This imposes an increased strain on the viable heart muscle, and afterload is increased. The relationship between afterload (tension), radius and wall thickness for a sphere is described by the following equation (Laplace's law):

$$\text{Tension} \propto \text{pressure} \times \text{radius/thickness}$$

More tension is required to contract a big sphere than a small sphere (Fig. 3). The same applies to the heart. Decreasing preload may improve myocardial performance because of the associated decrease in afterload (radius). From the above equation, the reason for left ventricular hypertrophy as a compensatory mechanism for hypertension and aortic stenosis is clear. Thick heart muscle is associated with decreased tension or afterload. Unfortunately, hypertrophy is also associated with diastolic dysfunction and increased oxygen requirements.

Contractility is the intrinsic ability of the heart muscle to generate contractile force independent of loading conditions. Increased contractility is associated with increased stroke volume.

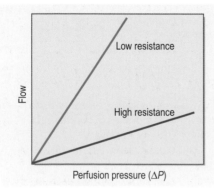

Fig. 1 **Flow = pressure/resistance.**

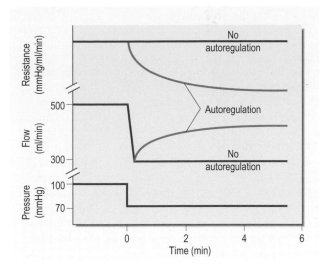

Fig. 2 **How various vital organs autoregulate.** Flow is maintained relatively constant with changes in perfusion pressure by varying the local resistance.

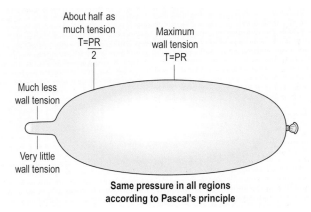

Fig. 3 **A balloon is a useful model to illustrate Laplace's law.**

Shock on the ICU

Hypovolaemic shock

Acute hypovolaemia, such as occurs with major surgery, burns, sepsis and haemorrhage, mandates aggressive resuscitation. Chronic intravascular volume depletion frequently occurs in critically ill patients, even when there is increased total body water. This may be secondary to low albumin or to leaky capillaries allowing fluid to accumulate in the interstitium. There is no gold standard for measuring volume status, and the reader is referred to p. 18 for further discussion. Pulse pressure variation and systolic pressure variation (pulsus paradoxus) are useful indicators of intravascular hypovolaemia. But these may be misleading, for example when there is obstructive shock.

Cardiogenic shock

Many ICU patients have myocardial dysfunction, whether owing to underlying heart disease or related to their critical illness. Severe sepsis is associated with multiple organ dysfunction. It is hypothesised that among the mediators released as part of the inflammatory response are myocardial depressant factors. Echocardiography is a non-invasive means of detecting myocardial dysfunction on the ICU. It is important to understand that positive pressure ventilation provides a degree of myocardial support. This is probably because the increased intrathoracic pressure decreases the radius of the heart, thereby decreasing afterload. Discontinuing positive pressure ventilation may precipitate cardiac decompensation.

Obstructive and restrictive shock

The most common cause on the ICU is inappropriate mechanical ventilation leading to dynamic hyperinflation of the lungs and compression of the capacitance vessels. The treatment is disconnection of the ventilator allowing air to escape from the lungs. Identifying patients at risk (e.g. those with asthma or chronic obstructive pulmonary disease) and allowing sufficient time for expiration are important in preventing this. Other causes of obstructive shock include bronchospasm, pulmonary embolism, tamponade and tension pneumothorax. Obstructive shock may be misdiagnosed, for example as hypovolaemia. It is frequently reversible, and missing the diagnosis may have devastating results. Pulmonary hypertension and right heart failure may lead to shock by decreasing blood return to the heart.

Distributive shock

This form of circulatory collapse is frequently encountered in the ICU setting. With the release of inflammatory mediators and cytokines, increased capillary permeability results, and there may be massive extravasation of fluid as well as vasodilatation and venodilatation. In the initial management of systemic inflammatory response syndrome (SIRS) and sepsis, large-volume fluid resuscitation is often necessary. With the loss of vascular tone, pressor agents such as noradrenaline (norepinephrine) and vasopressin (or terlipressin) may be required to restore pressure. Anaphylaxis is an important cause of distributive shock. Patients on the ICU receive multiple drugs and blood components. Anaphylaxis should always be considered in the differential diagnosis when a patient presents with distributive shock.

Clinical case

A 63-year-old woman underwent a hemicolectomy 1 week ago. She was fit prior to her admission, apart from having hypertension. She has become ill over the past 2 days and was admitted to the ICU with a diagnosis of pneumonia.

A central venous catheter, an oesophageal Doppler probe and an arterial line were inserted. She had a blood pressure of 90/30 with a heart rate of 110/min. The pulsus paradoxus was 14 mmHg, and she had a marked pulse pressure variation. The central venous pressure was 7 mmHg. She had a temperature of 39.7°C. She had bounding peripheral pulses with warm peripheries. The cardiac output was 6.5 L/min (cardiac index = 2.6 L/min/m²). Transthoracic echocardiography showed an 'empty looking' heart with mildly impaired function (ejection fraction = 40%). From what type of shock is she suffering?

Summary points

- Shock occurs when flow is insufficient to meet the needs of individual organs or of the whole organism.
- Pressure gradient determines flow.
- ICU patients' vital organ systems' autoregulation may be impaired or set at a higher pressure.
- Decreasing the size (radius) of the heart decreases its workload.
- Different types of shock frequently coexist in critically ill patients.

Oxygen delivery

The heart, lungs and blood work synergistically to deliver oxygen (O_2) to the tissues and vital organs. Many critically ill patients have insufficient oxygen delivery to meet their metabolic requirements. Shock is the condition in which inadequate oxygen supply leads to hypoxia at a tissue level. This supply–demand imbalance can, if prolonged, lead to organ dysfunction. Consequently, much of critical care is aimed at restoring and maintaining adequate oxygen delivery.

Physiology

Most of the oxygen in the blood is carried by haemoglobin. When haemoglobin is fully saturated with oxygen, as reflected by a pulse oximeter reading approaching 100%, each gram of haemoglobin carries about 1.34 mL of oxygen. The proportion of unbound oxygen is small, as oxygen does not dissolve well in blood. The total oxygen delivered to the body is the oxygen content of the blood multiplied by the cardiac output.

The amount of oxygen used by the body (VO_2) is the difference between arterial and mixed venous (pulmonary arterial) oxygen content multiplied by the cardiac output. Dividing the oxygen consumption by the oxygen delivery yields the oxygen extraction ratio (OER). As oxygen delivery decreases, the body increases oxygen extraction to maintain a constant VO_2. Normal OER is 20–30%. Under stress, the body can increase oxygen extraction to approximately 60%. Trained athletes can reach 80%. Important equations are shown in Box 1.

The amount of O_2 carried by haemoglobin depends on how much haemoglobin there is and the extent to which the haemoglobin in saturated with oxygen. The relationship between haemoglobin's oxygen saturation and the partial pressure of oxygen in arterial blood (P_aO_2) is described by the oxyhaemoglobin dissociation curve (Fig. 1). The sigmoid shape of the curve has important implications:

1 If $P_aO_2 > 60$ mmHg (8 kPa), the amount of additional O_2 bound to haemoglobin is rather small. Increasing P_aO_2 increases the blood oxygen content slightly by increasing the dissolved O_2.
2 The shape of the dissociation curve is advantageous, as O_2 affinity is high at high P_aO_2 (e.g. in the lungs) and relatively unaffected until P_aO_2 drops below 50–60 mmHg (6.57–8 kPa) [e.g. in the tissues, $P_aO_2 = 40$ mmHg (5.33 kPa)]. This facilitates the loading of oxygen to haemoglobin in the lungs and the offloading of oxygen to the tissues.

Several factors affect the curve:

1 Increased affinity for O_2 (shift left): alkalaemia, hypothermia, decreased 2,3-DPG, fetal haemoglobin, carboxyhaemoglobin, methaemoglobin.
2 Decreased affinity for O_2 (shift right): acidaemia, hyperthermia, increased 2,3-DPG, increased carbon dioxide partial pressure (Pco_2).

When oxygen delivery (DO_2) drops and oxygen extraction is maximal, oxygen utilisation (VO_2) becomes supply dependent. The DO_2 at which this happens is called the *critical oxygen delivery* (Fig. 2). This restriction in oxygen

supply leads to impairment in cellular production of adenosine triphosphate (ATP). The point of critical oxygen delivery in critically ill patients varies from 150 to 1000 mL/min/m².

Box 1. Important equations

Blood O_2 content (C_aO_2) = $(1.34 \text{ mL/g} \times \text{Hgb (g/L)} \times S_aO_2/100)$ + $(0.03 \times P_aO_2)$

O_2 delivery (DO_2) = blood O_2 content × cardiac output = $[1.34 \text{ mL/g} \times \text{Hgb g/L} \times \%S_aO_2) + (0.03 \times P_aO_2)] \times Q$ (L/min)

Oxygen utilisation (VO_2) = $Q \times (C_aO_2 - C_{mv}O_2)$ (Fick equation) = $Q \times 1.34 \times \text{Hgb} \times (S_aO_2 - SVO_2)$

Oxygen extraction ratio (OER) = $VO_2/DO_2 \times 100$

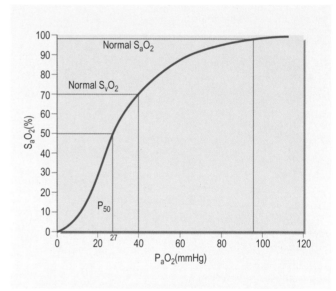

Fig. 1 **Oxyhaemoglobin dissociation curve** (divide by 7.5 to convert mmHg to KPa).

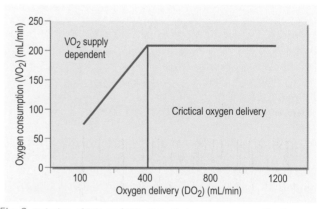

Fig. 2 **Relation of DO₂ and VO₂.** Note that oxygen consumption is constant until the level of critical oxygen delivery is reached (in this figure, 400 mL/min). Below this point, compensatory mechanisms are maximal, and oxygen consumption becomes dependent on the amount of oxygen supplied.

Monitoring oxygen delivery

Mixed venous O_2 saturation (SVO_2) is a useful parameter that, taken with other data, can indicate global oxygen balance. Continuous SVO_2 monitoring via oximetric pulmonary artery catheters is available. The central venous oxygen saturation provides a good approximation of SVO_2 and may also be useful in tracking whether the body's oxygen needs are being met. Intermittent measurements of mixed venous or central venous oxygen saturation can be achieved by sending blood specimens for laboratory co-oximetry measurement. Mixed venous oxygen saturation monitoring is a crude screen for adequacy of global oxygen delivery. When the SVO_2 is low, typically $< 60\%$, this suggests that oxygen delivery is insufficient to meet the body's metabolic needs. An important exception to this occurs in situations where oxygen does not reach the tissues or aerobic metabolic pathways are dysfunctional. Examples of this are sepsis and cyanide poisoning. If oxygen is not utilised, SVO_2 can be high even though global oxygen utilisation is impaired. SVO_2 does not provide information about specific oxygen utilisation. Lactic acid is produced during anaerobic glucose metabolism. Metabolic acidosis and elevated lactate ($> 2\,mmol/L$) may also be indicative of tissue hypoxia.

Optimising oxygen delivery

Hypoxia results when insufficient oxygen gets into the body, when the lungs are unable to achieve effective gas exchange, when the oxygen is not delivered to the tissues, when the cells are unable to use oxygen and when the tissues' demands exceed the supply of oxygen (Table 1).

DO_2 can be improved by increasing arterial saturation, cardiac output or haemoglobin (Fig. 3). There is a point beyond which increasing the haemoglobin concentration does not improve oxygen delivery owing to increased blood viscosity. Acceptable haemoglobin concentrations vary, but are widely held to be 7–8 g/dL unless patients have ischaemic heart disease, in which case the target haemoglobin may be as high as 12–13 g/dL. Increasing cardiac output may typically be achieved by increasing preload, decreasing afterload or increasing contractility. The problem with inotropes, such as dobutamine, is that they increase oxygen consumption as well as delivery.

Global versus regional hypoxia

The above discussion refers to total-body delivery of oxygen. Many clinical situations involve regional supply–demand imbalances that can lead to specific organ dysfunction even with adequate global oxygen delivery (Table 2). Examples of such situations include myocardial infarction and stroke.

Table 1 Causes of hypoxia and clinical examples

Cause	Example
Hypoxic inspired gas	High altitude
Dead space	Pulmonary embolism, COPD
Shunt (intrapulmonary)	Atelectasis, pneumonia, pulmonary oedema, ARDS
Shunt (extrapulmonary)	Cyanotic congenital heart disease
Hypoventilation	Opioid treatment, postoperative patients
Impaired carriage of O_2	Anaemia, carbon monoxide poisoning, methaemoglobinaemia
Histotoxic hypoxia	Cyanide poisoning (e.g. sodium nitroprusside)
Stagnant hypoxia	Congestive heart failure, cardiogenic and hypovolaemic shock
Hypermetabolism	Malignant hyperthermia, thyroid storm, phaeochromocytoma

ARDS, acute respiratory distress syndrome: COPD, chronic obstructive pulmonary syndrome.

Table 2 Evaluating individual organ function

Organ	Measures of dysfunction
Heart	ECG, echocardiography, cardiac output, troponin concentrations
Kidney	Urine output, creatinine concentration
Brain	Mental status, jugular venous saturation
Gut	Lactic acid levels, gastric tonometry

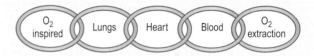

Fig. 3 **Oxygen delivery as a chain.** Efficient delivery of oxygen to the tissues depends on a chain of events. Any broken link in the chain can compromise oxygenation.

Clinical case

A 74-year-old man with a history of coronary artery disease presents to the ICU postoperatively following open abdominal aortic aneurysm repair. His vital signs include: pulse 94 bpm, arterial blood pressure 97/55 mmHg, arterial oxygen saturation 92% with 50% inspired oxygen concentration ($F_iO_2 = 0.5$). Cardiac output is 3.4 L/min. His mixed venous oxygen saturation is 50%. His haemoglobin is 65 g/L. Arterial blood gas values are: pH 7.32, PCO_2 32 mmHg (4.27 kPa), pO_2 65 mmHg (8.67 kPa). What is his global oxygen delivery? Is it adequate? What interventions can be undertaken to improve oxygen delivery to his tissues? How would one identify increased oxygen delivery?

Summary points

- Oxygen delivery is dependent on cardiac output and carriage by haemoglobin.
- Metabolic acidosis, elevated lactate and decreased venous oxygen saturation may all reflect inadequate global oxygen supply.
- Impaired oxygen delivery to individual vital organs may occur even when global delivery is sufficient.

ICU acid–basics

The concept of pH (Box 1) is complex and counterintuitive, but acid–base management in the intensive care unit (ICU) has become more rational in recent years. A solid understanding of acid–base often leads to watchful observation in preference to aggressive intervention (Fig. 1).

Basics

Important concepts are:

- The body tries to keep pH in the narrow range of 7.36–7.44.
- The respiratory system and kidneys play vital roles in pH regulation, the former by 'blowing off' carbon dioxide or 'retaining it' to lower or raise pH, and the kidneys by balancing their excretion of ions to keep pH in the normal range.
- Several 'buffer systems' exist in the body, which tend to damp down alterations in pH – there is a complex interaction between these systems, the fully dissociated ions ('strong ions') and the aqueous medium in which they exist.

Why is pH so important? Mainly because *all* metabolic processes within the body depend on pH. One explanatory theory is the 'alpha-stat' hypothesis – that the body maintains the ionisation state of protein components rather than pH itself.

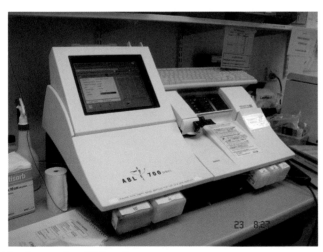

Fig. 1 **A modern ABG analyser.**

Measurement of pH in the ICU

Modern *ion-sensitive electrodes* are used to determine pH and concentrations of ions such as sodium (Na^+), potassium (K^+) and calcium (Ca^{2+}). It is the *activity* of these ions that is measured, but our laboratories and blood gas analysers automatically convert from activity to concentration.

A convenient checklist

In assessing disturbances of acid–base, consider the following.

The clinical context
An *apparent* derangement in one individual may represent 'normality' for them. For example, a pH of 7.34, P_{CO_2} of 8 kPa (60 mmHg) and serum bicarbonate of 35 mmol/L may represent baseline values in somebody with obstructive airways disease and carbon dioxide retention, or might represent gross derangement in a patient with acute pneumonia. The one patient might be sitting chatting to you, the other might be critically ill needing ventilation.

Current management
Most forms of therapy interfere with acid–base balance. In the ICU, we have ventilatory support, renal support and administration of fluid and drugs, especially diuretics.

The pH
If the pH is low, the patient is *acidaemic*; if it is high, *alkalaemia* is present.

The P_aCO_2
If the partial pressure of carbon dioxide in arterial blood is above the reference maximum for your laboratory (at sea level, often about 45 mmHg = 6 kPa), hypercapnia is present. Such carbon dioxide retention can be due to tiring and muscle weakness, *or* compensation for a metabolic alkalosis. The body *never* overcompensates.

Conversely, low P_{CO_2} values (under about 33 mmHg = 4.4 kPa) are termed hypocapnia. Both compensation for metabolic acidosis and primary hyperventilation (due to pain, anxiety or inappropriate ventilatory management) will cause hypocapnia.

The implications
It is easy to cause harm in the ICU by overzealous management of an acid–base 'disorder' (see the clinical case).

Managing the problem

Substantial derangements of acid–base balance will be encountered in the ICU. Several models partially explain such findings.

The traditional approach
The traditional approach of Siggaard-Andersen and others emphasises the centrality of the Henderson–Hasselbalch (HH) equation shown in Box 2.

Table 1 **The Boston formulae**			
State	Rule	Formula	Range
Metabolic acidosis	1.5 + 8	P_{CO_2} (mmHg) = 1.5 * bicarbonate + 8	± 2
Metabolic alkalosis	0.7 + 20	P_{CO_2} (mmHg) = 0.7 * bicarbonate + 20	± 5
Acute respiratory alkalosis	2 for 10	Bicarbonate (mmol/L) drops 2 mmol/L per 10-mmHg P_{CO_2} drop	?
Chronic respiratory alkalosis	5 for 10	Likewise, but 5 mmol/L	?
Acute respiratory acidosis	1 for 10	Bicarbonate (mmol/L) increases 1 mmol/L per 10 mmHg	?
Chronic respiratory acidosis	4 for 10	Likewise, but 4 mmol/L	?

Values are after Brandis, K. Acid–base physiology. URL: http://www.qldanaesthesia.com/AcidBaseBook/ABindex.htm.

Complex derived quantities such as 'base excess' are used to make pronouncements about acid–base balance. This approach makes several assumptions, such as normal serum albumin concentration, which are often untenable in the ICU setting.

The 'Boston School'

The 'Boston school', in addition to the traditional approach, emphasises the utility of several empirically derived equations (see Table 1).

It is not clear whether these equations are applicable across the spectrum of disease seen in modern ICUs.

The Stewart approach

Peter Stewart applied well-established chemical principles to human plasma and produced an elegant and satisfying analysis of how acid–base works. His approach is frequently misunderstood or criticised for reasons that seem quite divorced from logic, mathematics or clinical reasoning!

Stewart pointed out that there are many *dependent* variables that change as a consequence of acid–base disturbances (e.g. bicarbonate concentration, pH and concentration of hydroxyl ions). There are, however, only three important *independent* variables in human plasma: partial pressure of carbon dioxide, concentration of weak acids (mainly albumin) and something called the strong ion difference or SID. The SID is the difference in concentration between the completely dissociated cations (mainly sodium and potassium) and the anions (mainly chloride). It is normally about 42 mmol/L.

Only alterations in the three *independent* variables can have an influence on this chemical system described by six simple equations. The equations are easily solved using a computer to provide values for the *dependent* variables.

Stewart's approach has several merits:

1 It is a sound model of what is happening in plasma.
2 It alerts us to the effects of albumin concentration on acid–base balance, especially the masking effect of low albumin on a high anion gap (AG) (Box 3).
3 It easily explains such phenomena as 'dilutional acidosis', where the administration of large quantities of unphysiological fluids with a SID of zero is associated with the development of acidosis.

Box 3. The anion gap

For the commonly measured ions in plasma, Na^+, K^+, Cl^- and HCO_3^-, the sum of the concentrations of the positive ions is greater than that of the negatively charged ions. To maintain charge balance, there must be hidden negative ions – the *anion gap*, which is normally about 8–12 mmol/L. Hidden anions such as ketones and lactate increase the AG; a low albumin may conceal such ions.

Clinical case

A poorly controlled asthmatic stopped taking her inhaled steroids 2 weeks previously. She collapsed at home with severe bronchospasm and is now in the ICU on a ventilator. She has a normal build and weighs 70 kg. On maximal therapy, her ventilator settings (with a short inspiratory time) are as follows:

Respiratory rate 6/min; tidal volume 300 mL; plateau pressure 30 cmH$_2$O; F_iO_2 90%.

Haemodynamics are good and there is 4 cmH$_2$O of auto-PEEP. Arterial blood gas analysis reveals:

pH 7.16; P_{CO_2} 10 kPa (75 mmHg); HCO_3^- 25 mmol/L; P_{O_2} 8 kPa (60 mmHg).

What should be done? (From the text, you can guess the answer, but also see Appendix 2.)

Box 2. The Henderson–Hasselbalch equation

One of the several equations governing acid–base balance in human plasma is that describing the formation of hydrogen ions and bicarbonate from carbon dioxide and water:

$$CO_2 + H_2O \Leftrightarrow H_2CO_3 \Leftrightarrow H^+ + HCO_3^-$$

The law of mass action tells us that at equilibrium:

$$[H_2CO_3] = Ka * [HCO_3^-] * [H^+]$$

Taking the logarithm of both sides of the equation, we get the familiar HH equation:

$$pH = pKa + \log [HCO_3^-]/[H_2CO_3]$$

Replacing $[H_2CO_3]$ by 0.03 * P_aCO_2 is usually quite reasonable.

Summary points

- The body tightly regulates pH.
- pH in plasma largely depends on the partial pressure of carbon dioxide, the amount of weak acid (albumin) and the difference in concentration of positively and negatively charged strong ions.
- Although there are several different approaches to acid–base, there is much common ground.
- Hidden anions can increase the anion gap.

Carbon dioxide

In billions of cellular internal combustion engines, the body oxidises substrates such as glucose to build its energy stores. The fuel provided by this process is converted to the universal power currency of adenosine triphosphate (ATP), which drives the energy-consuming activities of the cells. Water and CO_2 are produced through this cellular respiration. CO_2 is an acidic metabolic byproduct, which is churned out at a whole-body rate of about 200 mL/min or 288 L/day (Fig. 1)! This amount may increase up to six times in the face of critical illness. When CO_2 delivery to and expulsion by the lungs is impaired or when CO_2 production soars, the body's buffering systems may be overwhelmed, resulting in respiratory acidosis.

Carbon dioxide has important effects on every organ system within the human body. Many health workers are aware of the potentially harmful effects of acidaemia and hypercapnia, including myocardial depression and arrhythmias. Surprisingly, there is often less concern about hypocapnia and alkalaemia, although the results may be catastrophic with impaired perfusion to vital organs.

CO_2 in critical care

At sea level, the normal range for P_{CO_2} is 36–44 mmHg (4.8–5.9 kPa). When the P_{CO_2} is low, this may represent appropriate compensation for metabolic acidosis or overzealous mechanical ventilation. Patients may hyperventilate when they are in pain or if there is a neurological injury. Pain should be treated, and iatrogenic hyperventilation should be avoided. Patients on the intensive care unit (ICU) frequently have lung pathology, which results in impaired ventilation. In order to blow off CO_2, high ventilation pressures and tidal volumes may be required. Further damage to the lungs may result. Permissive hypercapnia has therefore evolved as a treatment paradigm for patients with lung injury, such as pneumonia and acute respiratory distress syndrome (ARDS). The damage inflicted on the lungs with the mechanical ventilator in trying to achieve normal P_{CO_2} may outweigh the harm associated with mild hypercapnia. Increasingly, evidence is emerging that mild hypercapnia is well tolerated and not associated with bad outcome.

Benefits of mild hypercapnia

Hypercapnia shifts the oxyhaemoglobin dissociation curve rightward. This promotes oxygen offloading to the tissues. This may be advantageous during critical illness when the peripheral tissues are relatively deprived of oxygenation. Hypercapnia depresses actomyosin interactions resulting in decreased myocardial O_2 consumption. This combined with increased O_2 availability may result in cardioprotection. Hypercapnia results in decreased systemic vascular resistance, increased heart rate and increased cardiac output. From a neurological standpoint, there are experimental data showing that hypercapnia results in less free radical formation during brain ischaemia. It is speculated that this will result in better neurological outcomes for patients who have suffered cerebral ischaemia. Likewise, animal models have demonstrated that respiratory acidosis prevents increased capillary permeability after acute lung injury, possibly halting the progression to ARDS. At a cellular level, respiratory acidosis decreases cellular respiration and oxygen consumption. This may protect cells generally from hypoxic injury. Hypercapnia attenuates free radical production and decreases lipid peroxidation and inflammation.

Hazards of hypercapnia

In certain settings, hypercapnia may worsen patients' disease processes. With raised intracranial pressure, acute hypercapnia may result in a dangerous further increase in cerebral blood flow and pressure. Hypercapnia increases pulmonary vascular resistance and may precipitate acute right heart failure; it should be avoided when patients have pulmonary hypertension or right heart dysfunction. As CO_2 is an activator of the sympathetic nervous system, hypercapnia should be prevented when there is active ischaemic heart disease or susceptibility to arrhythmias (Fig. 2).

Dangers of hypocapnia

With few exceptions, hypocapnia is detrimental. Hypocapnia causes a leftward shift in the oxyhaemoglobin dissociation curve, thereby decreasing O_2 offloading and rendering vital organs and peripheral tissues prone to ischaemia. Hypocapnia increases myocardial sensitivity to calcium, which increases myocardial O_2 consumption. Additionally, coronary vasoconstriction may occur. So hypocapnia may well predispose to cardiac ischaemia. On a similar note, hypocapnia has negative effects on the pulmonary system. Hypocapnia results in dysfunctional surfactant production, decreased lung compliance, bronchospasm and increased microvascular leakage from the bronchopulmonary tree. This

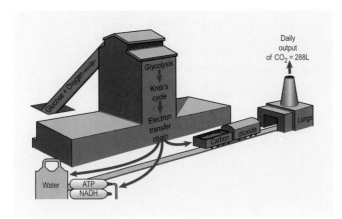

Fig. 1 **CO_2 production.**

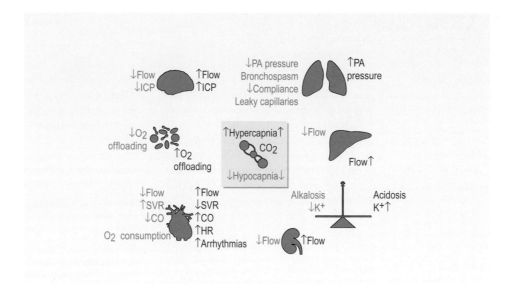

Fig. 2 **The effects of high and low CO₂.**

predisposes the critically ill patient to ARDS or to the worsening of ARDS. From a neurological standpoint, hypocapnia has been associated with a worse neurological outcome in both acute head injury as well as in patients who have suffered an ischaemic stroke (Fig. 2).

Conclusion

Carbon dioxide has many varied and complicated effects. Despite mounting evidence in experimental models showing that hypercapnia may be beneficial in the setting of myocardial ischaemia, lung injury and brain injury, the notion of therapeutic hypercapnia in the ICU remains hypothetical. Before moving from the bench to the bedside, we must discover the target population that may benefit from therapeutic hypercapnia. Likewise, a dose–response curve must be elucidated, as it is clear that severe hypercapnia is detrimental. Whatever the future holds for therapeutic hypercapnia, it is clear that carbon dioxide plays an important, and not fully understood, role in the physiology and pathophysiology of the critically ill.

Clinical cases

Comment on mechanical ventilation.

Case 1: An 80-kg adult male, was admitted following a Whipple's procedure. The ICU doctor set the mechanical ventilator to deliver a tidal volume of 12 mL/kg (960 mL) at a rate of 14 breaths/min. The fraction of inspired oxygen was 100%. An ABG drawn 2 h later revealed a pH of 7.58 with a $P\text{CO}_2$ of 23 mmHg (3 kPa) and a $P\text{O}_2$ of 370 mmHg (49.3 kPa).

Case 2: An 80-kg adult male, was admitted with severe pneumonia. Intubation and mechanical ventilation were deemed necessary. The ICU doctor set the mechanical ventilator to deliver a tidal volume of 6 mL/kg (480 mL) at a rate of 16 breaths/min. The fraction of inspired oxygen was 60%, the positive end-expiratory pressure (PEEP) was set at 10 cmH₂O and the inspiratory to expiratory ratio was 1:1. An ABG drawn 2 h later revealed a pH of 7.23 with a $P\text{CO}_2$ of 56 mmHg (7.37 kPa) and a $P\text{O}_2$ of 75 mmHg (10 kPa). The patient was haemodynamically stable.

Summary points

- Concerns about mild hypercapnia should not prevent the administration of adequate analgesia or weaning of mechanical ventilation.
- Hypocapnia is almost always deleterious.
- Inappropriate mechanical ventilation often results in hypocapnia.
- Mild hypercapnia is well tolerated and may be associated with improved outcome in some settings, such as ARDS.
- Hypercapnia may increase intracranial pressure, worsen pulmonary hypertension and precipitate cardiac arrhythmias.

Thermal disorders

Every process and every biochemical reaction within the body is influenced by temperature, usually profoundly so.

Normal temperature regulation (thermoregulation)

The body uses multiple mechanisms to both sense and control temperature. These are shown in Fig. 1.

Humans maintain body temperature within a range of 0.2°C, outside of which thermoregulatory processes kick in (Fig. 2). The narrow width of this interval, the *interthreshold range*, suggests that precise maintenance of body temperature is crucial to optimal long-term survival of the organism.

Flow of heat through the body is complex and difficult to conceptualise (Fig. 3); fairly simple mathematical models exist that divide the body up into segments and look at *radiative*, *conductive* and *convective* heat loss from each segment. With some success, these models predict temperature and fluid losses in burn victims, and have been used to calculate optimal environmental temperature for burns of various areas. Loss of thermal energy from burn wounds is substantial (50–120 W) and, if *evaporative loss* (sweating) also occurs, several hundred watts may be removed (Box 1)!

Fever

Fever is a common response to infection and/or inflammation (see p. 158).

Common sense suggests that in the critically ill patient we should not interfere with a febrile response unless we strongly suspect that the temperature rise is harming the patient. In most cases, there is no evidence that allowing the fever to persist is harmful. Despite this, in many intensive care units (ICUs), it is routine practice to administer antipyretic agents to anyone with fever (Table 1). With a marked inflammatory response *in the absence of infection*, it seems unlikely that fever has a survival benefit. Management of fever in the ICU patient is tricky. Indications for managing fever are given in Table 1. Options are listed in

---

Box 1. More mathematical gymnastics

Heat is usually measured in joules, and the heat flow of a joule per second is called a watt. An older measure is the calorie, a calorie being approximately 4.2 J.

Sweating results in enormous removal of heat from the body, as the evaporation of a single gram of sweat removes 2260 J from the skin, but at the cost of substantial fluid losses.

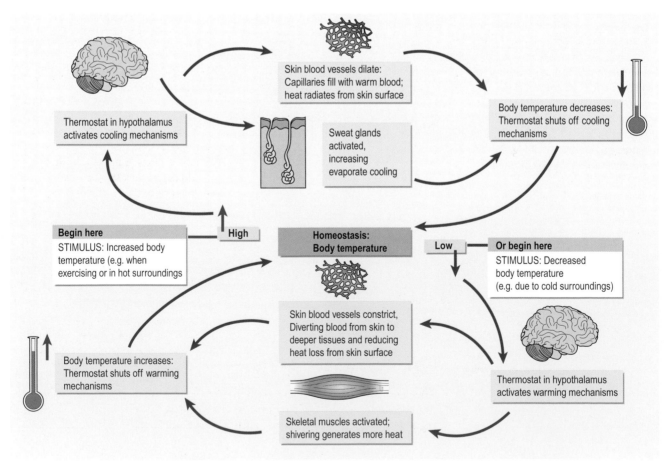

Fig. 1 **Methods for sensing and controlling body temperature.** http://fig.cox.miami.edu/~cmallery/150/physiol/c44x10thermo-reg.jpg

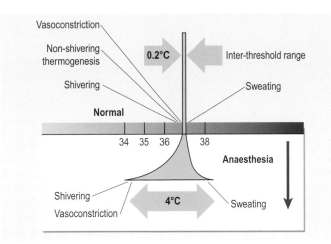

Fig. 2 **Normal and abnormal interthreshold thermoregulatory range showing difference in gain.** Agents such as anaesthetic volatiles, propofol and opiates profoundly affect thermoregulation by widening the interthreshold range from 0.2°C to ~ 4°C and decreasing the gain.

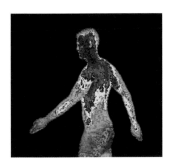

Fig. 3 **Body temperature can be measured at many sites including the tympanic membrane, intravascular, intravesical, rectal and skin.** It is important to distinguish between core body temperature, core brain temperature and peripheral temperatures, which will not necessarily correlate well. From www.athleteproject.com, with permission.

as putting on warm clothing! A more marked *fall* in temperature results in vasoconstriction and, finally, shivering. The muscular activity of shivering results in a substantial increase in metabolic demand, from 40% to over 100%.

Hypothermia is common postoperatively. There is convincing evidence that even mild degrees of hypothermia (under 36°C) are associated with dramatically worse outcomes.

Forced air warming is vitally important, as are measures such as warming of fluids and a high but tolerable environmental temperature.

Electric blankets and water-based convection heaters are obsolete and dangerous and should never be used.

Below 32°C, shivering ceases and ventricular fibrillation usually occurs when the core temperature drops to 27°C. Rewarming methods are controversial, with cardiopulmonary bypass being most effective. Do not attempt repeated defibrillation or give adrenaline in the profoundly hypothermic patient (under 30°C).

Table 2 and strong indications to manage fever in Table 3.

Hyperthermia

In contrast to fever, which is a physiological response to infection, *hyperthermia* is *failure* of normal autoregulatory control. Hyperthermia should always be managed aggressively, usually with external cooling. 'Why?' is a key question with hyperthermia, as failure to treat the *underlying cause* may well result in death. Causes are listed in Table 3.

Table 2 **Options for management of fever**
Paracetamol
Non-steroidal anti-inflammatories
Corticosteroids
Active external cooling
Haemodialysis
Do nothing

Table 3 **Causes of hyperthermia**
Environmental heat stress, 'heat stroke': *CNS dysfunction must be present to diagnose heat stroke*
Salicylate poisoning
Neuroleptic malignant syndrome
'Serotonin syndrome'
Thyroid storm
Brainstem injury
Cocaine
Amphetamine
'e' (ecstasy = MDMA = 3-4 ; methylenedioxymeth-amphetamine)
Malignant hypermetabolic syndrome (MH, malignant hyperthermia)

CNS, central nervous system.

Hypothermia

Minor changes in temperature result in our most effective form of temperature regulation – changes in behaviour such

Table 1 **Indications to manage fever aggressively**
With brain injury, outcomes are far worse if fever is allowed to persist
In the patient with markedly impaired oxygenation, high fever may be associated with further desaturation and deterioration
With *marked* fever (temperatures substantially above about 39.5–40°C), we can expect enzyme and organ system dysfunction and death, if the fever is not treated promptly. In man, the critical thermal maximum temperature is about 41.6–42°C; if this temperature lasts for 45 min to 8 h, death is likely.

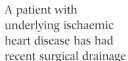

Clinical case

A patient with underlying ischaemic heart disease has had recent surgical drainage of a subphrenic abscess and develops postoperative fever. The patient is intubated, but awake and cooperative, feeling cold, and the temperature is 38.2°C. How do you manage this patient?

Summary points

- Do no tinker lightly with fever.
- Hyperthermia must be fixed – and the underlying cause found.
- Mild postoperative hypothermia can be very harmful.
- Following brain injury, avoid high temperatures and consider mild hypothermia.

Food, salt and fluids

Feeding and starving in the ICU

The commonest nutritional failing in intensive care units (ICUs), and generally in hospitals, is simply starvation. Often we delay feeding in the naive anticipation that 'things will get better'. Patients may miss feeds for a variety of other reasons, including repeated attempts to feed enterally where the bowel is simply not working, and starvation before anaesthesia.

In the well-nourished person who has moderate or minor illness, starving for several days is often of little consequence. Conversely, in someone who is nutritionally compromised with the added insult of major trauma or surgery, short periods of starvation may tip the balance between survival and death.

Where possible, it is preferable to feed patients enterally – via the gut. This preference is largely because enteral feeding is less costly, although some have argued that there are immune and survival benefits of enteral feeding. Competently delivered total parenteral nutrition (TPN) can completely replace enteral feeding, as has been shown outside the ICU where people carefully selected into expensive home TPN programmes live for years on TPN alone.

In many ICU patients, if a feeding tube can be placed in the jejunum, either a nasojejunal tube or a feeding jejunostomy (Fig. 1), then enteral feeding can be achieved, despite 'ileus' affecting the stomach and colon. The catch is that, unless anticipated and performed at the time of surgery, placement of such a jejunal tube may be technically difficult.

The consequences of starvation and refeeding

A short fast depletes the body's glycogen stores. Then muscle starts being broken down and, after about 4 days of starvation, the person's whole metabolism switches to fat utilisation. Protein catabolism decreases, and fat stores are broken down to free fatty acids, which are moved to the liver from which they are exported as ketones. The brain, which must normally have sugar, changes its metabolism to burn ketones for energy. When the starving person runs out of fat, usually at a point where their body mass declines to about 60% of their ideal weight, they die.

If the person is refed before they have passed the 'point of no return', dramatic metabolic changes occur. Aggressive refeeding can result in metabolic chaos, including life-threatening lowering of potassium and phosphate, as these are moved into metabolically active cells. In extreme cases of the 'refeeding syndrome', there may be gross electrolyte disturbance and myocardial dysfunction, culminating in pulmonary oedema and death. Gradual refeeding, vigilant management of electrolyte disturbance and provision of ample amounts of thiamine by infusion may be life saving in such circumstances.

Recovery from starvation can take over 6 months; even when 'normal' body mass has been regained, body composition will still remain abnormal, as muscle takes more time to recover than fat. It is common for nutritional depletion to continue for some time after discharge from the ICU and, indeed, after discharge from hospital; some such patients will still die.

Normal food requirements and how the ICU alters things

The work of Harris and Benedict provided reasonable estimates of *energy* requirements in normal adults. Unfortunately, their equations are inapplicable in the ICU setting, and literally hundreds of competing equations have been proposed. Many such equations are derived from regression analyses of requirements versus other factors 'thought to be of relevance', have no physiological basis and are not even dimensionally correct! In the past, some enthusiasts have applied 'correction factors' for a variety of ICU states, under the misapprehension that metabolically stressed patients might require 'more food' to compensate for such stresses. Such approaches can result in gross overfeeding, and consequent hyperglycaemia, which may be harmful. We know that patients in the ICU often have insulin resistance resulting in grossly impaired glucose tolerance (see p. 124).

A variety of strategies has been used to assess the 'metabolic need' of ICU patients, but the physiological basis for such assessments is usually questionable, and surrogate endpoints are often used rather than 'hard' ones, such as survival or duration of stay. Metabolic carts have been proposed as a solution, but these are unreliable at high F_iO_2 (where they are most needed) and, in addition, the metabolic rate of the ICU patient often varies considerably with time. There is no evidence that replacing a patient's daily energy expenditure in the ICU with an equivalent amount of calories is better than providing say 80% of this requirement ('permissive underfeeding'). In many ICUs, actual provision of food is commonly only about 80% of the target! One good use of the metabolic cart is to provide clear evidence of overfeeding (see Clinical case).

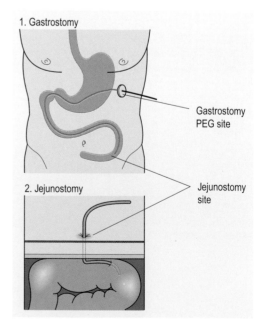

Fig. 1 **Different methods of obtaining access to the jejunum.** A gastrostomy can be used to feed a tube through the stomach and pylorus into the jejunum (1) or a tube can be placed in the jejunum surgically via the abdominal wall, the preferred method (2). PEG, percutaneous endoscopic gastrostomy.

A good basic approach

There are several prerequisites for good nutrition in the ICU (Box 1). Good basic strategies for energy provision include:

1 In a patient of average weight, give 25 kcal/kg/day (multiply by 4.2 for joules).
2 Use actual patient weight, but beware of the very fat and very tiny -- allometric scaling (feeding based on weight raised to the power of three-quarters) is one solution in such patients.
3 Balance energy provision between fat and carbohydrate. Most patients will not tolerate more than about 4 mg/kg/min glucose. One strategy is to increase energy as lipid, watching for lipaemia.
4 Protein at 1–1.5 g/kg/day is adequate but, with many conventional feeds, 1.5 g/kg protein results in excessive calorie provision!
5 Give sufficient (but not excessive) water, electrolytes and micronutrients, trying to avoid the latest fads.

Nutritional assessment

Many different methods have been used to assess nutritional state, but none is superior to the time-hallowed 'subjective global assessment', in which a skilled physician categorises the patient into one of three nutritional states (A, B or C – well nourished, mildly to moderately malnourished or severely malnourished).

In the critically ill, the albumin level is *totally unreliable* as an indicator of nutritional state. Early on in critical illness, small vessels becomes leaky – albumin leaks out. Administration of intravenous albumin is a practice of dubious merit from both a nutritional and a financial point of view.

Important things to monitor in the nutritionally compromised are shown in Box 2.

Box 1. Prerequisites for good nutrition in the ICU

1 Assess and document the patient's nutritional status.
2 Weigh the patient (and continue to do so daily, an appropriate hoist and scale is a vital and often neglected component of ICU equipment).
3 Plan your nutritional strategy.
4 Monitor the response to feeding, and adjust feeding as described below.
5 Competent and safe delivery of food is essential:
- Reliable pumps
- Access ports for enteral nutrition must be a different size and shape from parenteral access ports
- Meticulous attention to asepsis
- Never add anything to TPN (see p. 12)
- TPN must be given through a separate, dedicated line
- Have ICU protocols and clear guidelines for the provision of TPN and enteral feeds.

Box 2. Monitoring nutrition

- Monitor and manage blood sugar
- Balance intake and requirements for energy and protein daily
- Watch renal function and electrolyte levels (Na, K and Mg/PO$_4$ where relevant)
- Watch for hyperlipidaemia with TPN
- Ask 'Are we winning?' Abnormalities in tests that are not traditionally seen as 'nutrition related' (e.g. arterial blood gas analysis, liver 'function' tests or platelet count) may signal problems with nutrition
- Look out for infection.

Clinical case

A 135-kg 1.7-m man who is not normally diabetic is receiving 30 kcal/kg/day, and the team is having 'difficulty weaning the patient' with tachypnoea and hypercarbia, despite otherwise adequate organ function (apart from some derangement in liver function tests, with mild elevation of alkaline phosphatase and transaminases). In addition, he is hyperglycaemic requiring substantial amounts of insulin. Metabolic evaluation shows a respiratory quotient of 1.2. What is happening and how would you fix the problem?

Myth debunked: bowel sounds

The absence of bowel sounds is an extremely poor predictor of the ability to feed enterally, and should *not* preclude such feeding. Bowel sounds will only be heard if the bowel contains swallowed air, which may not be present in ICU patients.

Myths debunked: organ-specific diets and immunonutrition

Immunonutrition and tailoring nutrition for specific organs still have adherents, but good evidence of benefit is lacking. For example, the old-fashioned approach of limiting protein intake in renal failure is likely to be harmful.

Summary points

- Starvation is common in hospital.
- Feeding is largely common sense mixed with attention to detail.
- Early TPN is required if enteral feeding is impossible in the nutritionally compromised.
- Weigh the patient!

Electrolyte abnormalities: sodium, potassium, calcium

Introduction

Electrolytes play a variety of essential roles in cellular function. Electrolyte disturbances occur frequently in critically ill patients. These disturbances reflect underlying pathologies and therapy needs to be directed towards treating these conditions. However, electrolyte imbalances may be acutely life-threatening, necessitating urgent management while underlying conditions are treated.

Sodium

Sodium is the primary cation in extracellular fluid (ECF) and is a crucial determinant of ECF volume. Sodium is freely filtered in the kidneys and mostly reabsorbed; the fractional excretion of sodium (FeNa) is normally less than 1%. A direct relationship exists between the mean arterial pressure (MAP) and natriuresis; a decrease in MAP results in increased production of angiotensin and aldosterone, both of which lead to increased retention of sodium in an effort to increase the MAP. at the same time, hypothalamic nuclei measure serum osmolality and regulate the release of anti-diuretic hormone (ADH) in response to increased serum osmolality. Pathologies rarely affect sodium metabolism directly. Rather, disturbances in water matabolism lead to secondary changes in sodium concentrations.

Hyponatraemia

Hyponatraemia is the most common electrolyte disorder. It usually reflects an underlying disturbance in water balance and can be divided into three categories. Hyponatraemia with hypovolaemia [i.e. decreased total body water (TBW) and decreased Na but a relatively greater loss of Na] results from either renal or extra-renal loss of sodium and water. Hyponatraemia with euvolaemia (i.e. increased TBW with near-normal total Na) can result from excess ADH production, diuretic use or primary polydipsia. Hyponatraemia with hypervolaemia (i.e. increased TBW and increased Na but a relatively greater increase in water) occurs with congestive heart failure, cirrhosis and renal failure. Iatrogenic hyponatraemia occurs when patients receive infusions of low-sodium fluid, such as 5% dextrose.

Features of hyponatraemia reflect CNS dysfunction and include nausea, vomiting, cognitive impairment, lethargy, confusion, seizures and coma. Management depends on the rate at which the hyponatraemia developed. In the face of hyponatraemia the brain decreases the salt content of its own interstitial fluid. It follows this with a reduction in osmotically active intracellular substances, such as potassium, amino acids, polyols and methylamines. This rapid adaptation decreases the extent of brain oedema. A rate of decrease of more than 0.5 mmol/L/hour exceeds the capacity of these adaptive mechanisms. Acute hyponatraemia may be corrected rapidly, whereas chronic hyponatraemia should be corrected gradually; one rule of thumb is no more 8–12 mmol/L/day. Excessively rapid correction of chronic hyponatraemia can result in central pontine myelinolysis, a devastating and irreversible loss of brainstem function, resulting in problems ranging from dysarthria to locked-in syndrome (Fig. 1). Normal saline, sodium bicarbonate or hypertonic saline may be used to correct hyponatraemia. Serum sodium *must* be checked frequently during correction.

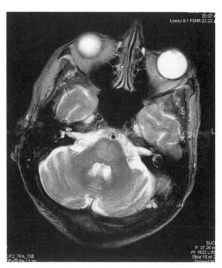

Fig. 1 **MRI scan showing central pontine myelinolysis.**

Hypernatraemia

Hypernatraemia reflects either the loss of fluids or increased intake of sodium. Thirst usually prevents the development of hypernatraemia, but this autoregulation is often compromised in critically ill patients. Patients typically exhibit anorexia, weakness, restlessness, nausea and vomitting. More serious hypernatraemia can result in altered mental status, lethargy, stupor, coma or brain shinkage and consequent cerebral haemorrhage. Hypernatraemia of brief duration can be corrected rapidly. For chronic hypernatraemia, gradual correction (no more than 0.5 mmol/L/hour) is required. With hypovolaemia, 0.45% NaCI or 5% dextrose may be used. Patients on ICU frequently have excess body water with intravascular dehydration and hypernatraemia. Correcting this with hypotonic fluids may simply exacerbate fluid overload and oedema. This hypernatraemia tends to resolve with resolution of critical illness.

Potassium

Potassium is the primary intracellular ion and plays a key role in membrane electrical activity. Serum levels are often affected by shifts between intra- and extracellular compartments rather than changes in total potassium stores. The distribution across the cell membrane is largely controlled by the Na-K ATPase; increased activity of this transporter in response to insulin or beta-adrenergic signalling results in potassium uptake by cells. Acidosis results in potassium efflux from cells in exchange for proton uptake by cells. Long-term potassium regulation is determined largely by renal processing, particurlarly under the influence of aldosterone, which causes potassium loss in exchange for sodium retention.

Hypokalaemia

Chronic hypokalaemia most often reflects either renal or gastrointestinal loss. Common causes of excess loss include diarrhoea, laxative use and diuretic use. Acute hypokalaemia can reflect a transcellular shift of potassium, often in response to insulin or beta-adrenegic agonists. Mild hypokalaemia

(3.0–3.5 mmol/L) is usually asymptomatic. However, serum potassium in this range is often associated with increased cardiac arrhythmias in patients with cardiovascular disease. It is advisable to maintain serum potassium in these patients above 4.0 mmol/L. Severe hypokalaemia manifests as cardiac arrhythmias, muscular weakness, paralytic ileus and rhabdomyolysis.

Hypokalaemia is often evident from ECG changes, including flat or inverted T waves, ST segment depression and prominent U waves (Fig. 2). Mild hypokalaemia may require no therapy. Diuretic induced hypokalaemia may be managed by either the addition of a potassium-sparing diuretic such as spironolactone or by prophylactic potassium replacement. Oral potassium replacement is favoured owing to the slower uptake. In severe cases, parenteral replacement can be used, but careful monitoring is required. Rapid potassium infusion causes diastolic cardiac arrest and death.

Hyperkalaemia

Hyperkalaemia most often results from decreased renal excretion, secondary to renal failure or drugs [including angiotensin-converting enzyme (ACE) inhibitors, non steroidal anti-inflammatory drugs (NSAIDs), and spironolactone] or from increased potassium release from cells, secondary to cell lysis or transcellular potassium shifts. Symptoms include weakness, paraesthesias and palpitations.

ECG changes include peaked T waves, decreased P waves, prolonged PR interval and QRS prolongation (Fig. 3). Prior to the onset of ventricular fibrillation, the ECG trace may have a sine wave appearance. Hyperkalaemia in the presence of ECG changes is an emergency. Calcium antagonises the pro-arrhythmic effects of hyperkalaemia. Serum potassium is lowered by promoting an intracellular shift with bicarbonate, insulin (with glucose) or a beta-agonist such as albuterol. Excretion of potassium may be promoted by increasing gastrointestinal loss with kayexelate, a potassium-binding resin, or by increasing renal potassium loss with a loop or thiazide diuretic. In extreme cases, haemodialysis can be instituted.

Calcium

Calcium plays a variety of crucial roles in cellular signalling, neural function, muscle contraction and blood coagulation. Ninety-eight per cent of body calcium is located in bone while the circulating calcium is tightly regulated by parathyroid hormone and vitamin D. In the extracellular fluid, 50% of calcium is bound either to albumin and other anions. Laboratory values frequently reflect total calcium concentration. Only the free, ionised form is clinically relevant.

Hypercalcaemia

The most common cause of hypercalcaemia is hyperparathyroidism. In the hospitalized patient, the most common cause is malignancy, especially lung, breast and renal cancer, and multiple myeloma. The classic symptoms of hypercalcaemia are shooting pains associated with renal stones, lethargy and impaired cognition, nausea and abdominal pain, and polyuria/polydipsia (Fig. 4). Treatment should be aimed at the underlying pathology. In severe cases, calcium may be decreased by enhancing renal clearance with fluids and forcing diuresis with a loop diuretic. Bisphosphonates help arrest bony destruction in malignancy.

Hypocalcaemia

Often the ionised calcium fraction is within normal limits. The most common cause of genuine hypocalcaemia is hypoparathyroidism, often secondary to surgery. The clinical hallmark of hypocalcaemia is tetany, including Trousseau's sign (carpal spasm after inflation of a sphygmomanometer cuff) and Chvostek's sign (facial twitching as a result of tapping the facial nerve). Management of acute hypocalcaemia includes slow administration of intravenous calcium. It is crucial to monitor magnesium and to administer magnesium if needed as hypomagnesaemia renders hypocalcaemia resistant to therapy. If hyperphosphataemia is present, the phosphate should be reduced with a binding agent prior to delivery of calcium to prevent calcium precipitation. Mild, asymptomic or chronic hypocalcaemia can be treated with oral replacement.

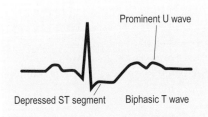

Fig. 2 **ECG features of hypokalaemia.**

Prominent U wave

Depressed ST segment   Biphasic T wave

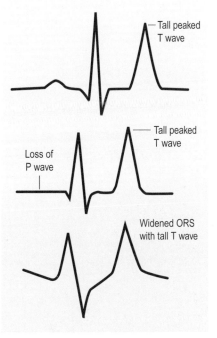

Tall peaked T wave

Loss of P wave

Tall peaked T wave

Widened QRS with tall T wave

Fig. 3 **ECG features of hyperkalaemia**

> *Practice point*
>
> With diabetic ketoacidosis, loss in urine leads to potassium depletion. The acidosis, however, results in elevated serum potassium. With administration of insulin, the serum potassium decreases dramatically and dangerous hypokalaemia may result.

Electrolyte abnormalities: magnesium, phosphate

Magnesium

Magnesium is a predominantly intracellular ion with important roles as a cofactor for various enzymes, phosphate transfer, muscle contractility and neuronal transmission. Isolated disturbances in magnesium are rare; hypomagnesaemia is frequently accompanied by hypokalaemia and hypocalcaemia. Prolongation of the QT interval on the ECG may occur with these derangements (Fig. 5). Cardiac arrhythmias (especially torsades de pointes), tremor, choreiform movements and mental status changes can result from magnesium depletion. Causes of magnesium depletion include gastrointestinal and renal losses.

Hypomagnesaemia is common with alcohol abuse. Oral supplementation is of little benefit; in severe depletion intravenous magnesium should be corrected to prevent cardiac arrhythmias and to facilitate correction of other electrolyte deficiencies.

> ### Practice point
> If magnesium depletion is not treated, coexisting potassium and calcium deficiencies may be refractory to correction.

Phosphate

Most phosphate is stored in the bony skeleton; the remainder is intracellular, where it plays an essential role in cellular energy processes and signalling. Acute hypophosphataemia usually reflects a shift of phosphate from plasma into the cells in association with insulin-stimulated carbohydrate metabolism or as a result of alkalosis. Hypophosphataemia also results from hyperparathyroidism, which decreases renal reabsorption of phosphate. Hyperphosphataemia most often results from renal failure or massive cell necrosis.

Hypophosphataemia results in weakness, cardiac arrhythmias, confusion, hypercalciuria, and hypermagnesuria. Treatment focuses on the underlying condition. Sustained, severe hypophosphataemia (<0.48 mmol/L) requires oral replenishment such as milk or oral supplements. Hyperphosphataemia

(>1.6 mmol/L) can lead to secondary stimulation of parathyroid glands, metastatic calcification and pruritis.

In particular, a combination of hypercalcaemia and hyperphosphataemia (such that the

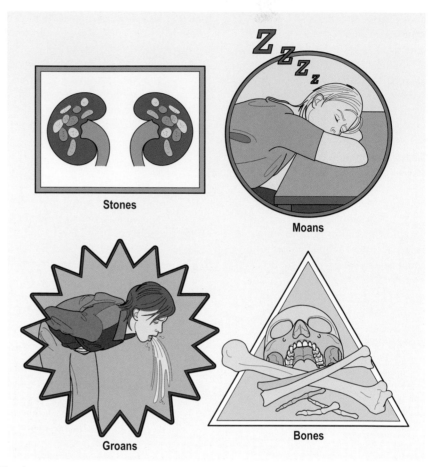

Fig. 4 **Hypercalcaemia.**
Stones – renal stones
Moans – lethargy and impaired cognition
Groans – nausea and abdominal pain
Bones – bony destruction

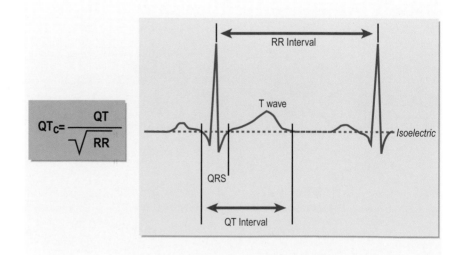

$$QT_C = \frac{QT}{\sqrt{RR}}$$

Fig. 5 **Hypocalcaemia and hypomagnesaemia may be associated with a prolonged corrected QT** (QTc) interval on the ECG (> 460 ms).

product of the two is greater than 5–6 mmol^2/L^2) often leads to calcium phosphate precipitation and results in calcification and tissues damage. Acute, life-threatening hyperphosphataemia requires haemodialysis in conjunction with the administration of dextrose and insulin to shift phosphate into the intracellular compartment. Chronic hyperphosphataemia is treated by reduced phosphate intake and the use of phosphate-binding agents (Table 1).

Table 1	**Emergency management of electrolyte derangement**	
Electrolyte	**Decreased**	**Increased**
Sodium	Use normal saline (154 mmol/L Na), bicarbonate or hypertonic saline Increase ≤ 8–12 mmol/L/day If severe CNS symptoms are present, increase at up to 1–2 mmol/L/hour	Infuse IV 5% dextrose or water flushes through a feeding tube If acute, decrease at 1 mmol/L/hour If chronic, decrease at 0.5 mmol/L/hour Use isotonic saline if hypovolaemic
Potassium	Continuous ECG monitoring. KCl up to 20 mmol/L/hour IV. Magnesium repletion. Oral replacement is safer.	Continuous ECG monitoring. 50 mL 8.4% sodium bicarbonate IV 10–20 ml 10% calcium gluconate over 2–5 min 10 U regular insulin with 50 mL 50% dextrose 10–20 mg nebulised albuterol Furosemide 40–80 mg IV Kayexalate 20 g every 4–6 hours
Calcium	200 mg elemental Ca IV over 10–20 min Infuse 0.5–1.5 mg calcium/kg/hour Continue oral replacement Replete magnesium	Isotonic saline and furosemide Bisphosphonates Consider calcitonin and haemodialysis
Magnesium	4– mmol Mg IV over 5–10 min. 25 mmol Mg IV over 12–24 hours	IV Ca if concern for cardiac arrhythmias
Phosphate	Do not exceed 0.08 mmol phosphate/kg over 6 hours Switch to oral replacement when possible	Haemodialysis

CNS, central nervous system; ECG, electrocardiogram; IV, intravenously.

Clinical case

Twenty-four hours following a total thyroidectomy for cancer, a 63-year-old man bled into his neck. He started experiencing difficulty breathing and he was taken to the ICU where a tracheal tube was placed and positive pressure ventilation ensued. He had a mild metabolic acidosis and a haemoglobin of 8 g/dL. The junior doctor on the ICU ordered a rapid transfusion of 2 units of packed red cells and increased the tidal volume and respiratory rate on the ventilator. Shortly thereafter, the patient was noted to have increased muscle tone with facial twitching. There is a prolonged QT interval on the ECG. What should be done?

Summary points

- Administration of low-sodium maintenance fluid is a common cause of hyponatraemia
- Acute electrolyte derangements may be treated more rapidly than chronic derangements.
- Rapid correction of hyponatraemia may result in central pontine myelinolysis.
- Electrolyte derangements frequently co-exist; correction of one disorder may be refractory unless others are treated simultaneously
- Diarrhoea, diuresis, alcoholism and malnutrition are associated with electrolyte deficiencies.

Fluid therapy in the ICU

Tempers fray and passions flare when disputes arise about fluid management on the intensive care unit (ICU). There is often conflict among physicians with different perspectives, all of whom have cogent arguments supporting their views. Many intensivists live by the mantra, 'Run them dry and watch them die'. Dehydration leads to renal failure, which is associated with significantly increased mortality. On the other hand, evidence is mounting that excessive fluid administration worsens pulmonary function with conditions such as acute respiratory distress syndrome (ARDS). Even for patients having major abdominal surgery, where established wisdom has dictated that liberal perioperative fluid administration is advisable, recent evidence contradicts this, suggesting that restrictive fluid administration is associated with improved outcome. Proponents of conservative fluid replacement therapy point out that acute tubular necrosis (ATN) is not fatal owing to the availability of renal replacement therapy, whereas there is currently no long-term means of providing pulmonary replacement therapy. Furthermore, renal function may recover for up to several months after ATN has occurred. One of the biggest problems associated with fluid therapy is that, while ICU patients frequently have intravascular volume depletion, they also tend to have 'leaky' capillaries or low plasma oncotic pressure, so that much of the fluid that is administered does not remain in the intravascular space. The net result is that many ICU patients retain fluid, develop anasarca and have an appearance likened to that of the 'Michelin Man' (Fig. 1).

(Total body) hypervolaemia

Hypervolaemia
Many ICU patients have a tendency to hypervolaemia. Fluid accumulates especially in the interstitial space owing to increased hydrostatic pressure in the vasculature, decreased plasma oncotic pressure and loss of capillary integrity. When patients have heart failure, increased venous pressure results, and fluid leaks from the vessels. Additionally, in response to low cardiac output, renal sodium absorption increases, resulting in a net increase in extracellular volume.

Albumin is important to maintain oncotic pressure. Many chronically ill patients have hypoalbuminaemia, which contributes to fluid loss into the interstitial space. With inflammation, sepsis and systemic inflammatory response syndrome (SIRS), damage to the endothelium occurs. Fluid and albumin leak from the vessels into the interstitial space. The accumulation of protein in the interstitial space increases its oncotic pressure and draws further fluid from the vessels (Fig. 2). When this occurs in the lungs, gas exchange may become compromised and lung function deteriorates. Tissue oedema in general may lead to impaired microcirculation, decreased tissue oxygenation, poor delivery of nutrients, decreased wound healing and increased susceptibility to infection.

Diagnosis
Oedema, ascites, pleural effusions, pulmonary oedema (crackles, wheezes, radiograph features) and worsening oxygenation may be suggestive of fluid overload. Daily chest radiographs are valuable tools in monitoring fluid status. Additionally, changes in total body water can be followed by daily measurement of body weight as well as meticulous recording of input and output.

Management
In the absence of pulmonary compromise, fluid overload may not require urgent treatment. Fluid restriction or diuretic therapy with a daily net negative fluid balance goal is usually appropriate. With severe fluid overload, haemodialysis, ultrafiltration or other renal replacement therapy can be used to reduce total body water.

(Intravascular) hypovolaemia

Hypovolaemia is defined as a real or effective decrease in intravascular volume. The decreased intravascular volume results in symptoms that reflect reduced organ perfusion, including altered mental status, cold skin and extremities, endorgan dysfunction, orthostatic changes, thirst, decreased stroke volume and resulting tachycardia, and decreased urine output.

Pathophysiology
Hypovolaemia in conjunction with total body water depletion reflects total loss of fluids from the body. This can result from loss of blood or fluids and/or inadequate replacement, and is most commonly seen as a result of bleeding, diarrhoea, vomiting, sweating, burns or inappropriate urinary losses with renal disease, adrenal insufficiency, diuretics or hyperglycaemia.

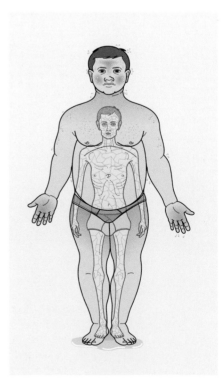

Fig. 1 **Intravascular volume depletion despite total-body volume overload.** Dry on the inside, wet on the outside.

concluded that skin turgor and capillary refill are not useful in the evaluation of adults. Orthostatic tachycardia (an increase of > 30 beats/min) is strongly suggestive of hypovolaemia, as is supine tachycardia.

Urine output is often used as an index of organ perfusion, especially in postoperative patients. Normal urinary output is 0.5–1 mL/kg/h or 30–60 mL/h.

Daily monitoring of total input and output for all critically ill patients as well as measurement of daily weight facilitates detection of fluid imbalance.

Critically ill patients often have continuous haemodynamic monitoring, including arterial pressure lines and central venous catheters. Filling pressures, either of the right heart (central venous pressure or right atrial pressure) or of the left heart (pulmonary capillary wedge pressure), are often used to determine whether fluid resuscitation is indicated. However, dynamic parameters have been shown to correlate better with fluid status. One simple index is the measurement of the pulsus paradoxus; a decrease in systolic arterial pressure of more than 10 mmHg with spontaneous inspiration. In mechanically ventilated patients, changes in pulse pressure and the expiratory decrease in systolic arterial pressure have been shown to correlate with a response to fluid resuscitation.

Choice of fluids

A seminal study, the SAFE study, compared saline with albumin in critically ill patients. Both were equally efficacious, and mortality did not relate to which fluid was administered. The ratio of crystalloid to colloid required for resuscitation was found to be about 1.14:1. There appears to be no scientific support for the popular notion that, for resuscitation, three times more crystalloid is required than colloid to achieve a comparable result.

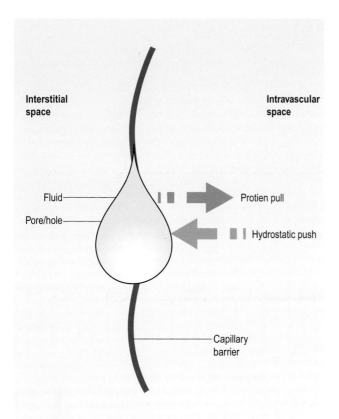

Fig. 2 Factors affecting the distribution of intravascular fluids.
Proteins – especially albumin – are responsible for oncotic pressure. When these are low or when they leak into the interstitial space, fluid leaks out. When hydrostatic pressure is elevated – typically with heart failure – fluid is pushed into the interstitial space. When the capillary barrier is leaky, fluid can more easily enter the interstitial space.

Interstitial space

Intravascular space

Fluid

Pore/hole

Protien pull

Hydrostatic push

Capillary barrier

Appropriate treatment includes correction of the underlying problem as well as concurrent aggressive fluid or blood resuscitation.

Hypovolaemia with normal or increased interstitial fluid volume occurs with failure of vascular integrity or decreased plasma oncotic pressure. There is no net shortage of fluid; the fluid shifts from the intravascular space to the interstitial space. Leaky capillaries are present with sepsis and ARDS. The fluid management is controversial in such cases. Typically, fluid is administered in the early phase and is subsequently restricted. However, there is no consensus about the optimum fluid management strategy. With cirrhosis and nephrotic syndrome, albumin is decreased, as is plasma oncotic pressure. This is difficult to treat because any fluid administered tends to distribute freely to the interstitium. In some patients, the best approach to such problems in the ICU setting may be to use pressor agents such as noradrenaline, phenylephrine or vasopressin to maintain blood pressure to prevent the administration of excessive amounts of fluid.

Diagnosis

A variety of clinical signs have been used to evaluate volume status, particularly hypovolaemia. Orthostatic hypotension, tachycardia, poor skin turgor, slow capillary refill and dry mucous membranes or axillae have been used to identify hypovolaemia. A recent review of the utility of these signs

Clinical case

A patient underwent lung transplantation for chronic obstructive pulmonary disease (COPD). This was complicated by a reperfusion injury; 70% inspired oxygen is required to achieve oxygen saturation > 95%. The chest radiograph shows bilateral patchy opacification. The urine output is 30 mL/h, the blood pressure is 85/45, the heart rate is 110/min and there is a pulsus paradoxus of 12 mmHg. The creatinine has not increased from baseline and is within normal limits. Should this patient receive fluid resuscitation?

Summary points

- Many ICU patients have generalised oedema coupled with intravascular volume depletion.
- For pulmonary impairment, run them dry.
- For renal impairment, ensure adequate hydration.
- Urine output of > 0.5 mL/kg/h is usually sufficient.
- There is no proven benefit of colloids over crystalloids.
- Daily fluid balance review and weight measurement facilitate more accurate assessment of a patient's fluid status.

Blood and blood components

Between 15% and 25% of intensive care unit (ICU) patients receive blood transfusions every day. The hazards of transfusion are not appreciated, and the benefits are ill defined. Liberal transfusion is associated with increased mortality. For the majority of patients, blood transfusion is contraindicated unless the haemoglobin decreases below 7 g/dL. There are various blood components with indications for specific component transfusions (Table 1).

Packed red blood cells

Haemoglobin is necessary to maintain the oxygen-carrying capacity of blood. However, stored blood is not very effective in restoring oxygen delivery. Red cells stored for longer than 2 weeks are depleted of 2,3 DPG. This curtails their ability to offload oxygen. Adenosine triphosphate (ATP) concentrations decrease in stored blood, and red cells change from disc to sphere shape. This results in capillary sludging and tissue ischaemia. Stored cells lose protective antioxidants. Haemoglobin is converted to met-haemoglobin, which does not bind oxygen. There is a trend towards increased morbidity and mortality with increased storage time of transfused red cells.

Red cell transfusion increases the likelihood of infection. Bacteria require iron for growth; red cells whet their appetites. Coupled with this, transfusion results in immunosuppression. Arginase, which is released from stored red cells, has been implicated. Soluble human leucocyte antigen (HLA) class I antigens are associated with transfusion-induced immunomodulation (TRIM). Transfused red cells introduce inflammatory cytokines, bactericidal permeability-increasing protein and tumour necrosis factor. Transfusion results in neutrophil activation and may trigger systemic inflammatory response syndrome (SIRS).

Red cell transfusion is associated with febrile reactions, dilutional coagulopathy and the risk of life-threatening incompatible transfusion reactions (Table 2). The independent mortality with red cell transfusion is estimated at 1:125 000. There is controversy about patients with coronary artery disease; transfusions may be considered for a haemoglobin less than 10 g/dL. But studies report conflicting results even for this patient population. The above patient, following coronary revascularisation, should not require transfusion with a haemoglobin > 7 g/dL.

Platelets

Platelets are necessary components for coagulation. Platelet counts of $< 5 \times 10^9$/L are associated with spontaneous bleeding. A cutoff of 50×10^9/L at the time of elective surgery is usually an adequate guideline for transfusion. A platelet count $> 100 \times 10^9$/L is preferred for those undergoing major surgeries, such as cardiac surgery. In addition to the risks of platelet transfusions, such as alloimmunisation and non-cardiogenic pulmonary oedema, the independent risk of mortality from platelet transfusions is 1:30 000. In view of the high risks, other strategies should be tried (p. 132) before resorting to platelet therapy. The surgeon may be wrong about the lack of a surgical problem.

Table 1 **Indications for blood component transfusions**

Blood component	Indications
Packed red blood cells	Haemorrhagic shock, surgical blood loss, trauma, symptomatic anaemia
Platelets	Control bleeding from decreased platelet count or function
Fresh frozen plasma	Restore the levels of multiple clotting factors in massive blood loss, liver failure, warfarin therapy requiring reversal
Cryoprecipitate	Restore fibrinogen levels and certain clotting factor levels (e.g. factor VIII) in those with dysfunction or deficiency, such as massive transfusions, fibrinogen deficiency

Table 2 **Risks that arise from transfusions and their prevention**

Type	Risk	Prevention
Immunological complications	Haemolytic transfusion reaction: acute and delayed	Match ABO and Rh groups, check compatibility
	Immune-mediated platelet destruction	Minimise platelet transfusions
	Febrile non-haemolytic reaction	Prophylaxis with paracetamol and/or diphenhydramine, if recurrent – use leucocyte-reduced components
	Allergic reaction (urticaria, anaphylaxis)	Prophylaxis with paracetamol and/or diphenhydramine, if recurrent – use plasma-free components
	'Non-cardiogenic' pulmonary oedema or transfusion-related acute lung injury (TRALI)	Use leucocyte-reduced components
	IgA deficiency	IgA-deficient or leucocyte-reduced components
	Post-transfusion purpura	Minimise transfusions
	Alloimmunisation	Minimise transfusions, use single donor platelets for platelet transfusions
	Graft versus host response	Irradiate transfusions for the immunocompromised
Non-immunological complications	Bacterial infection	Effective storing techniques, infuse within 4 h
	Infections (human immunodeficiency virus, hepatitis B and C, human T-cell lymphotropic virus, syphilis, cytomegalovirus, etc.)	Screening of blood products and donors, minimise transfusions
	Volume overload	Intravenous furosemide in between transfusions, effective fluid management
	Haemorrhagic diathesis (dilutional thrombocytopenia or clotting factor deficiency)	Platelet, fresh frozen plasma and/or cryoprecipitate transfusions as needed
	Iron overload	Minimise transfusions
	Air embolism	Careful infusions, minimise air in tubing
	Metabolic abnormalities (e.g. citrate toxicity/hypocalcaemia, hyper- or hypokalaemia, metabolic alkalosis or acidosis)	Minimise transfusions
	Hypothermia	Fluid warmer, minimise transfusions

Unlike other blood components, platelets must be stored at room temperature to prevent aggregation. The growth in platelet bags of virulent bacteria, such as Streptococci and Staphylococci, is common. Platelets should not be transfused beyond 5 days of storage or if there is suspicion of contamination, such as a cloudy appearance.

Fresh frozen plasma

The excessive chest drain output and elevated INR suggest a deficiency of clotting factors from surgery, cardiopulmonary bypass and volume replacement. Fresh frozen plasma (FFP) may replenish these factors. However, there are no randomised studies showing that FFP decreases bleeding. FFP also replenishes anti-clotting proteins, such as antithrombin, protein C and protein S. If there is residual heparin, the addition of antithrombin may exacerbate bleeding. FFP is not indicated if the PTT is prolonged and the INR normal. Protamine in small increments may correct the PTT.

Cryoprecipitate

Cryoprecipitate is the cold-insoluble precipitate that separates with thawing of FFP. It contains acellular large-molecular-weight plasma proteins such as fibrinogen, factor VIII and von Willebrand factor. A fibrinogen level < 144 mg/dL (4.23 µmol/L) is a reasonable cutoff for transfusion.

Compatibility

There is a risk of incompatibility with transfusion. Mismatch of the ABO and Rh(D) systems leads to life-threatening haemolysis (Fig. 1). Antibodies to A and B occur without prior exposure. Sensitisation is required for Rh(D) antibodies. There are over 400 red blood cell (RBC) antigens to which one can develop antibodies with transfusions. It is therefore important to run tests prior to transfusions.

- Type: type patient's blood (ABO, Rh)
- Screen: check for antibodies against non-ABO antigens (e.g. Kell)
- Cross-match: mix recipient's sera with potential donor RBCs to look for cross-reaction.

With red cells, the major danger is antibodies to the donor cells. Therefore, O-negative blood is the 'universal donor' – the least antigenic. With other components, the risk of graft versus host reactions is more important. Therefore, AB components are the 'universal donors' – the least likely to have antibodies. Rh-negative patients should receive Rh-negative products, especially women of childbearing age. The more exposures one has, including transfusions and pregnancies, the higher the likelihood of atypical antigens and antibodies occurring. With every exposure, the risks increase!

Leucocyte reduction

Morbidity and mortality may be decreased by the use of leucocyte-reduced components. Complications with leucocytes include febrile reactions, graft versus host disease, refractoriness to platelets, immune suppression and delayed autoimmune diseases. Leucocyte reduction may decrease the likelihood of variant Creutzfeldt–Jakob disease (CJD) transmission.

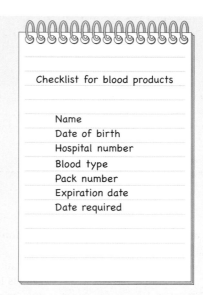

Fig. 1 **Clerical errors and mismatch transfusions may be reduced if two health professionals check the blood product against the patient's hospital card.**

Checklist for blood products

Name
Date of birth
Hospital number
Blood type
Pack number
Expiration date
Date required

Transfusion-related acute lung injury (TRALI)

Non-cardiogenic pulmonary oedema, also known as TRALI, is a serious reaction that results from the donor's antibodies targeting recipient leucocyte HLA antigens or priming lipids. It is the third most common cause of death associated with transfusion. Antileucocyte immunoglobulin (Ig)G antibodies are directed against recipient leucocytes, resulting in pulmonary sequestration, complement activation and acute lung injury (ALI).

Clinical case

A 67-year-old patient underwent abdominal surgery for small bowel obstruction and was 'oozing' from his surgical sites. He received 6 units of red cells. The haemoglobin following transfusion was 9.5 g/dL, platelet count was 75×10^9/L, the INR was 1.65 and the PTT was 51 s. He was given 4 units of fresh frozen plasma and 1 unit of pooled platelets. The patient complained of shortness of breath and was distressed. He deteriorated and tracheal intubation was required. What is the initial differential diagnosis?

Summary points

- Restrictive transfusion decreases mortality.
- Massive transfusions can cause coagulopathies, hypothermia and metabolic derangements.
- Prolonged storage increases morbidity.
- Leucocyte reduction decreases morbidity.
- With every transfusion, the risk of morbidity increases.

Central nervous system

Neurological assessment

If, through our efforts in the intensive care unit (ICU), we save all the endangered organ systems at the expense of the brain, this is truly a Pyrrhic victory. Assessing and tracking changes in neurological function is one of the priorities of intensive care. It is important to distinguish between localising neurological signs and generalised alterations in mental status.

Basic concepts

The most common abnormal neurological finding in the ICU is an altered level of consciousness. The severity of the derangement can be described using a spectrum of terms ranging from alert to comatose. Within that range are lethargy, stupor and obtundity. Frequently, the level of consciousness is intentionally, although perhaps inappropriately, altered with sedative and hypnotic drugs.

History and physical examination

History of head or spine injury, seizure, drug use, headache, vertigo, nausea, vomiting and visual changes should be sought. Past history of epilepsy, hypertension, diabetes, renal failure, stroke, drug abuse, cancer or neurosurgery can be helpful.

The complete neurological examination contains six components: mental status, cranial nerves, motor function, sensation, reflexes and cerebellar function. A more succinct examination is practical in the initial ICU evaluation. This should include confirmation of stable vital signs, pupil responses to light and eye movement, response to noxious stimulus, plantar response and exclusion of 'psychogenic' coma by dropping the patient's hand over the face.

When time allows, a more thorough evaluation should be completed. In the comatose patient, specific assessments include a Glasgow Coma Scale score, brainstem reflex response (such as 'doll's eyes', corneal and gag reflexes), spontaneous eye movements, deep tendon reflexes and a search for external evidence of trauma or drug use. Neck stiffness evaluation and lumbar puncture may be indicated once a spine injury is ruled out. Finally, a general medical examination should be completed.

Diagnostic studies

Computerised tomography (CT), magnetic resonance imaging (MRI) and electroencephalography can all be helpful in early assessment.

Initial laboratory tests should include arterial blood gas analysis, electrolytes and glucose, toxicology screen, and cerebrospinal fluid (CSF) evaluation.

CT is helpful for the identification of acute haemorrhagic events and mass lesions that may be amenable to surgical treatment. CT is usually more readily available and faster than MRI. Nonetheless, in the more stable patient, MRI is especially helpful in evaluating the posterior fossa and is more sensitive for acute ischaemic changes and disruption of the blood–brain barrier.

Electroencephalography is the best tool for evaluation of seizure activity. It can also be useful in the evaluation of coma resulting from toxic or metabolic disorders such as viral encephalitis, drug overdose or hepatic failure. Electroencephalography can detect and assist in the management of non-convulsive status epilepticus.

Basic monitoring

Frequent neurological examination is essential. Commonly employed ICU monitors such as electrocardiography, pulse oximetry, end-tidal carbon dioxide partial pressure, core body temperature, invasive blood pressure, central venous pressure and frequent blood gas analysis may all be useful in the setting of central nervous system (CNS) disorders.

More specific monitoring devices include intracranial pressure (ICP) monitors or ventriculostomy catheters (Fig. 1). The former allows for more accurate use of treatments of elevated ICP, while the latter allows for assessment and direct treatment of intracranial hypertension by the removal of CSF.

Continuous monitoring of arterial blood pressure [specifically mean arterial pressure (MAP)] and ICP allows for continuous assessment of cerebral perfusion pressure (CPP). Maintaining adequate CPP is one of the keystones of therapy in neurological intensive care (CPP = MAP–ICP).

Advanced monitoring

Jugular venous oximetry uses fibreoptic technology to monitor oxygen saturation in the jugular bulb. A jugular venous saturation of less than 50% suggests critical brain ischaemia. This may be useful in guiding therapy to avoid secondary brain injury following trauma.

A non-invasive method of evaluating cerebral blood flow is transcranial Doppler ultrasonography (TCD) (Fig. 2). Data from this instrument include flow velocities in the arteries at the base of the brain. An increase in the velocity can be indicative of vasospasm such as occurs with subarachnoid haemorrhage (Fig. 3).

Evoked potentials have been developed to help predict outcomes in neurological diseases. Evoked potentials determine the level of brain function in the comatose patient. By providing an auditory or somatosensory stimulus, evoked potentials can be recorded over time (Fig. 4). Patients with absent evoked potentials have a very poor prognosis for recovery of consciousness, although emergence from coma has been reported.

Monitoring pain and sedation

A common problem in the ICU is achieving adequate analgesia without overzealous sedation. Pain is frequently difficult to assess owing to impaired communication, but physiological signs of pain such as elevated heart rate or blood pressure may provide clues. In the patient who can communicate, a pain scale can be beneficial to optimise analgesia.

Sedation may be required for management of the ICU patient, although sedative medications are overused. An attempt to identify the cause of agitation is warranted before instituting sedative therapy.

Attempts to measure sedation include the use of raw electroencephalography data (Fig. 5).

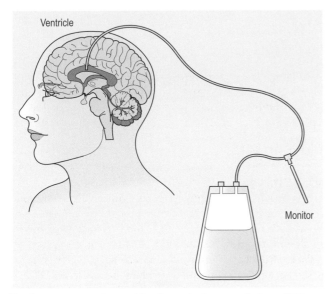

Fig. 1 **Illustration of a combined ventriculostomy drain and ICP monitor.**

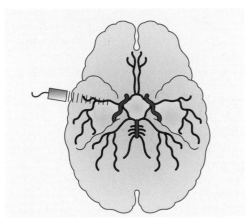

Fig. 2 **Transcranial Doppler probe placed over middle cerebral artery (MCA).**

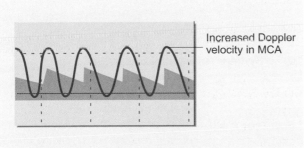
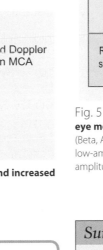

Fig. 3 **Doppler traces showing normal MCA velocities and increased MCA velocities.**

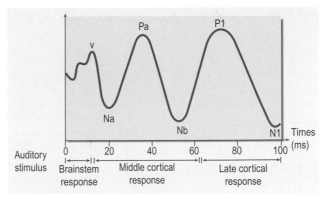

Fig. 4 **Auditory evoked potentials.** Brainstem and cortical recorded electrical responses following an auditory stimulus. Both latency and amplitude are important in evaluating auditory evoked responses.

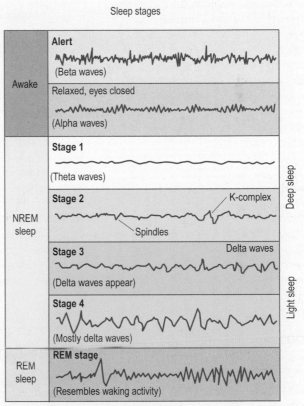

Fig. 5 **Changes in EEG patterns ranging from wakefulness to rapid eye movement (REM) sleep.** The EEG follows the sequence: BATtereD (Beta, Alpha, Theta, Delta). When a person is awake, the EEG has disorganised, low-amplitude, high-frequency activity (Beta). With deep sleep, there is high-amplitude, low-frequency activity (Delta).

Clinical case

A 40-year-old woman who suffered a head injury in a motor vehicle collision is admitted to the ICU. She is intubated, mechanically ventilated and extremely agitated. From a neurological point of view, what evaluation and management techniques are most important?

Summary points

- It is important to detect focal neurological signs.
- Targeted history and examination are useful.
- Electroencephalography may detect non-convulsant seizure activity.
- Absence of evoked potentials is associated with poor prognosis.
- Maintaining cerebral perfusion pressure is one of the keystones of therapy in neurological ICU.

Central nervous system injury

Central nervous system (CNS) trauma involves injury to the brain or spinal cord. Injury to either can be devastating to the patient and family. Both direct and indirect costs to society are large.

Brain injury

Traumatic brain injury accounts for approximately half of prehospital deaths from motor vehicle collisions. Late survival from brain injury is dependent on avoiding secondary brain injury due to hypoxia and hypotension.

Physiology

The skull is non-expandable after closure of the fontanelles. It contains the brain, cerebrospinal fluid (CSF) and blood. The Monro–Kellie doctrine states that intracranial pressure (ICP) is proportional to the volume of the contents of the skull. Consequently, ICP can be altered only by changing the volume of the intracranial contents. Resulting perfusion pressure to any organ is the difference between the driving pressure and the resisting pressure. For the brain, cerebral perfusion pressure (CPP) equals mean arterial pressure (MAP) minus ICP. Cerebral blood flow (CBF) equals CPP divided by cerebral vascular resistance (CVR).

$$CPP = MAP - ICP$$
$$CBF = CPP/CVR$$

CBF remains relatively constant between MAPs of 50 to 150 mmHg. This autoregulation is achieved through local release of mediators, such as nitric oxide and endothelins, which acutely alter CVR. Autoregulation is deranged in severe brain injury, and CBF becomes exquisitely sensitive to changes in MAP and ICP (Fig. 1). Additionally, ICP is frequently elevated with brain injury. Thus, increased MAP may be required to maintain adequate CPP.

Pathology

Intracranial abnormalities related to trauma can be classified according to involvement of the brain (intra-axial) or the potential spaces around the brain (extra-axial). Of these lesions, space-occupying extra-axial subdural and epidural haematomas are most amenable to surgical therapy (Table 1).

Glasgow coma scale

The Glasgow Coma Scale is widely used for early assessment of the severity of brain injury (Table 2). A score of eight or less is usually referred to as 'coma'. These patients have severe brain injuries and are at high risk of mortality and/or long-term disability.

Initial management

Immediate priorities include securing the airway, supporting ventilation and oxygenation, and optimising circulation and organ perfusion. Patients with severe brain injury from blunt trauma often have associated injuries, particularly of the spine and spinal cord. Computerised tomography (CT) of the brain and spinal cord is useful in evaluating patients with suspected head injury, allowing diagnosis of many of the intra- and extra-axial pathologies (Table 1).

Table 1 Types of brain injury

Intra-axial injuries:	Extra-axial injuries:
Contusion	Subarachnoid haemorrhage
Intraparenchymal haematoma	Subdural haematoma
Diffuse axonal injury	Epidural haematoma
Intraventricular haemorrhage	

Table 2 Glasgow Coma Scale

	Points
Eye opening:	
Spontaneous	4
To speech	3
To pain	2
None	1
Verbal communication:	
Oriented	5
Confused conversation	4
Inappropriate words	3
Incomprehensible sounds	2
None	1
Motor response:	
Obeys commands	6
Localises to pain	5
Withdraws to pain	4
Abnormal flexion	3
Abnormal extension	2
None	1
Total points*	

*Best score is 15 points; worst score is 3 points.

Treatment

Treatment of brain injury hinges upon avoidance of secondary hypoxic injury. Important goals are maintaining adequate CPP (60–70 mmHg) and blood oxygen content while striving to minimise cerebral metabolic requirements. CPP may be maintained by increasing MAP with drugs such as phenylephrine and noradrenaline (norepinephrine) or by decreasing ICP. An ICP monitor may be inserted. ICP can be decreased by evacuation of space-occupying lesions such as epidural and subdural haematomas, drainage of CSF with a ventriculostomy catheter, removal of a portion of the skull (craniectomy), osmotic diuresis with mannitol to decrease brain oedema and supporting ventilation to maintain $P_a\text{CO}_2$ between 35 and 40 mmHg. Sedation and neuromuscular blockade may decrease metabolic requirements. Barbiturate- or propofol-induced coma (electroencephalography burst suppression) may be beneficial in the first 24–48 h. Mild hypothermia (35–36°C) has shown promise in several

Fig. 1 **Cerebral blood flow as a function of mean arterial pressure for the injured and uninjured brain.** Autoregulation (the plateau) is lost with acute brain injury, and flow is exquisitely sensitive to changes in perfusion pressure.

studies, but remains an experimental intervention. Maintaining normoglycaemia has been associated with improved neurological outcome.

Spinal cord injury

Evaluation in the ICU

Pertinent historical points include mechanism of injury, time course and extent of neurological deficits, and treatments already initiated. Physical examination should include an attempt to determine the level of injury based upon sensory and motor deficits. A map of myodermatomes can be helpful (www.asia-spinalinjury.org).

Classification

Spinal cord injuries are either complete, with loss of all sensory and motor function distal to the injury, or incomplete. Incomplete lesions can be divided either functionally or pathologically. Functional injury scales are based on the degree of loss of sensory and motor function.

Initial management

If tracheal intubation is required, in-line stabilisation of the cervical spine must be maintained. Patients with cervical spinal cord injuries are unable to breathe if the level of injury is above C3–C5. Even with lower lesions, respiratory compromise can be important owing to denervation of the intercostal musculature and paradoxical chest wall motion with negative pressure ventilation.

Parenteral infusion of corticosteroids should be initiated as soon as spinal cord injury is suspected following the improved neurological outcomes demonstrated in the NASCIS studies. The recommended regimen is methylprednisolone 30 mg/kg over 1 h within 8 h of injury followed by continuous infusion of 5.4 mg/kg/h over the next 23 h. Recently, the benefit of routine administration of corticosteroids has been questioned. Spinal immobilisation should be maintained until spinal column and cord injury are ruled out or stabilising devices or operative procedures are implemented.

Complications

Spinal cord injury can affect many organ systems. Neurogenic or spinal shock may occur with high thoracic lesions where sympathetic outflow is interrupted. This should be treated with peripheral vasoconstrictors and adequate fluid resuscitation. This problem typically resolves within 72 h of injury. Pulmonary and urinary tract infections are common, the former because of difficulty clearing secretions and frequent need for tracheal intubation and the latter secondary to indwelling urinary catheters or frequent bladder catheterisations. Prophylactic administration of proton pump inhibitors or histamine receptor blockers may decrease the occurrence of stress ulcers. Dysphagia and gastroparesis may necessitate surgical enteral access and long-term enteral nutritional support. Decubitus ulcer formation is a pernicious problem, which should be prevented by frequent position changes or rotating beds once the spine is stabilised. Deep venous thrombosis and pulmonary embolism are frequent and potentially lethal complications of paralysis. Pharmacological and mechanical deep vein thrombosis (DVT) prophylaxis measures are warranted in all patients with spinal cord injuries. Patients who develop thromboembolism despite prophylaxis should have an inferior vena cava filter placed.

Clinical case

A 32-year-old male is involved in a motor vehicle collision. He is admitted to the ICU after craniotomy for evacuation of a right subdural haematoma. He is intubated and mechanically ventilated. He does not open his eyes. He withdraws his right arm to stimulation. What is this patient's Glasgow Coma Score? A ventriculostomy catheter has been placed intraoperatively. The ICP is 28 mmHg. Arterial blood pressure is 120/60 (MAP = 80). What is the CPP? What can be done to increase CPP?

Summary points

- Intracranial pressure increases if there is an increase in blood, CSF or brain volume.
- Autoregulation of CNS blood flow is lost with CNS injury.
- Increase blood pressure to maintain adequate CNS perfusion pressure.
- Mild hypothermia and normoglycaemia may be associated with improved neurological outcome.
- Prevent stress ulcers, pressure sores and DVTs.

Weakness in the ICU

Neuromuscular disorders may be categorised as muscular diseases that lead to intensive care unit (ICU) admission and those that are acquired in the ICU (Table 1, Fig. 1). A variable loss in muscle mass and strength is inevitable following all but the briefest stays in ICU. In a study of patients ventilated for more than 7 days with no prior neuromuscular abnormalities, the incidence of weakness was 25%. Mechanical ventilation is a major contributor to muscle wasting. Prolonged use of drugs, including steroids and muscle relaxants, produces myopathy and prolonged paresis. Muscular weakness and atrophy in critically ill patients has long been attributed to a combination of immobilisation and catabolism. It has recently become apparent that specific injuries to the peripheral nerve, the neuromuscular junction and the muscle are more likely causes of weakness. Clinically, delayed weaning from the ventilator and prolonged rehabilitation are the most important consequences. Detailed electrodiagnostic examination is necessary for accurate diagnosis. A combined muscle and nerve biopsy may be helpful. Features associated with different causes of weakness on the ICU are shown in Table 2.

Table 1 **Differential diagnosis of weakness on ICU**	
Category	**Examples**
Critical illness	Critical illness polyneuropathy Myopathy of intensive care
Autoimmune	Guillain–Barré syndrome Myasthenia gravis Dermatomyositis/polymyositis
Nutritional	Increased catabolism and wasting Undernutrition
Electrolyte disorders	Phosphate, magnesium, potassium, calcium, sodium
Endocrine	Hyperthyroidism, hypothyroidism
Infection	Botulism, poliomyelitis, tetanus, diphtheria, HIV, West Nile, Creutzfeldt–Jacob
Toxins	Organophosphates, lead, tick paralysis, belladonna
Drugs	Muscle relaxants, steroids, magnesium, aminoglycosides, dapsone
CNS injury	Stroke Spinal cord damage
Congenital	Muscular dystrophy, periodic paralysis, motor neurone disease, spinal muscular atrophy, Tay–Sachs, lower motor neurone syndromes, myotonia, porphyria
Metabolic	Alkalaemia
Paraneoplastic	Eaton–Lambert syndrome, proximal myopathy

Critical illness polyneuropathy and myopathy of intensive care

Among patients who develop weakness, there is a predominance of organ transplant recipients and patients with systemic inflammatory response syndrome (SIRS) and multiorgan dysfunction.

Severe critical illness polyneuropathy has the following features: limb weakness, amyotrophy and reduced deep tendon reflexes. Motor signs tend to be more important than sensory. The mixed motor and sensory disturbance of critical illness polyneuropathy may be explained by a combination of the pure motor syndrome and the mild sensory neuropathy. The electromyogram (EMG) may remain abnormal years after ICU discharge.

Myopathy occurs frequently on the ICU. Three main types have been identified: critical illness myopathy, myopathy with selective loss of myosin filaments and acute necrotising myopathy of intensive care. These histological types probably represent variable expressions of a toxic effect. Candidates for such myotoxic effects are the mediators of the systemic response in sepsis and high-dose administration of steroids and muscle relaxants. The influence of these latter agents appears to be particularly important in the pathogenesis of myosin loss and myonecrosis. Axonal damage attributable to critical illness neuropathy may be an additional factor triggering myopathies in the ICU. Muscle membrane inexcitability has been identified as an alternative mechanism of severe weakness in ICU patients.

Anterior spinal artery syndrome

Patients who undergo thoracic aortic surgery are at risk of spinal cord ischaemia. The anterior spinal artery arises from the aorta and supplies most of the anterior spinal segments of the spinal cord. Hypotension and increased intracranial pressure result in decreased spinal cord perfusion pressure and may precipitate this devastating complication. Paraplegia is the usual consequence.

Guillain–Barré syndrome (GBS)

GBS is an acute, inflammatory, demyelinating condition affecting nerve roots, cranial and peripheral nerves. The syndrome is frequently preceded by a viral or bacterial infection. Cytomegalovirus, herpes simplex virus, human immunodeficiency virus (HIV), Epstein–Barr virus, *Campylobacter* and *Chlamydia* have been implicated. Activation of the immune system is involved in the

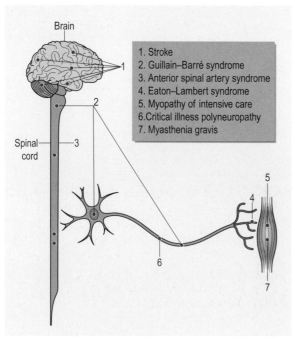

Brain

1. Stroke
2. Guillain–Barré syndrome
3. Anterior spinal artery syndrome
4. Eaton–Lambert syndrome
5. Myopathy of intensive care
6. Critical illness polyneuropathy
7. Myasthenia gravis

Spinal cord

Fig. 1 **Anatomy of weakness on ICU.**

Table 2 **Features associated with different causes of weakness on the ICU**

Disorder	Pathology	Reflexes	Muscle tone	Nerve conduction velocity/ EMG amplitude	Distinguishing features
Myopathy of intensive care	Myotoxicity and myonecrosis	Absent	Decreased	Normal Decreased	Elevated CPK
Critical illness neuropathy	Motor and sensory denervation	Decreased	Decreased	Normal Decreased	Multiorgan failure
Stroke	Focal insult/s to CNS	Increased	Increased	Normal Normal	Localising signs CT or MRI scan
Guillain–Barré syndrome	Demyelination and axonal damage	Decreased	Decreased	Slow Normal or decreased	High CSF protein
Myasthenia gravis	Antibodies to cholinergic receptors at NMJ	Normal	Normal	Normal Decreased	Ocular weakness Improves with edrophonium
Eaton–Lambert syndrome	Decreased release of acetylcholine	Normal	Normal	Normal Decreased	In association with malignancy

CNS, central nervous system; CPK, creatine phosphokinase; CSF, cerebrospinal fluid; CT, computerised tomography; MRI, magnetic resonance imaging; NMJ, neuromuscular junction.

pathogenesis (Fig. 2). The major feature is acute ascending and progressive weakness, which may result in respiratory failure. Improvement usually starts after 2–4 weeks. Autonomic dysfunction is an important component. Sensory involvement may occur with more severe forms of GBS. Excruciating pain is common. Management includes respiratory support, analgesia, physiotherapy, prevention and treatment of infection, treatment of autonomic instability and thrombosis prophylaxis. Plasmapheresis and human immune globulin therapy reportedly decrease the severity of the syndrome. The role of steroids is unclear.

Eaton–Lambert syndrome

Weakness may occur in association with malignancy, typically with small cell carcinoma of the lungs. There is decreased release of acetylcholine from the motor nerve at the neuromuscular junction. An important clinical difference between this condition and myasthenia gravis is that weakness improves with repeated muscle use, as opposed to the fatigability with myasthenia.

Myasthenia gravis

This is an autoimmune disorder in which there are antibodies to the nicotinic acetylcholine receptor at the neuromuscular junction. Involvement of muscles supplied by cranial nerves is usual, including ocular and bulbar muscles. Proximal muscles are more commonly affected. There is improvement following administration of an acetylcholinesterase inhibitor, such as edrophonium or pyridostigmine. Weakness is accentuated with repeated muscle contraction. There is no sensory component. Non-depolarising muscle relaxants result in profound weakness. Treatment options include plasmapheresis, intravenous human immune globulin, immunosuppression (corticosteroids, azathioprine, ciclosporin) and acetylcholinesterase inhibitors.

Clinical case

A 27-year-old woman presented with status asthmaticus. A tracheal tube was inserted, and mechanical ventilation was instituted. She was sedated for a week. She received nebulised albuterol and ipratropium at 4-hourly intervals. Intravenous hydrocortisone was given at 8-hourly intervals. Vecuronium was administered by continuous infusion for 4 days. After a week, she was weak and unable to breathe without assistance from the mechanical ventilator. To what is the weakness attributable?

Clinical tip

Avoid suxemethonium (succinylcholine) in patients with neurological injury or weakness. Hyperkalaemic cardiac arrest may follow its administration.

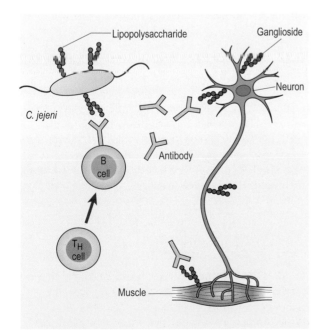

Fig. 2 **Possible mechanism of injury in Guillain–Barré syndrome.** Antibodies form to microbial antigen (e.g. lipopolysaccharide). These cross-react with ganglioside resulting in widespread inflammatory demyelination.

Summary points

- Critically ill patients frequently have ICU myopathies and polyneuropathy.
- Weakness is common with SIRS and organ transplantation.
- Steroids, muscle relaxants and prolonged ventilation increase risk.
- MRI or CT scan, EMG and muscle biopsy may guide diagnosis.

Seizures

In Shakespeare's *Julius Caesar*, Casca describes Caesar's epileptic seizure: 'He fell down in the market place and foamed at mouth and was speechless'. The key features of a generalised seizure typically include convulsions and loss of consciousness. An epileptic seizure results from abnormal hypersynchronous electrical firing by the cortical neurons in the brain, leading to uncontrollable behaviour. A 'seizure disorder' (epilepsy) is classified by a history of at least two seizures. Seizures can be classified into two major categories: epileptic seizures and non-epileptic (also known as pseudoseizures). Non-epileptic seizures do not stem from abnormal electrical firing in the cortex, but rather have physiological or psychological causes. Several physiological causes of seizures include cardiac arrhythmia, sudden changes in blood pressure, hypoglycaemia, infection or metabolic imbalance. A seizure may also result from severe psychological stress.

Epileptic seizures can be divided into simple (no change in consciousness) versus complex (change in consciousness) and generalised (whole brain affected) versus partial (part of the brain affected). While the majority of epileptic seizures have no identifiable cause, several causes are shown in Box 1.

Diagnosis

History of epilepsy, trauma and drugs or toxins is important. Electroencephalograms (EEGs) are used to characterise the electrical activity in the brain as normal versus abnormal. Magnetic resonance imaging (MRI) and computerised tomography (CT) are frequently employed to rule out a brain tumour, cancer or a stroke. Lumbar puncture may yield information, for example about meningitis or encephalitis.

Targeted laboratory data are important in ruling out non-neurological causes. Among these are blood sugar concentrations (hypoglycaemia), calcium levels, urea (blood urea nitrogen) and creatinine (renal function), liver function tests, white blood cell count, blood cultures and continuous electrocardiogram (ECG) monitoring to rule out cardiac

arrhythmia. Appropriate management involves treating the underlying cause of the seizure.

Treatment

Anti-seizure medication is generally prescribed to those individuals suffering from epileptic seizures with recurring episodes. An anti-epileptic regimen should not be prescribed after a single episode.

For post-traumatic seizures, the traditional medication regimen includes phenytoin, sodium valproate, carbemazepine and clonazepam. Newer anti-seizure medications, such as gabapentin, lamotrigine, tiagabine and topiramate, have fewer overall side-effects. Recurrent seizures are treated with polytherapy in order to control symptoms and prevent neurological damage.

When the symptoms are disabling and unresponsive to medications, other treatment options include extratemporal cortical resection, functional hemispherectomy and vagus nerve stimulation.

ICU management

Patients in the intensive care unit (ICU) are often critically ill with multiple organ dysfunction, increasing the likelihood of seizures secondary to numerous physiological causes. The extensive medications of these patients may also lower the seizure threshold as well as mask symptoms of a seizure, thereby impeding prompt and effective medical treatment. Patients in the ICU often present with neurological injuries that predispose them to seizures (see Table 1), with no guarantee that prophylactic anti-epilepsy drugs will have any effect.

Patients in the ICU often present with sepsis, metabolic disturbances and drug toxicity, all of which predispose an individual to seizures. Of these, metabolic disturbances are responsible for 30–35% of seizures in the ICU. Lorazepam (1–5 mg intravenously) has been found to be superior to both phenytoin and diazepam in the acute treatment of seizures in the ICU. After control is achieved with a short-acting benzodiazepine, long-term prophylaxis should be achieved with monotherapy, as anticonvulsant drug interactions present a major problem in the ICU. Phenytoin, carbamazepine and phenobarbital can affect the concentrations of a number of medications owing to their stimulation of hepatic cytochrome P450 enzymes.

Box 1. Causes of seizures

Bleeds: subarachnoid and intracranial
Alcohol and withdrawal
Space-occupying lesions (e.g. tumours)
Hypoxia
Epileptic focus
Drugs and withdrawal

Glucose: high or low
Eclampsia
Toxins
Stroke

Temperature (fever, heat stroke)
Infection (meningitis, encephalitis, abscess)
Genetic
Hyponatraemia (electrolyte abnormalities)
Trauma

Prognosis

The majority of seizures are not life threatening and do not result in permanent brain damage. The true danger in most seizures lies in the limitations imposed upon everyday activities such as driving. In fact, most fatalities occur secondary to the activity being performed at the time of seizure onset. If a seizure lasts for at least 5 min continuously or there are at least two events that occur without a complete intervening recovery period, this is known as status

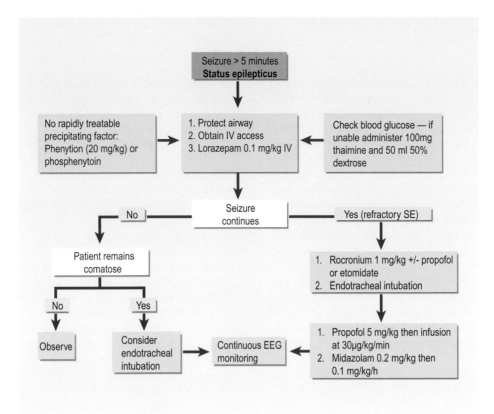

Fig. 1 **Algorithm for the management of status epilepticus** (adapted from *Chest* 2004; 126(2): 582–591, with permission).

Table 1 **Risk of seizures**	
ICU neurological pathology	**Risk of seizures (secondary to pathology)**
Stroke	6–12%
Intracranial tumour	> 25%
Traumatic head injury	≥ 4%

epilepticus. The onset of status epilepticus warrants urgent intervention (Fig. 1) owing to the risks of acidosis, fever, cardiac arrhythmias, neurogenic pulmonary oedema, hyperthermia, pulmonary aspiration, rhabdomyolysis and trauma. When these episodes last for more than 10 min, the mortality odds ratio increases to 10. The increased mortality is a result of cerebral damage secondary to excitotoxicity, calcium overload leading to apoptosis and decreased protein and nucleic acid synthesis.

When a patient presents with uncontrolled seizures or status epilepticus, there are a few steps to follow to increase the likelihood that neurological function is preserved:

1 ABCs (maintain airway, breathing and circulation).
2 Monitor vital signs for instability.
3 Administer oxygen, glucose and thiamine if needed.
4 Check electrolytes, glucose, renal function, liver function, myoglobin, creatine kinase, full blood count and blood cultures.
5 Take a history and conduct a physical examination with a focus on neurological examination.
6 Administer anti-epileptic drugs (lorazepam, phosphenytoin and propofol are common for status epilepticus).
7 Exclude other reversible causes, such as blood clots (CT scan or MRI scan).

8 Institute continuous EEG monitoring to detect seizure activity without convulsions (non-convulsive status epilepticus).
9 Consider lumbar puncture.
10 Treat complications of seizures, such as hyperthermia and hyperkalaemia.
11 Hydration and urinary bicarbonate may decrease the likelihood of myoglobin-induced renal failure.

Clinical case

A 72-year-old man presents with seizures 24 h after a motor vehicle crash. His most recent seizure began upon admission to the ICU and, 15 min later, the seizure has not resolved. What type of seizure does he have? What should be done in the ICU? What should be done next? (Describe the protocol for this variety of seizure.) What medications would you administer acutely? Recently, there was a patient who presented with a similar problem and had a 'reaction' to phenytoin and died. Taking this information into account, what would you do?

Summary points

- Seizures are characterised by spike waves on the EEG.
- Status epilepticus is a medical emergency.
- There are many reversible causes of seizures.
- Seizures without convulsions occur commonly in critically ill patients.
- Lorazepam is a useful drug for the acute treatment of seizures.

Altered mental states

Patients in the intensive care unit (ICU) are frequently confused or agitated. It may be difficult to distinguish between metabolic causes of neurological dysfunction and organic brain disease (Fig. 1). Altered neurological function may be a component of multiple organ dysfunction syndromes and critical illness in general. One of the biggest challenges facing ICU staff is the interaction with uncooperative patients. The temptation may be to provide sedation, but this may lead to further obtundity and even increased mortality. Much as it may be difficult for family members and staff to see patients apparently struggling and uncomfortable, this may be a stage through which some patients pass while they are recovering.

Cognitive impairment may be a signal of a life-threatening but treatable illness. Delirium is associated with a higher mortality and a longer hospital stay. Many sedatives and psychoactive medications are used in the ICU, but these can also adversely affect a patient's cognition, especially for those with pre-existing cognitive impairment.

Dementia

A large proportion of ICU patients are old. For those over age 65 years, 4–15% have mild dementia and 2–5% have severe dementia. This increases with age so that 15–20% of patients over the age of 80 years have severe dementia. A patient with dementia is at risk of delirium. Dementia consists of multiple cognitive defects including deficits in memory, aphasia, apraxia, agnosia, loss of abstract thought, behavioural and personality changes, and impaired judgement. Dementia itself is not associated with changes in the level of consciousness. The patient is typically alert and able to maintain eye contact. Dementia is of gradual onset and has steady progression. A collateral history from a close family member may be important in establishing pre-existing dementia.

Anxiety

Anxiety is usually attributable to worries about severe illness and the stress of being in an alienating ICU environment. A patient with anxiety reports excessive fears or worries and may have cognitive changes, physiological symptoms and restlessness. It is important not to confuse delirium with anxiety. Treatment consists of reassurance, honest communication and facilitating contact with family members and friends. Anxiolytic medications, such as benzodiazepines (lorazepam 1–2 mg) and clonidine (0.1–0.2 mg), may be useful for these patients.

Agitation

Agitation occurs in approximately 70% of patients in the ICU. It is defined as excess motor activity that may be dangerous. A patient may display continual movement, such as fidgeting and restlessness, and may be somewhat disoriented. The vital signs may be abnormal with an elevated blood pressure, heart rate and respiratory rate. Agitated patients may try to remove the tracheal tube, the urine catheter, intravenous catheters and arterial lines. Providing ventilatory assistance to agitated patients is difficult as they frequently breathe asynchronously with the mechanical ventilator. Life-threatening causes of agitation should be ruled out, including cerebral ischaemia, global hypoxaemia, hypotension, low cardiac output, drug-related causes (drug effects, drug interactions and withdrawal), infection, metabolic derangement and major organ failure. Other causes include discomfort or pain, sleep deprivation, fear, inability to communicate, anxiety and confusion. The aetiology is often multifactorial. When life-threatening causes have been excluded, analgesia should be considered and mild sedation may be an option. Haloperidol, in increments as low as 1 mg, is sometimes given in this setting. Patient restraint may be indicated to prevent them from harming themselves.

Delirium

As many as 70–80% of ICU patients experience delirium. It is the most common mental disorder among elderly patients in the ICU. Delirium is characterised by fluctuating disturbance of consciousness, cognition, concentration, memory and attention. The onset is rapid and is typically secondary to a general medical condition or medication. Other manifestations include shifting attention, lethargy, disorganised thinking, disturbances in wake–sleep cycles, delusions, hallucinations and cognitive dysfunction. There may be periods of lethargy with decreased activity as well as lucid intervals. The patient may become physically aggressive with anxiety and restlessness or may be hypoactive.

Important aetiologies of delirium are listed in Box 1. 'For assessment of acute confusion/delirium see Fig. 2'.

Opioid withdrawal

Opioid withdrawal occurs when there is abrupt cessation of opioids. The peak of withdrawal depends on the specific drug. For example, heroin withdrawal peaks at 36–72 h and lasts 7–10 days. Signs and symptoms include an influenza-like

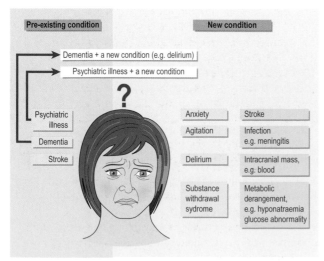

Fig. 1 **Causes of altered mental states.**

illness, mydriasis, lacrimation, rhinorrhoea, piloerection, yawning, sneezing, anorexia, nausea, vomiting, diarrhoea, anxiety, insomnia, sweating, stomach cramps, anxiety, restlessness, seizures, myalgias and dehydration. Treatment includes long-acting opioids, such as methadone, or infusions of fentanyl or morphine. Methadone (10–60 mg/day) may also help to wean patients who have been receiving opioids for a long time in the ICU. Clonidine may improve the symptoms of withdrawal.

Benzodiazepine withdrawal

Benzodiazepine withdrawal occurs when benzodiazepines are stopped abruptly. Signs and symptoms include rebound anxiety, fear, agitation, diaphoresis, seizures, tremors, insomnia, photophobia, palpitations, nausea, dysphoria, irritability, hypotension, tachycardia and hyperthermia. Withdrawal may be prevented with a slow wean, e.g. with oral lorazepam.

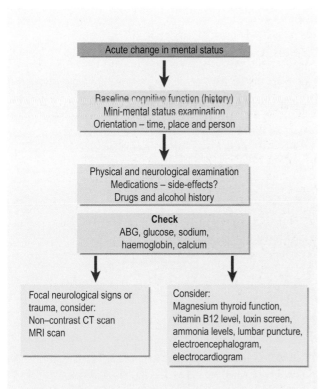

Fig. 2 **Steps in evaluating acute confusion.**

Alcohol withdrawal

Alcohol withdrawal atypically occurs about 72 h after the last alcoholic drink, but may manifest up to 2 weeks. The patient may experience tremors, tachycardia, hypertension, malaise, nausea, seizures, delirium tremens, tremulousness, agitation and hallucinations. A more serious withdrawal syndrome, delirium tremens, occurs in 5% of hospitalised patients with a history of alcohol abuse and carries a mortality of 1–15%. Delirium tremens peaks at 2–5 days after the last alcoholic drink. There is a progression of signs and symptoms. First, there is autonomic hyperactivity consisting of tachycardia, tremors and anxiety. Then psychotic symptoms, such as hallucinations and delusions, may occur. And, finally, confusion, seizures, coma and death may follow.

Treatment consists of pre-emptive long-acting benzodiazepines such as lorazepam or diazepam to decrease the severity of withdrawal symptoms and reduce the risk of seizures and delirium tremens. Very high doses are needed in the event of delirium tremens. It is also crucial to maintain electrolyte balance and administer glucose, thiamine (100 mg/day), vitamin B12 and folate to prevent Wernicke's encephalopathy and hypoglycaemia. Anticonvulsants such as carbamazepine, beta-blockers and clonidine may decrease the severity of withdrawal symptoms. The alpha2-agonist dexmedetomidine may have a role in this setting.

Prevention and management of delirium and agitation

Honest communication and simple reassurance may go a long way towards decreasing agitation and anxiety. Natural daytime lighting coupled with less activity and noise at night may help to promote cyclical sleep. Ensure that patients have access to their hearing and visual aids. Sensory stimulation may be very comforting, including touch, familiar voices, music and possibly television. Avoid unnecessary medications, especially in the elderly who metabolise drugs more slowly and are at higher risk of drug interactions and side-effects. Minimise sedative medications, which may exacerbate agitation and confusion.

Clinical case

A 65-year-old male is admitted to the ICU after Whipple's surgery. He is alert and oriented and is the tracheal tube is removed. His vital signs are within normal limits. On postoperative day 1, he becomes agitated and confused. He has tremors in his arms. The heart rate is 96/min and the blood pressure is 150/80 mmHg. His arterial blood gas, electrocardiogram, temperature, oxygen saturation and respiratory rates are within normal limits. How would you proceed?

Summary points

- Delirium is the most common mental disorder in the ICU.
- It is important to rule out underlying medical causes of neurological dysfunction.
- Minimise the administration of drugs, especially sedative agents.
- Consider withdrawal syndromes, which may manifest as delirium or agitation.

Analgesia in the ICU

People admitted to the intensive care unit (ICU) are very likely to be in pain. For many reasons, this pain may be missed if ICU staff are not supervigilant. The reasons for such errors are shown in Box 1.

Pain management in the ICU

A lot of pain management is common sense. With every ICU patient, it is wise to continually ask the question 'Is *this* patient in pain?' It is obvious that patients with major fractures or other injuries, or a major surgical wound such as a thoracotomy or laparotomy, are likely to require extremely good analgesia. Less evident is pain in patients who do not have obvious wounds, especially those with severe neuromuscular disease, for example, those with Guillain–Barré syndrome or Parkinson's disease.

In the ICU, assessment of pain often cannot be based on the patient's 'subjective report'. Fortunately, good nurses are usually sensitive to the patient's need for analgesia. In the ideal circumstance where caregivers can communicate well with the patient, a visual analogue scale, verbal reported score or even a face scale (Fig. 1) can be used to quantify the pain.

Modalities of pain relief

There are many different 'pains', and management of postoperative wound pain is clearly quite distinct from management of, say, neuropathic pain. Basic principles apply – the World Health Organization 'Pain Ladder', although designed for cancer pain, is generally useful (Fig. 2). We believe that most patients can and should be given baseline paracetamol, in addition to the other analgesics provided. The presence of liver disease is generally *not* a contraindication to the use of paracetamol in appropriate doses.

The ideal form of pain relief for acute surgical pain is clearly to block the transmission of pain impulses. There are many ways in which this can be done including regional infusion of local anaesthetic (with or without added agents) and *epidural* infusion of local anaesthetic and/or opioids, which we regard as the gold standard for pain relief. Thoracic epidural analgesia is

Box 1. Reasons why pain is missed in the ICU

1 *Ignorance.* Surveys of some ICUs indicate that some nurses and doctors attending to the critically ill are still unaware of the effects of the drugs they give. For example, they may believe that sedative agents such as benzodiazepines have analgesic properties!

2 *Losing the patient in among the technology.* All too often, ICU nurses and doctors get caught up in the technology of ICU and lose sight of the patient. It is easy to become reactive to individual parameters, so that when, for example, a patient develops tachycardia, one reaches for an 'appropriate' drug, rather than asking why the heart rate is so fast, and whether pain might be the cause.

3 *Intubation or inability to communicate.* If the paralysed patient is not receiving adequate analgesia, they may be in excruciating pain and completely unable to communicate their distress! Warning features may be tachycardia and hypertension, and even crying. Likewise for the patient who is blind, deaf or cannot speak.

4 *Head injury or impaired level of consciousness.* A patient with an impaired level of consciousness due to a head injury may have substantial pain (including a severe headache!) but be unable to communicate this pain. Their restlessness may well be due to severe pain.

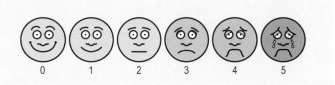

Fig. 1 **Wong & Baker faces scale.** Like all tools, this scale has its limitations, but is useful where other communication is limited, especially in children. From Hockenberry et al (2005) Wong's Essentials of Pediatric Nursing, p. 1259, with permission.

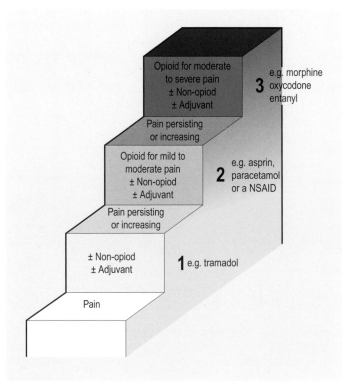

Fig. 2 **WHO pain ladder.**

often achievable in patients electively admitted to the ICU after major abdominal surgery but, in other patients, especially those with coagulation disturbances, another method of pain relief must be sought.

If an epidural is in place, we must be vigilant for complications of the therapy. Such complications include hypotension, nerve damage or even, on rare occasions, an epidural haematoma. Loss of motor function in someone with an epidural means that the infusion should be stopped immediately and, if function does not return promptly, mandates urgent magnetic resonance imaging (MRI) scanning to exclude epidural haematoma. Regional analgesia should be sited and managed by staff with expertise, with prior informed consent and meticulous documentation of pre-existing neurological status.

Opiates and patient-controlled anaesthesia

Where epidural infusion cannot be achieved, or is contraindicated, the next best therapy is the use of intermittent boluses of opiates such as morphine or fentanyl. If the patient can press the button of a patient-controlled analgesia (PCA) system, well and good, but administration by a concerned nurse is equally effective.

If the use of PCA or nurse-controlled analgesia is impossible or is considered inappropriate, infusions of opiates are possible, but those prescribing such therapy must always be aware of the likelihood of excessive sedation and respiratory depression. In addition, morphine has an active metabolite, morphine 6-glucuronide, which accumulates in renal failure and can cause prolonged sedation. Fentanyl is considered more appropriate in the presence of substantial renal dysfunction.

Tramadol is a weaker analgesic than morphine, with several analgesic actions independent of its opioid effect. It is useful for mild to moderate pain. Other opiates such as codeine, sufentanil and remifentanil are less used in ICU for various reasons.

The most dangerous side-effect of opiates in patients who do not have a protected airway and ventilatory support is respiratory depression, with decreased rate and depth of breathing, as well as a tendency to obstruct their upper airway. The most distressing side-effect is nausea (with vomiting), which can be diminished by administration of anti-emetics.

Those who prescribe opiates should be aware of their tendency to cause constipation and even ileus. This problem is most marked in association with recent bowel surgery, where tramadol may cause less ileus, but is a less potent analgesic.

Other agents with analgesic properties

Opiates such as oxycodone and methadone may be particularly useful in patients with renal dysfunction. There is a vast array of non-opioid agents which are potentially useful

for pain. These include clonidine, ketamine, non-steroidal anti-inflammatory drugs (with potential for renal and gastric side-effects) and dexmedetomidine. For a brief discussion of neuropathic pain, see Box 2.

Box 2. Neuropathic pain

Neuropathic pain arises from within the neural pathways that normally transmit painful stimuli. There may be a clear prior nerve injury, or no injury may be identifiable. Neuropathic pain is often dramatically different from pain associated with tissue injury, and is frequently severe and poorly responsive to conventional methods of analgesia. A complex problem, it may respond to the administration of anti-epileptic agents and other drugs that interfere with neuronal transmission, such as carbamazepine, gabapentin and mexiletine. Antidepressants such as amitriptyline or nortriptyline may be useful, especially where there is evidence of 'central sensitisation' (central mechanisms that worsen pain or contribute to its persistence). One indicator of central sensitisation is the presence of *allodynia*, where a stimulus that is usually not painful, such as light touch, elicits the sensation of pain. Neuropathic pain often antedates ICU admission, but some authorities believe that poor perioperative pain control predisposes to chronic, complex pain states.

Myth debunked

It is commonly stated that opiates cause hypotension but, in the ICU setting, it is more common for the opiates to reveal hypovolaemia which has been masked by the vasoconstriction associated with severe pain. If a patient becomes hypotensive when given analgesia, always consider the possibility that you have underassessed their volume status!

Clinical case

A patient recently admitted to the ICU following a motor vehicle accident has had a laparotomy and pinning of a fractured neck of femur. He is on naltrexone for management of chronic alcoholism and took his last dose just prior to the crash. How would you manage his pain?

Summary points

- Pain is often missed in the ICU – continually look for pain!
- Regional blocks are ideal but often not achievable.
- PCA or nurse-administered analgesia works well.
- Watch for opiate-induced sedation.
- Neuropathic pain differs from pain associated with tissue injury and can be tricky to manage.
- Poor pain control in the ICU may predispose to chronic pain.

ICU sedation

Why sedate?

Sedative agents are widely used in the intensive care setting. Goals of sedation are often poorly defined. There are few good studies of sedation in the intensive care unit (ICU), and we do not know the long-term effects of use of such agents (if any).

In the ICU, we often administer a variety of agents that are commonly used during conventional anaesthesia but, in contrast to the brief and controlled use of these agents in the operating theatre, we sometimes administer them for days or weeks on end. ICU management can resemble a 'prolonged and badly run anaesthetic'! It behoves us to justify the use of such agents, and carefully monitor patients under ICU sedation.

There seems to be compelling upfront justification for aggressive use of sedation in ICU, in order to minimise the 'stress' of being on a ventilator and the discomfort of having an endotracheal tube, as well as other invasive management. However, it is worth noting that many patients tolerate current modalities of ventilation very well with minimal or no sedation, especially if they have a tracheostomy.

Often what people being managed in the ICU require more than sedation is appropriate analgesia, combined with good care from a concerned nurse who is willing to attend to their needs and repeatedly explain what is happening. Where memories of intensive care have been studied, there has been no correlation between retention of memories and the amount or type of sedation used (see 'Myth debunked').

Some patients undoubtedly do require sedation, which should be given for the minimum time necessary, with appropriate monitoring, just as for any other drug. Reasons for sedation include the confused and uncooperative patient (where other agents such as neuroleptics may be of use), and patients who are so ill that it is believed by the attending physician that the added demands placed on them by being awake and alert will compromise their outcome. Sedation is mandatory in patients on neuromuscular blocking agents (NMBAs; see Box 1). A reason that is commonly provided as justification for sedation is the mere fact that the patient is on a ventilator, or 'dyssynergy' between the patient's breathing and the ventilation. With appropriate adjustment of the modern ventilator, it is often possible to minimise or abolish such 'dyssynergy'.

Sedation policies differ widely from ICU to ICU. Blanket policies that require the use of heavy sedation in the ICU (sometimes even with aggressive use of NMBAs for paralysis) are either a relic of the past or based on the unsubstantiated belief that all patients on ventilators should be 'spared' the 'stress' of being awake and aware in the ICU. Some experts have expressed concern that heavy sedation may be used to facilitate understaffing of ICUs.

Assessment of sedation

Many different rating scales have been proposed for the assessment of sedation, but the most commonly used is the Ramsay scale (Box 2). Such a formal rating scale should be used regularly in all sedated patients, in concert with ongoing careful clinical assessment and a lot of common sense.

Although the Ramsay scale refers to 'sleep', we must be aware that this is a bad term, with few similarities between sedation and normal physiological sleep.

Sedation goals and management

If sedative medication is required, the ongoing need for such therapy should be continually assessed. Wherever possible, management should probably include daily (preferably morning) interruption of infusions, with assessment of the patient's response. Sedatives are best given by continuous

---

Box 1. Neuromuscular blocking agents (NMBAs)

In the modern ICU, neuromuscular blockade is infrequently required. Even tetanus, which used to be a cast-iron indication for the use of NMBAs, can now often be managed with large doses of benzodiazepines (some add high-dose magnesium with appropriate monitoring). The occasional patient with severe acute respiratory distress syndrome or other causes of severe respiratory failure requiring 'unphysiological' and poorly tolerated ventilatory strategies *will* require short-term use of NMBAs. Other indications for the use of NMBAs include their brief employment during *procedures* with, of course, appropriate analgesia and sedation/anaesthesia, and for suppression of shivering during *induced hypothermia*. NMBAs may be required in some asthmatics and the odd case of central hyperventilation.

Use of neuromuscular blockade puts the patient at greatly increased risk of harm if monitoring for ventilator disconnection is not meticulous. There is also the risk of *awareness* if appropriate sedation is discontinued at any time. In addition, long-term nerve or muscle damage may be seen (so-called 'critical illness polyneuropathy', which can be difficult to distinguish from the myopathy that often also occurs). In the twenty-first century, it is inappropriate ever to administer NMBAs in the ICU for more than brief periods without appropriate, regular use of a nerve stimulator (Rudis et al 1997).

Box 2. Ramsay scale

'Awake'
1 Anxious and/or agitated
2 Cooperative, orient(at)ed and tranquil
3 Respond to commands

'Asleep'
4 Quiescent with brisk response to light glabellar tap or loud auditory stimulus
5 Sluggish response to light glabellar tap or loud auditory stimulus
6 No response

(See Ramsay et al 1974) Many other scales have been proposed, including Riker SAS, MAAS and VICS.

infusion, and the infusion rate should be titrated to achieve the minimum amount of sedation required, ideally Ramsay level 2.

Non-pharmacological methods of resting the ICU patient

The agitated patient in the ICU is often dysphoric because of a variety of influences (Box 3). Appropriate provision of circadian daylight and darkness of sufficient degree, 'quiet times' during which interventions including monitoring are appropriately kept to a minimum and external stimuli such as music or television may all do a vast amount to ameliorate the patient's distress. Simple measures such as sitting the patient at 60° and informing them what is going on may be more valuable than a truckload of medication, quite apart from the salutary effect of the semi-erect posture on pulmonary and gastrointestinal function.

Drugs for sedation and their side-effects

Commonly, agents for sedation include benzodiazepines and propofol. Other agents such as etomidate and ketamine have appropriately fallen into disfavour, the former because of its adrenal suppressive effect (and one study showing an association with increased mortality), the latter because of its tendency to induce hallucinations and even psychosis.

Benzodiazepines

Commonly used benzodiazepines include lorazepam, midazolam and diazepam. Each has its own merits and demerits (Box 4). Problems with benzodiazepines are several. Tolerance tends to occur with time, necessitating the use of industrial quantities of the agents on occasion. Withdrawal may occur rapidly, especially with the shorter acting benzodiazepines, and is often missed or misidentified. Hypotension may be seen in some patients, but it is usually mild unless they are grossly volume depleted. Awakening from sedation with benzodiazepines is slower than with propofol.

Propofol

This drug should only be used for short-term sedation (under 48 h) where it is extremely effective. The patient wakens rapidly following cessation, but propofol is associated with several problems including a large lipid load on those receiving high infusion rates, and hypotension in some. In addition, prolonged infusion of high doses in children has been associated with the development of metabolic acidosis and death; a few similar cases have been described in older patients.

> ## Box 3. Some causes of ICU agitation
>
> 1 Sleep deprivation (which is almost invariably present in ICU patients)
> 2 Pain
> 3 Sensory deprivation (especially in elderly patients deprived of their normal environment, daylight, spectacles and hearing aid)
> 4 Intercurrent disease (local cerebral insults as well as organ dysfunction, infection and more)
> 5 Withdrawal states.

> ## Box 4. Advantages and disadvantages of commonly used benzodiazepines
>
> 1 *Lorazepam* Effective agent, may accumulate with severe liver dysfunction. Also good for seizure disorders (as are the other two). No active metabolite, a major advantage, but contains polyethylene glycol and propylene glycol, which may contribute to metabolic acidosis (Mullins and Barnes 2002).
> 2 *Midazolam*. Tends to accumulate with prolonged use, especially if not titrated by having a daily 'sedation holiday'. The principal metabolite (1-hydroxymidazolam) accumulates in renal failure and, without careful monitoring, the patient can sleep for a week (see also p. 12).
> 3 *Diazepam*. Extremely long half-life, with active metabolite (oxazepam) with an even longer half-life. The drug is very alkaline, precluding intramuscular use, and potentially irritates veins if given peripherally.

> ## Myth debunked: sedation does not influence memories of the ICU
>
> 'The lack of memory of intensive care is present in one third of patients and is influenced more by length of stay in ICU than by the sedation received. Sedation does not influence the incidence of factual, sensation, and emotional memories of ICU admitted patients.' (Capuzzo et al 2001)

> ## Summary points
>
> - Sit the patient up and tell them what's going on!
> - Sedation is often applied with poor justification in the ICU.
> - Sedation is not a substitute for analgesia.
> - Sedation is mandatory in the patient paralysed with NMBAs.
> - Daily interruption of sedation (with careful assessment) should be used wherever feasible.

Organ donation

Intensivists are aware of the benefits of organ transplantation for transplant recipients, and that outcomes are improving despite increasing recipient co-morbidity and severity of illness. The success of transplantation has increased the demand for organs, while the epidemiology of brain death is changing, with changes in the opportunity for organ donation and the nature of donated organs. Many transplant waiting lists are growing. Transplant professionals report increases in 'time on the waiting list' and 'death on the waiting list' and call for an 'increase in the organ donation rate'. However, intensivists have been slow to examine the processes of organ donation within the intensive care unit (ICU) (Streat 2004), and transplant professionals have been reluctant to examine the appropriateness of increasing access to waiting lists in the absence of parallel growth in organ availability. Intensivists should ensure that, on every occasion when organ donation is a possibility, this is recognised and the process of donation is professionally and compassionately supported. It must be recognised that deceased donor organ donation cannot meet the demand for organ transplants, and so transplant professionals should continually re-examine the appropriateness of widening access to potential recipients with increasing case complexity (Frigerio et al 1997).

Responsibilities of the intensivist and the process of organ donation

Intensivists must accept responsibility for organ donation because they are caring for dying patients (and their families) in the ICU and organ donation occurs in this context. Intensivists must ensure that the organ donation process is carried out to an exemplary standard, (Box 1) and is seen to be so.

The required knowledge and skills are subtle and specific and must be acquired through specialised education, supported by best practice reference documents and ongoing clinical experience.

Recognition of the potential for organ donation to occur

Absolute contraindications to organ donation – transmissible malignancy or infection – are uncommon. Most extracerebral malignancies and certain infections will probably remain absolute contraindications, but other donor characteristics are no longer absolute contraindications. An appropriate authority (e.g. coroner or medical examiner) may legally interdict organ donation under certain circumstances (e.g. homicide). An early discussion with the appropriate organ procurement or equivalent agency is recommended to clarify the issue of absolute contraindications (see Box 2).

Determination of brain death

This is a clinical responsibility of the intensivist and must be carried out according to nationally appropriate codes of practice. Although there is no worldwide consensus definition of brain death (Wijdicks 2001), all codes of practice require these three essential components:

- The presence of a condition known to produce severe and irreversible structural brain damage
- The exclusion of possible confounding factors
- The determination by clinical examination that there is profound, persistent, unresponsive coma and absence of brainstem function.

Some codes of practice include specific tests (e.g. electroencephalography). Where clinical examination is confounded (e.g. by barbiturate coma), then absent cerebral blood flow must be documented by angiography or other reliable imaging. The determination of brain death is facilitated by a proforma which, when completed, should be included in the medical record.

Offering the option of organ donation to the family

Whoever offers the family the option of donation must be skilled at communicating with grieving people. An existing strong relationship, established over previous family meetings, facilitates the intensivist fulfilling this role in Australia and New Zealand – although this practice varies widely around the world.

Box 1. Organ donation process

- Care of the dying patient and the family (p. 170)
- Recognition of the possibility that organ donation could occur
- Determination of brain death
- Liaison with the appropriate organ retrieval services
- Discussing the option of donation with the family
- Maintaining physiological stability and good organ function until organ retrieval
- Providing aftercare for the family of the deceased, irrespective of whether organ donation took place.

Box 2. Information likely to be required by organ procurement organisations and transplant teams

- Age, sex, weight, approximate height
- Previous medical history (including co-morbidity, surgery, medication, alcohol, smoking, illicit drug use and allergies)
- Detailed history of fatal illness (including infection, cardiac arrest, hypotension or hypoxia)
- Current clinical status (including ventilatory and inotropic support and physiological parameters)
- Current investigations (including blood group, arterial blood gases, chest radiograph, electrocardiogram, urea, creatinine, electrolytes, glucose, bilirubin, transaminases, alkaline phosphatase and gamma glutamyl transpeptidase, prothrombin ratio, activated partial thromboplastin time, haemoglobin, white cell count, platelets and all microbiology).

Organ donation modifies human rituals surrounding death, even death in the ICU. The fact of brain death and its medical and legal implications must first be conveyed to the family. It can be difficult for families to accept brain death as death, given the life-like appearance of the skin, the rise and fall of the chest and the warmth of the hands that are preserved by ventilatory and circulatory support. For some family members, the opportunity to view a clinical examination for brain death, (or the cerebral arteriogram when clinical examination is confounded) may help them to understand brain death. Intensivists should offer these options if they would assist the family and should ensure that the family have understood and accepted the finality of brain death before discussing organ donation.

In offering the option of organ donation, the intensivist should ensure that the discussion is neither coercive nor discouraging and that the family are supported during this time. Families and circumstances vary widely, and a prescriptive approach to the discussion is not appropriate. The intensivist should be informed about and prepared to discuss these issues:

- That this is a circumstance in which organ donation and subsequent organ transplantation is possible
- That organ donation is an option, not an obligation
- The nature and timing of organ retrieval processes in the operating room
- Subsequent possible (usually multiple) transplantation processes
- A general account of expected recipient outcomes
- The views and wishes of the now-deceased towards organ donation, if these are known, and any such discussion that they may have had with the family
- The views and wishes of the family
- Any other issues that the family might wish to discuss.

Some families have little knowledge or understanding of organ donation and transplantation. Discussion of organ donation and willingness to be part of it vary widely in the community. Although organ retrieval is carried out in a respectful manner in the operating room with identical surgical processes to those usually used on living people, it can be thought of by some as 'mutilating'. Some people have strong personal views against organ donation, which may or may not be based on religious, spiritual or cultural beliefs. Even in countries that legally allow the previously expressed wishes of the deceased to determine whether organ donation may take place, usual practice continues to involve the family and not to proceed with organ retrieval if there is family objection. This practice acknowledges the legitimate interest of family members in what happens to their loved one after death and recognises that organ donation requires a very high level of public trust in the process and the professionals involved, which would probably be jeopardised if the family were excluded from the process. In the absence of organ donation, it is appropriate to remove ventilatory support soon after brain death, allowing time for family needs.

The intensivist must ensure that extracranial physiological stability and optimal organ function is preserved during the several hours until organ retrieval takes place, and should facilitate the family spending time at the bedside during this time if they wish. Some tests (e.g. echocardiography or bronchoscopy) may occur during this time, and the family should be informed about the reasons for these. The intensivist should also ensure that the family is offered an opportunity to spend time with the deceased after organ retrieval if they wish.

Maintenance of extracerebral physiological stability (Wood et al 2004)

Immediately prior to brain death, there is usually a short episode of hypertension and tachycardia (occasionally tachydysrhythmia). Pulmonary oedema, biventricular dysfunction and myocardial injury may rarely occur. If treatment of these phenomena is necessary a short acting beta-blocker (esmolol) should be used. Hypotension follows soon after this event and may be profound in the presence of hypovolaemia or cardiac dysfunction. Hypotension can rapidly impair donor organ viability and should be treated promptly with volume expansion and inotropic support. Low-dose noradrenaline is safe, effective and most commonly used to achieve a mean arterial pressure around 70 mmHg. Diabetes insipidus usually occurs, manifest by brisk water diuresis, which can rapidly lead to hyperosmolality and hypovolaemia. Intermittent low-dose DDAVP or very low-dose vasopressin infusion is effective. (Other hormone abnormalities do not have serious implications.) Oxygen consumption and carbon dioxide production fall by ~ 25%, and minute volume should be correspondingly reduced to maintain normocarbia. The fall in energy expenditure (heat production) along with loss of vasomotor tone (with no possibility of shivering-induced thermogenesis) increase the risk of hypothermia developing. Spontaneous movements and spinal motor reflexes commonly persist in brain death. Sympathetic responses may justify the use of opioids during surgical stimulation in the operating room.

Aftercare of the donor family

The literature has focused on the needs of the donor family, and there may be specific issues that need to be addressed, sometimes by way of a family meeting with an intensivist at some later stage. Most organ donation agencies and transplant programmes facilitate limited anonymous communication between recipients and donor families, but direct contact is not recommended. However, routine aftercare for the families of all patients dying in ICUs is increasingly recommended. Such programmes (Cuthbertson et al 2000) are well received and have the potential to improve the care of subsequent families by revealing areas of inadequate or inappropriate communication.

Summary points

- Intensivists should recognise all opportunities for organ donation, and support this process professionally and with compassion.
- Specialised education of intensivists is required to address organ donation appropriately.
- Determination of brain death must be consistent, and confounding factors must be rigorously excluded.
- The skilled communicator who *offers the option* of organ donation to the family must have previously established a strong relationship in previous meetings.
- It is wise to acknowledge the legitimate interest of the family members in what happens to their loved one after death.
- Skilful maintenance of extracerebral stability is required around the time of brain death.
- Routine aftercare of donor families is recommended.

Cardiovascular system

Monitoring the cardiovascular system

Why monitor the cardiovascular system (CVS)?

Cardiovascular malfunction often occurs as a consequence of the stresses of trauma, surgery, fluid deficits or excesses, and drugs administered by doctors. The primary function of the CVS – movement of oxygen and nutrients to tissues throughout the body and removal of waste products – is difficult to assess in its entirety, so we use measurement of 'proxies' (Box 1).

Complex tests of CVS function

Much ingenuity has been focused on the assessment of overall oxygen delivery to and consumption by the critically ill patient, despite a lack of good evidence that aggressive manipulation of such parameters does anything but harm. Understanding of the mechanism of cardiovascular disease may, however, facilitate management.

Echocardiography

Transthoracic echocardiography (TTE) is possibly the single most useful way to assess the heart and whole CVS in the ICU (see Box 3). TTE *may* be inadequate, especially in those with substantial lung disease, where transoesophageal echocardiography (TOE = TEE) may be of value. TEE is of particular merit in diagnosing infective endocarditis and visualising thrombus in the left atrium.

Pulmonary artery catheterisation (PAC)

Fig. 1 shows a PAC. Although popular in the past, PACs have not convincingly been shown to help in improving patient outcomes and should be deployed selectively. Information provided by a PAC includes (Box 2):

- Cardiac output (by thermodilution)
- Mixed venous saturation
- Pulmonary 'capillary' wedge pressure
- Central venous temperature
- Pulmonary arterial pressures
- Calculation of systemic and pulmonary vascular resistances.

Other methods of monitoring

Table 1 lists newer methods of monitoring, some of which show promise. All provide an automated estimate of cardiac output on a near-continuous basis.

Box 1. Proxies for assessing CVS function

1. Clinical assessment: attach less weight to abnormal measurements in the face of good organ function. Malnutrition is a powerful predictor of poor outcome. A tachycardia of over 130/min in the absence of fever is worrying
2. Blood pressure and pulse pressure (Fig. 1)
3. Measures of cardiac output (Table 1)
4. Assessment of myocardial function, particularly using echocardiography
5. Microcirculatory assessment.

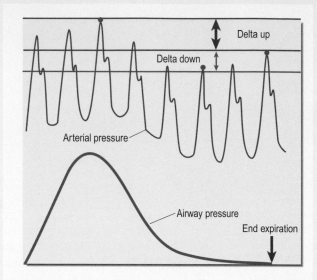

Fig. 1 **Fluctuations in arterial blood pressure and pulse pressure.** Looking at a single ventilator breath, delta down is the maximum drop in systolic arterial pressure from the pressure at end-expiration. Delta up is the maximum rise, and systolic pressure variation (SPV) is the sum of the two.

The microcirculation

In the past, some physiologists have accorded the heart a central role it does not deserve! The heart is largely a slave to the demands of the rest of the body, which takes what it needs. A convincing argument can be made that, in order to assess circulatory function, one should look not at the heart, but at the opposite end of the circulation – the microcirculation, where oxygen delivery is actually occurring. Previously, gastric intramucosal pH (pHi) looked promising but, recently, interest in such measurement has waned.

Table 1 **Methods of monitoring cardiac output**	
Method	**Notes**
Pulse contour analysis	Stroke volume variation indicates hypovolaemia
PiCCO (pulse contour + thermodilution) LiDCO (pulse contour + lithium dilution)	Use dilution methods to calibrate. Assume constant flow, no loss of indicator and complete mixing
Transoesophageal Doppler	Gives aortic blood flow, not cardiac output. Limitations
Perturbation of inspired [CO_2], e.g. 'NICO'	Shows lung perfusion, affected by V/Q mismatch
Bioimpedance	Small varying signals limit reliability

The 'guesstimate' cardiac output

CO = pulse pressure * heart rate * 2

The assumption is that a 1-mmHg change in pressure occurs if 2 mL of volume are added to the circulation. This 'guesstimate' output (which should not be relied upon in practice, as it makes unwarranted assumptions about the compliance of the aorta) is only useful in exploring the 'believability factor' of a machine-acquired number for cardiac output!

Preliminary research suggests that assessment of microcirculatory function in the tongue may be of value in predicting outcome.

Box 2. High school physics: an approximation of cardiovascular relationships!

1 $CO = HR * SV$
2 Peripheral resistance = mean pressure/CO
3 CaO_2 = arterial oxygen content = Hüffner's constant * [Hb] * S_aO_2
4 Oxygen delivery = $CaO_2 * CO$
5 $\dot{V}O_2 = CO (CaO_2 - CvO_2)$ = the Fick principle of 'what goes in must come out'.

CO, cardiac output; HR, heart rate; SV, stroke volume; S_aO_2, arterial oxygen saturation; [Hb], haemoglobin concentration; $\dot{V}O_2$, oxygen consumption; CvO_2, venous oxygen content. Hüffner's constant is theoretically calculated at 1.39 mL of oxygen per gram of haemoglobin. Toxins (e.g. carbon monoxide) binding to haemoglobin decrease its efficiency in carrying oxygen (Fig. 2).

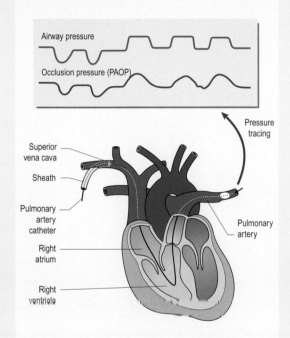

Airway pressure

Occlusion pressure (PAOP)

Pressure tracing

Superior vena cava

Sheath

Pulmonary artery catheter

Right atrium

Right ventricle

Pulmonary artery

Fig. 2 **Reading pulmonary artery occlusion pressure (PAOP).** A pulmonary artery catheter in position with the balloon inflated so that PAOP pressure might be measured. The red tracing shows airway pressure, which is closely tracked by the PAOP pressure (shown in blue). The PAOP reflects left atrial pressure. The first two breaths are spontaneous breaths, the next three are machine delivered. Two red arrows show end-expiration, the first for a spontaneous breath, the second for a machine breath. The balloon should not be left inflated, and *never* inflated if resistance is encountered. For clarity, the catheter is shown in the left pulmonary artery, but more often floats into the right!

Box 3. Utility of echocardiography in the ICU

Echocardiography quickly tells us about:

- Volume status
- Systemic vascular resistance
- Myocardial contractility
- Presence of pericardial fluid.

Clinical case

A 29-year-old woman, previously well, is being ventilated for 'severe acute respiratory distress syndrome (ARDS)', but no underlying cause has been found on extensive investigation. Clinically, she has a soft apical holosystolic murmur, with no third heart sound. A technically difficult transthoracic echocardiography shows 'mild mitral regurgitation'. She has mild renal dysfunction and mildly abnormal liver function tests. What is your approach to management?

Myth debunked

- There is an inconstant relationship between tachycardia and fever, despite older 'rules' specifying values of about 18 beats/min/°C.life.

Practice point

Don't try this at home! Before users can start making confident assessment based on TTE, they should have at least 20, and preferably 50, supervised TTEs under their belts. There are pitfalls, even for the expert.

Clinical pearl

Fluid status and postural change in blood presure: If the blood pressure doesn't drop when the patient is tilted head-up, they are almost certainly volume replete!

Summary points

- Assess the *whole* patient.
- 'Normal' values vary in different patients and circumstances.
- Marked variation in blood pressure with respiration suggests volume depletion.
- Echocardiography is useful
- Read pressures at *end-expiration*.

Ischaemic heart disease

Ischaemic heart disease is a significant public health problem and the leading cause of death for men and women in industrialised nations. It is becoming an increasing problem in developing regions of the world. Major risk factors for the development of coronary artery disease (CAD) and targets of primary prevention include smoking, hypertension and unfavourable lipid profile. Patients with a family history of premature cardiac disease are at increased risk and should be identified for close follow-up and management of modifiable risk factors. Diabetes mellitus and chronic kidney disease should be considered risk equivalents to the known presence of CAD, and secondary prevention efforts should be aimed at patients with these conditions.

The typical patient with an ischaemic event presents complaining of chest tightness, pressure or heaviness, although up to half of all myocardial infarctions (MI) may be silent and unrecognised by the patient, especially in women and the elderly. Other associated symptoms may include nausea, vomiting, shortness of breath, diaphoresis, weakness or profound fatigue (Fig. 1). A variety of cardiac and non-cardiac conditions must be included in the differential diagnosis for patients presenting with these non-specific complaints including myocardial ischaemia, aortic dissection, pericarditis, peptic ulcer disease, gastro-oesophageal reflux, pulmonary embolism, pneumothorax, acute cholecystitis, oesophageal perforation and mediastinitis. Early, prompt recognition and management of acute coronary syndrome (ACS) is critical because as many as one-third of patients with ST elevation MI will die within 24 h from the onset of ischaemia, often due to ventricular fibrillation (Table 1). A brief, focused history and physical examination will help to identify patients at risk of ACS and any conditions for which antiplatelet, antithrombin or fibrinolytic therapy might be contraindicated (Box 1).

Table 1 Complications of acute myocardial infarction
Post-infarction angina and infarct extension
Pericarditis
Ventricular free wall rupture
Ventricular septal rupture
Ventricular wall aneurysm
Acute mitral regurgitation
Right ventricular infarction
Heart failure and cardiogenic shock
Dysrhythmias
Ventricular fibrillation
Atrial fibrillation

Box 1. Focused history and examination for patients with chest pain

History
Characteristics of chest 'pain', timing, associated symptoms
History of cardiovascular disease (hypertension, stroke, transient ischaemic attack, aneurysm, claudication)
History of cardiac risk factors (family history, diabetes, smoking, hyperlipidaemia)
Neurological symptoms
Risk of bleeding

Examination
Airway, breathing, circulation
Vital signs (check left and right extremities)
General appearance (pale, diaphoretic)
Pulmonary evaluation for rales, wheezing
Cardiac evaluation for rubs, murmurs, gallops, irregular beats
Peripheral pulses, capillary refill
Jugular venous distension
Focal neurological findings

Anatomy of acute coronary syndrome

Acute coronary syndromes are part of a spectrum of conditions that include unstable angina (UA), non-ST elevation MI (NSTEMI) and ST elevation MI (STEMI). They are generally due to disruption of high-risk plaques, they occur in areas of turbulent flow (i.e. branching points) and are associated with abundant inflammatory cells. Disruption of the plaque exposes substances that promote platelet aggregation and development of thrombus. The extent of injury depends on the presence of collateral flow in the area of occlusion and the relationship between myocardial oxygen supply and demand.

Even at rest, the heart works at near-maximal oxygen extraction, having the highest metabolic rate and the highest arteriovenous oxygen difference of all organ systems. Myocardial oxygen demand is determined by heart rate, contractility and wall tension. Unmatched myocardial oxygen demand to supply results in ischaemia and possible infarction with myocardial necrosis, culminating in myocardial diastolic dysfunction, regional systolic wall motion abnormalities, ST segment changes on electrocardiogram (ECG), chest pain and elevation of serum markers of myocardial injury. Transient myocardial

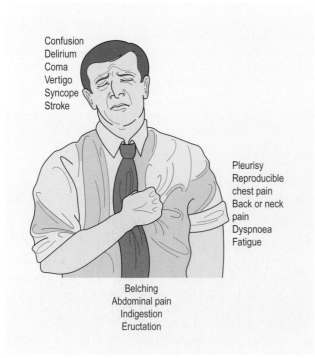

Confusion
Delirium
Coma
Vertigo
Syncope
Stroke

Pleurisy
Reproducible chest pain
Back or neck pain
Dyspnoea
Fatigue

Belching
Abdominal pain
Indigestion
Eructation

Fig. 1 **Angina equivalents.**

dysfunction following reperfusion is coined stunning, whereas hibernation is characterised by a prolonged decrease in contractility in hypoperfused areas. Myocardial contractile reserve is preserved in both entities and may improve with time or revascularisation.

Diagnosis

All patients presenting with symptoms consistent with ACS should be triaged with high priority and placed on continuous cardiac monitoring. A 12-lead ECG should be performed rapidly and will determine the next appropriate course of action.

The presence of ST elevation, new left bundle branch block (LBBB) or true posterior MI, as suggested by ST depression in leads V1 to V4 with tall R waves in the right precordial leads, identifies patients who may benefit from early reperfusion therapy. In cases where the ECG is normal or non-diagnostic but clinical suspicion is high, repeat ECG at frequent intervals and assessment for biochemical markers may detect the development of an injury pattern. Bedside ECG may also help determine the aetiology of chest discomfort in patients suspected of having ACS with non-diagnostic initial studies.

Biochemical markers

A number of biochemical markers such as creatine phosphokinase (CK), lactate dehydrogenase and cardiac troponins increase in response to myocardial tissue damage. Patients with STEMI are diagnosed on the basis of the 12-lead ECG, and results of biomarker testing should not delay reperfusion therapy. Cardiac troponin I (cTnI) and cardiac troponin T (cTnT) levels may begin to rise 3–6 h after the onset of ischaemia, and may persist for as many as 7–10 or 10–14 days respectively. On account of its more rapid rise and fall, the CK-MB isoenzyme is the preferred biomarker for patients with STEMI to assess effectiveness of reperfusion therapy and to diagnose reinfarction.

Management

The general goals of management are to re-establish coronary blood flow in less than 120 min after the onset of chest pain for patients with STEMI, and to minimise myocardial oxygen demand in patients with compromised myocardial oxygen supply, including those with UA and NSTEMI. Reperfusion therapy in patients with STEMI can be accomplished either by pharmacological (fibrinolysis) or catheter-based (primary percutaneous coronary intervention, PCI) methods.

All patients should receive supplemental oxygen to keep the oxygen saturation at least at 90%. Intravenous access should be established. Continuous ECG monitoring for arrhythmias and ST segment deviation and frequent vital sign assessment for haemodynamic instability should be performed. Defibrillation capability should be available.

All patients with ACS should receive antiplatelet and antithrombin therapy. Relief of chest pain may be accomplished with a combination of opiate analgesics, nitrates and beta-adrenergic antagonists. Opiate analgesics such as morphine not only provide pain relief, but are useful in reducing sympathetic autonomic nervous system activity. Beta-adrenergic antagonists decrease myocardial oxygen demand by lowering heart rate and contractility. By slowing the heart rate, diastole is relatively increased, allowing for greater time for coronary perfusion. Patients with hypotension or bradycardia may not be candidates for nitrates or beta-adrenergic antagonists. Hypotension should be managed first with fluid administration unless there is evidence of congestion. Vasopressor agents may be necessary if blood pressure does not respond to fluid resuscitation. While the use of inotropic agents may be considered in order to improve ventricular performance and low cardiac output states, their use may precipitate worsening ischaemia due to increases in the primary determinants of myocardial oxygen consumption, i.e. heart rate, contractility and wall tension. Intra-aortic balloon counterpulsation is a useful therapy in these settings and works by increasing diastolic blood pressure (DBP) during balloon inflation, termed 'diastolic augmentation', thereby improving coronary perfusion pressure (CPP). It also reduces left ventricular wall tension with properly timed balloon deflation, 'systolic augmentation'.

Secondary prevention

Secondary prevention efforts are aimed at reducing the risk of reinfarction and improving mortality and morbidity in patients with coronary artery disease. Smoking cessation, blood pressure control, reducing and improving lipid profile, diabetes management, weight control and daily use of aspirin, beta-adrenergic antagonists and angiotensin-converting enzyme (ACE) inhibitors (unless contraindicated) are recommended interventions with demonstrated benefit.

> ### Clinical case
> During morning ward round you observe that a 68-year-old male patient, now 48 h status post repair of an aortic abdominal aneurysm, becomes agitated, confused and distressed, complaining his chest feels 'heavy'. His vital signs are pulse 114 bpm and irregular, arterial blood pressure 87/55 mmHg, and arterial oxygen saturation 90%. Physical examination reveals diaphoresis, bibasilar rales and diminished peripheral pulses. A 12-lead ECG reveals new-onset atrial fibrillation (AF) and a new LBBB. What is your differential diagnosis? What are your immediate diagnostic and therapeutic interventions?

> ### Clinical pearl
> CPP = DBP–LVEDP
> (LVEDP, left ventricle end-diastolic pressure)

> ### Summary points
> - Beware of atypical presentation of myocardial ischaemia.
> - Time to reperfusion is crucial.
> - Always consider aspirin, heparin and beta-blockade.
> - Remember right-sided precordial leads to detect right ventricle infarct.
> - Avoid beta-blockers in patients with cocaine-induced ischaemia to avoid unopposed alpha-effects.

Heart failure in the ICU

Congestive heart failure (CHF) is a significant health problem and poses a tremendous burden to society in health care costs. In contrast to favourable trends for most cardiovascular conditions, the incidence, prevalence, morbidity and mortality of CHF are increasing. Causative factors have shifted from hypertension and valvular heart disease to coronary artery disease, an increasing prevalence of diabetes and ageing of the population. Despite advances in therapy, hospitalisations for CHF remain high, and survival rates after development of symptoms remain poor. Admission to an intensive care unit (ICU) is responsible for more than 30% of the costs associated with the management of acute decompensation of chronic heart failure.

Heart failure: a clinical syndrome

Heart failure is a clinical syndrome characterised by dyspnoea, fatigue and fluid retention that is caused by the inability of the heart to maintain adequate blood circulation to the peripheral tissues and the lungs. Structural or functional disorders result in impaired ventricular filling and/or ejection. Left ventricular (LV) dysfunction is generally progressive with changes in LV geometry and architecture, 'cardiac remodelling', sustaining altered mechanical performance. Reduced cardiac output activates the neurohormonal system, leading to increased circulating levels of noradrenaline (norepinephrine), angiotensin II, aldosterone, endothelin and vasopressin, among others. These factors contribute to salt retention, increased peripheral vascular resistance, altered renal blood flow and function, and ventricular remodelling, all factors that perpetuate the vicious cycle of cardiac failure (Fig. 1).

Systolic versus diastolic heart failure

While heart failure has traditionally been thought of in terms of reduced LV ejection fraction, many patients (up to 40% in some series) presenting with symptoms of heart failure have preserved LV systolic function. This clinical syndrome is known as diastolic heart failure. LV relaxation is an active, energy-requiring process. Derangements in cellular energetics, intracellular calcium homeostasis or passive elastic properties of ventricular muscle may contribute to decreased ventricular relaxation and distensibility, leading to elevated filling pressures, inadequate ventricular filling during diastole and increased risk of congestion. Diastolic heart failure can occur alone or in conjunction with systolic heart failure. Differentiation between systolic and diastolic heart failure cannot be made on the basis of history, physical examination, electrocardiogram (ECG) or chest radiograph alone.

Right heart versus left heart failure

The RV is a thin-walled chamber designed to eject into the low-resistance pulmonary vascular circuit. As such, it responds poorly to acute increases in afterload. It has a complex contractile mechanism, and LV contraction contributes significantly to RV ejection. RV free wall perfusion correlates with mean arterial pressure (MAP), so maintenance of adequate RV perfusion pressure may be at odds with goals of reducing afterload for LV failure. RV failure and distension causes a leftward shift in the interventricular septum, reducing LV cavity size, compliance and filling.

In the patient presenting with heart failure, it is important to assess both right and left ventricular function as the management goals may vary. The signs, symptoms and other diagnostic findings for right and left heart failure often differ and are summarised in Table 1 – a note of caution, however, as many patients may exhibit signs and symptoms of biventricular failure.

Assessment

A careful history and physical examination are critical first steps in the evaluation of the patient with known or suspected heart failure. While ischaemic heart disease is causally linked to the majority of heart failure cases and should be included in the differential diagnosis, a number of other important causative or contributing factors must be considered (Box 1). Assessment of cardiac function should include evaluation of heart rate and rhythm, preload, afterload and contractility because any disturbance in one may result in altered function in another. One of the most useful diagnostic tools used for both initial workup and follow-up is two-dimensional echocardiography with Doppler flow studies.

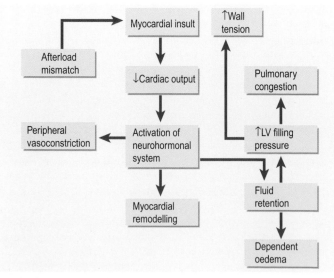

Fig. 1 **Pathophysiology of heart failure.**

Management of heart failure in the ICU

The management of heart failure in the ICU starts with determining the aetiology of the heart failure and correcting any derangements in heart rate, rhythm, preload, afterload and contractility. Management goals and therapeutic options for *acute* left and right heart failure are listed in Tables 2 and 3. The reader is referred to the following link for the American Heart Association (AHA)/American College of Cardiology (ACC) 2005 guideline update for the diagnosis and management of *chronic* heart failure: http://content.onlinejacc. org/cgi/reprint/46/6/e1.

Table 1 **Signs, symptoms and other diagnostic findings for right and left heart failure**

	Left heart failure	Right heart failure
Symptoms	Decreased exercise tolerance	No congestion
	Dyspnoea/orthopnoea	Fatigue
	Non-productive cough	Decreased appetite
Signs	Bibasilar crackles/± wheezing	No crackles
	3rd or 4th heart sounds	Elevated JVD
	Decreased pulse strength	Loud P2 heart sound
	Poor peripheral perfusion	Hepatomegaly and tenderness
		Peripheral oedema
ECG	LV hypertrophy	RV hypertrophy/strain
	Signs of ischaemia	P-pulmonale
	Arrhythmias	Arrhythmias (atrial fibrillation)
Chest radiograph	Cardiomegaly	Right heart enlargement
	Pulmonary oedema	'Pruned' pulmonary vessels
	Pleural effusions	
Echocardiography	Restrictive mitral valve inflow	RV hypertrophy ± dilatation
	LV dilatation ± hypertrophy	Decreased RV function
	Decreased LV function	D-shaped IVS
	Regional wall motion abnormalities	Tricuspid regurgitation
	Ischaemic mitral regurgitation	↑ Pulmonary artery pressures
Angiography	± Coronary artery disease	Pulmonary embolic disease

IVS, interventricular septum; JVD, jugular venous distension; LV, left ventricle; RV, right ventricle.

Table 2 **Goals for management/support of left ventricular failure**

Optimise preload	Fluids for hypovolaemia
	Diuretics if LVEDP elevated
Control heart rate/rhythm	Beta-blockers if LVEF normal
	Amiodarone if LVEF reduced
	Biventricular pacing if QRS > 0.12 s
Reverse ischaemia	ASA, heparin, nitrates
	Percutaneous coronary intervention
	Surgical revascularisation
Reduce afterload	ACE inhibitors
	Angiotensin II receptor blockers
	Intravenous arterial vasodilators
Improve LV contractility (acute)	Beta1-adrenergic receptor agonists
	Phosphodiesterase III inhibitors
	Calcium sensitiser agents (still in clinical trials in USA)
Anticoagulation	EF ≤ 20% at risk for thrombus
	Atrial fibrillation

ASA, aspirin; EF, ejection fraction; LVEDP, left ventricular end-diastolic pressure; LVEF, left ventricular ejection fraction.

Table 3 **Goals for management/support of right ventricular failure**

Optimise preload	Fluids for hypovolaemia … remember higher filling pressure (CVP) often necessary
	Diuretics if RV distended and LV filling compromised
Reduce pulmonary vascular resistance	Avoid hypoxaemia, hypercarbia, acidosis, ↓ temperature
	Judicious PEEP, avoid ↑ mean airway pressures
	Provide adequate analgesia
	Inhaled vasodilators (nitric oxide, prostaglandins)
	Systemic vasodilators
	Endothelin antagonists
Maintain RV blood flow/perfusion	Maintain adequate MAP for RV free wall perfusion (alpha-agonists, vasopressin, IABP)
	Coronary revascularisation for ischaemia
Improve RV contractility (acute)	Beta1-adrenergic receptor agonists
	Phosphodiesterase III inhibitors
	Calcium sensitiser agents (still in clinical trials in USA)
Anticoagulation	EF ≤ 20% at risk for thrombus
	Pulmonary thromboembolic disease
	Atrial fibrillation

CVP, central venous pressure; EF, ejection fraction; IABP, intra-aortic balloon pump; LV, left ventricle; MAP, mean arterial pressure; PEEP, positive end-expiratory pressure; RV, right ventricle.

Box 1. Factors contributing to the development of heart failure

Ischaemic heart disease: diabetes, dyslipidaemia, family history, smoking, obesity

Hypertension

Valvular heart disease

Congenital heart disease

Sleep-disordered breathing

Cardiotoxic agents: alcohol, chemotherapy agents

Thyroid disorder

Phaeochromocytoma

Myocarditis

Mediastinal irradiation

Conduction system disease (need for pacemaker)

Cardiomyopathy (hypertrophic, idiopathic)

Skeletal myopathies

Clinical case

A 63-year-old patient is admitted with recent-onset respiratory distress and oxygen saturation of 89% on 6 L of oxygen administered via nasal cannula. He underwent femoral–popliteal bypass surgery 3 days previously for severe claudication. He has a medical history significant for longstanding hypertension, smoking, peripheral vascular disease, mild obesity and diet-controlled diabetes. On presentation, his pulse is irregular 116 bpm, blood pressure 186/89 mmHg, he has good peripheral pulses with rales and mild wheezing on chest auscultation. What are your diagnostic considerations? How will you proceed?

Summary points

- The incidence and morbidity/mortality of CHF is increasing.
- CHF may be due to systolic or diastolic dysfunction or both.
- The presentation and management challenges for right heart and left heart failure differ.
- Echocardiography is one of the most valuable diagnostic aids for assessing patients with CHF.

Arrhythmias

Critically ill patients are vulnerable to arrhythmias, especially when there is multisystem dysfunction.

Factors predisposing to arrhythmias include:

- **I**nfarction and **I**schaemia
- **S**urgery (cardiac/thoracic/vascular/neurological)
- **T**rauma (hypovolaemia)
- **A**ngioplasty (reperfusion)
- **R**enal failure
- **T**emperature (hypo-/hyperthermia)
- **M**etabolic (acidaemia/alkalaemia/hypoxaemia/hyper-/hypocapnia)
- **E**lectrolyte disturbances (especially potassium and magnesium)
- **D**rugs (e.g. haloperidol/digoxin/beta-agonists/theophylline/tricyclics, etc.)
- **S**hock

Anatomy and physiology

Automaticity is the property of heart cells to depolarise spontaneously. The sinoatrial node (SAN) is usually the heart's pacemaker. When this fails, the role falls to other areas that typically have a slower intrinsic rate than the SAN (Fig. 1). Within the system, there are physiological delays to conduction, such as occurs in the atrioventricular (AV) node. When pathways are disrupted, heart blocks and bradycardia may result. When there are accessory or re-entrant pathways, tachyarrhythmias may result.

Diagnosis

Diagnosis of arrhythmias in the intensive care unit (ICU) may be difficult owing to a rapid heart rate, low-voltage electrocardiogram (ECG) complexes and competing paced rhythms. A 12-lead ECG, a rhythm strip or an atrial ECG may aid in diagnosis. Adenosine may slow conduction through the AV node, illuminating differences among sinus tachycardia, atrial fibrillation and atrial flutter. When atrial epicardial leads are present (following heart surgery), an atrial ECG (Fig. 2) allows comparison of atrial activity with a simultaneous standard ECG rhythm strip.

Questions to ask when assessing arrhythmias:

1 Is the arrhythmia fast or slow?
2 Is the origin of the rhythm disturbance ventricular or supraventricular?
3 Is the patient haemodynamically compromised?
4 Does the arrhythmia need urgent management?
5 What is the underlying cause that predisposed to the arrhythmia?
6 What triggered the arrhythmia?
7 Will the arrhythmia recur?

Tachyarrhythmias

A tachy- or fast arrhythmia is characterised by a ventricular rate exceeding 100/min. Narrow QRS complex tachyarrhythmias are associated with supraventricular origins. Wide complex tachycardias may be associated with ventricular origin. However, underlying conduction defects, such as bundle branch blocks, may be associated with wide QRS complex arrhythmias with supraventricular origins. For all arrhythmias, cardioversion (or defibrillation) may be urgently required when there is haemodynamic instability. When there are recognisable QRS complexes (i.e. not ventricular fibrillation), the 'shock' should be synchronised. This ensures that the 'shock' coincides with the QRS complex. If an unsynchronised 'shock' is delivered, it can occur during the T wave when the heart is vulnerable (relative refractory period). This may trigger a more malignant

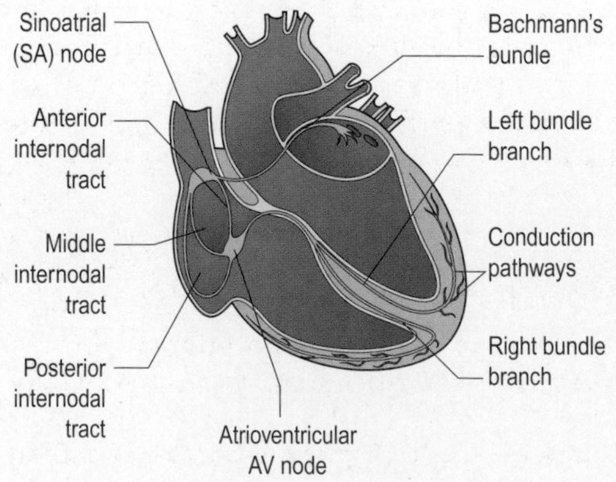

Fig. 1 The paths by which electrical impulses normally travel through the heart. The intrinsic rate of automaticity slows with downstream passage.

Sinoatrial (SA) node
Anterior internodal tract
Middle internodal tract
Posterior internodal tract
Atrioventricular AV node
Bachmann's bundle
Left bundle branch
Conduction pathways
Right bundle branch

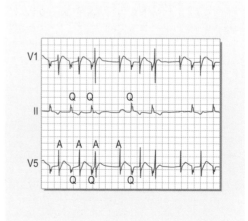

Fig. 2 **Atrial ECG.** Lead II is a standard ECG strip. Leads V1 and V5 are attached directly to the atrial pacing wires. An electrical spike (A) is a display of atrial activity. The occurrence of the QRS complex (Q) is visualised at the same time in all leads. In lead II, P waves are not appreciated. The atrial leads (V1 and V5) reveal P spikes, a long PR interval and show that not all atrial activity is conducted.

rhythm, such as ventricular fibrillation. Electrical cardioversion is painful and, if practical, a sedative such as propofol or midazolam should be given prior to delivering the 'shock'.

Supraventricular tachycardia (SVT)

The origin of the arrhythmia is above the ventricles. When QRS complexes are less than 0.12 s, this is suggestive of a SVT (Fig. 3). A decrease in ventricular rate in response to adenosine is also indicative that the origin of an arrhythmia is supraventricular, as adenosine transiently slows conduction through the AV node. Vagal stimulation may be attempted if there is no contraindication, such as carotid disease. Beta-blockers, calcium channel blockers and digitalis slow conduction through the AV node. These drugs may be counterproductive for ventricular arrhythmias or when there are aberrant conduction pathways, such as the bundle of Kent in Wolff–Parkinson–White syndrome. Amiodarone may be useful in treating SVTs.

Atrial fibrillation and atrial flutter

Atrial fibrillation is characterised by an irregularly irregular ventricular rate with the absence of P waves. A rapid ventricular rate is common and may lead to haemodynamic instability. Atrial flutter is characterised by flutter P waves, which are rapid successive P waves between QRS complexes. The ventricular rate is usually regular and is typically a fraction of 300/min (i.e. 150, 100, 75 or 60/min). Atrial flutter may progress to atrial fibrillation. Control of ventricular response rate and anticoagulation may be indicated for flutter or fibrillation. Transoesophageal echocardiography is useful to check that there is no clot (that may embolise with restoration of sinus rhythm) in the left atrial appendage prior to attempts at electrical or pharmacological (e.g. with amiodarone) cardioversion.

Ventricular tachycardia (VT) and ventricular fibrillation (VF)

VT is a ventricular originated rhythm with a rate between 100 and 250/min sustained for 30 s or longer. QRS complexes are broad (> 0.12 s). VT can be monomorphic (same QRS morphology) or polymorphic (different QRS morphologies). Polymorphic VT has a higher incidence of deterioration into VF. VT is poorly tolerated arrhythmia and may require immediate electrical or pharmacological (e.g. amiodarone)

cardioversion. VF is disorganised ventricular tachycardia that is incompatible with life. ECG shows irregular, indiscernible QRS complexes with rates as high as 400/min. Pulseless VT and VF mandate immediate defibrillation. There are syndromes, such as long QT and Brugada syndrome, that predispose people to ventricular arrhythmias. It is important that these are diagnosed. Implantable cardioverter/defibrillators prevent deaths in people who are prone to ventricular arrhythmias.

Bradyarrhythmias

Bradycardia is a ventricular rate less that 50/min and results from abnormalities anywhere in the conduction system. Symptomatic bradycardia may be treated temporarily with chronotropic drugs [e.g. atropine or isoprenaline (isoproterenol)]. Emergency pacing may be required.

Sick sinus syndrome is characterised by fluctuation in sinus-originated depolarisation. Failure to regulate heart rate to meet metabolic needs is a sign. Myriad arrhythmias may present, including sinus bradycardia, sinus arrest (> 3-s pauses) and tachycardia–bradycardia syndrome. A rate-adaptive permanent pacemaker is indicated.

Heart blocks can be first, second or third degree, with increasing severity. Conduction delay through the AV node presents with a prolonged PR interval (> 200 ms) on the ECG; this is a first-degree block. Second-degree blocks are divided into Mobitz type I (Wenckebach block) and Mobitz type II. Second-degree blocks occur when the atrial rhythm fails to conduct to the ventricle in a 1:1 ratio. With Mobitz type I, the ECG shows a progressive increase in the PR interval until a P wave fails to conduct. In Mobitz type II, there is no prolongation of the PR interval before an abrupt conduction failure. Third-degree atrioventricular block is referred to as 'complete heart block'. There is no relationship between atrial activity and ventricular activity.

⚕ Clinical case

A 58-year-old woman presents with acute myocardial infarction. ECG shows sinus tachycardia (110/min) with ST elevations in leads V3 to V6. Within a few minutes, she loses consciousness. The heart rate is now 160/min and the ECG strip reveals wide complex tachycardia. There is no pulse.

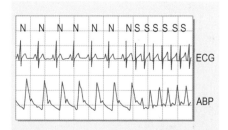

Fig. 3 **Abrupt onset of a narrow complex tachycardia that appears regular.** N, normal sinus rhythm; S, SVT; ECG, ECG rhythm strip; ABP, arterial blood pressure.

Summary points

- A 12-lead ECG and a rhythm strip aid in diagnosing arrhythmias.
- Underlying causes of arrythmias should be identified and treated.
- Amiodarone may be useful for treating ventricular and supraventricular arrhythmias.
- Amiodarone may result in chemical cardioversion.
- Electrical cardioversion may be required when patients are haemodynamically unstable.
- Symptomatic bradycardias require pacing.

Pacing

Many patients admitted to intensive care units (ICUs) have either temporary or permanent pacemakers in place, or may require placement of a temporary pacemaker as an emergency intervention. Cardiac pacing is frequently indicated following acute myocardial infarction and cardiac surgery. Critically ill patients are at heightened risk for suppression and irritability of the electrophysiological pathways that provide normal conduction governing synchronous contraction of the myocardium.

Every ICU should have the expertise and the wherewithal to institute temporary cardiac pacing. Depending upon the aetiology of the conduction abnormality, temporary pacing may be a bridge to a permanent pacemaker or may afford time for healing of the myocardium and the conduction pathways. During critical illness, pacemakers may function suboptimally and may require adjustment until illness resolves. Metabolic disturbances such as hypoxaemia, hypothermia and acidaemia, various drugs such as beta-blockers, and cardiac injury, oedema or pericardial effusion may all alter the pacing thresholds of cardiac tissue.

Modes

A three- or four-letter code is commonly used to describe a pacemaker's mode of function (Table 1). Selecting the mode with which to pace depends on the type of pacemaker and the electrophysiological and anatomical considerations specific to the patient. Apart from choosing a mode and setting a minimum heart rate, there are other important settings such as the PR interval with dual chamber pacing. Improper pacing can lead to suboptimal or deleterious results.

With temporary pacing, the sensitivity and stimulation output may be tested and reset by the clinician as needed. The greater the sensitivity, the more likely it is that the pacemaker will sense native conduction. However, if the pacer is too sensitive, it may 'oversense'. Oversensing leads to underpacing. On the other hand, undersensing can lead to inappropriately timed pacing spikes. If a spike occurs during the T-wave segment, it can trigger an arrhythmia such as ventricular tachycardia. This is referred to as the R on T phenomenon.

Stimulation, measured in milliamps (mA), is the electrical current administered to the myocardium via the pacing electrode. With stimulation, 'less is more'. Sufficient energy is needed to achieve capture, but prolonged pacing with high stimulation outputs can lead to higher stimulation thresholds, thus making capture more difficult over time. To avoid loss of capture, setting the stimulation output to 1.5 times the stimulation threshold is a reasonable approach to achieve continuous pacing while limiting the threshold tolerance.

Indications for pacemaker placement include:

- Sick sinus syndrome
- Symptomatic bradycardia
- Tachycardia–bradycardia syndrome
- Atrial fibrillation with a slow ventricular response
- Type IIb heart block
- Complete atrioventricular block (third-degree block)
- Long QT syndrome.

Relative indications for pacemaker placement include:

- Severe systolic dysfunction
- Hypertrophic cardiomyopathy
- Paroxysmal atrial fibrillation.

Permanent pacemakers

The ICU clinician should be aware of the reasons why the pacemaker was inserted and how it is expected to perform. If a pacemaker has a malfunction such as oversensing, emergency placement of a magnet overlying the pacemaker may convert the pacemaker mode into the VOO setting (asynchronous ventricular pacing at a fixed rate). A magnet may also be used to deactivate the automatic defibrillator function if it is delivering inappropriate shocks. Removal of the magnet does not necessarily restore the previous settings; a magnet should thus be used only in emergency situations. Electrophysiological interrogation of a permanent pacemaker performed at the bedside provides precise pacemaker settings and capabilities. Traditional sequential pacemakers pace the right atrium followed by the right ventricle. This results in a delay between right ventricular and left ventricular contraction, which can decrease cardiac output. This manifests as a left bundle branch block on the electrocardiogram (ECG). Biventricular pacing results in synchronous contraction of both ventricles and is useful for patients with severe systolic heart failure (Fig. 1).

Temporary pacemakers

Epicardial pacing

Epicardial pacing is most frequently used following cardiac surgery. Typically, epicardial pacing wires are sutured to the right atrium and the right ventricle. These wires exit through the skin and are attached to an external pulse generator or pacemaker box (Fig. 2). With optimal lead placement and healthy heart muscle, the output needed for capture ranges from 2 to 20 mA. The wires become less effective over time as lead position may change or myocardial scarring develops. When epicardial pacing is no longer needed or no longer effective, the wires are removed by gentle traction. Generally, this should not be done when there is a bleeding tendency or therapeutic anticoagulation.

Table 1 **Lettering system for pacemakers**			
Mode	Paced chamber	Sensed chamber	Response to sensed event
AAI	Atrium	Atrium	Inhibition
AAO	Atrium	Atrium	None
VVI	Ventricle	Ventricle	Inhibition
VOO	Ventricle	None	None
DDI	Dual	Dual	Inhibition
DDD	Dual	Dual	Triggered inhibition

Each letter denotes a pacemaker capability: first letter stands for chamber(s) paced, second letter stands for chamber(s) sensed, and third stands for response to sensed event. A fourth letter is sometimes seen and denotes rate-adaptive capabilities.

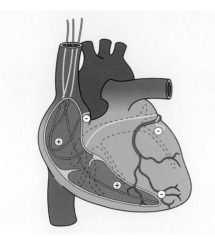

Fig. 1 **The location of pacer leads with a biventricular pacemaker.** Leads are evident in the right atrium and right ventricle. The third lead passes through the coronary sinus to reach a position where the left ventricle is paced.

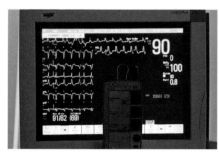

Fig. 2 **A pacemaker box attached to epicardial leads.** The pacing mode is VVI. The heart rate is set at 90/min. The ventricular output is 8 mA. The monitor shows multiple ECG leads demonstrating ventricular pacing spikes, wide QRS complexes and consistent capture.

Transvenous pacing

Transvenous pacing is accomplished by direct stimulation of the endocardial surface via an electrode-tipped venous catheter. The catheter is inserted with the Seldinger technique as is usual for central venous catheters. The right internal jugular vein provides the most reliable and direct passage to the heart. Catheter positioning may be directed by fluoroscopy when time, training and availability permit. ECG monitoring may guide tip positioning in the absence of fluoroscopy and must be used to confirm the efficacy of transvenous pacing. Along with ECG display of capture, haemodynamic stability should be assessed when implementing temporary pacing. The usual mode of transvenous pacing is VOO with the endocardium of the right ventricle as the target for the catheter tip. A pacing pulmonary artery catheter affords one of the easiest methods of achieving emergency transvenous pacing. The catheter is advanced into the pulmonary artery in the usual fashion. A pacing wire is then advanced through a dedicated lumen and is directed onto the endocardium of the right ventricle (Fig. 3).

Transcutaneous pacing

With sudden onset of a life-threatening bradyarrhythmia such as complete heart block, transcutaneous pacing provides a quick way to implement temporary pacing. Hands-free adhesive electrode pads are applied directly to the skin. These pads are most commonly placed in the anteroposterior or anterolateral positions.

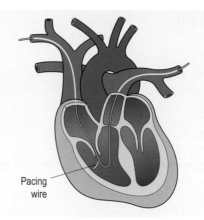

Fig. 3 **Pacing pulmonary artery catheter (PAC).** The tip of the PAC is in the left pulmonary artery. The pacing wire (arrow) can be seen emerging from a lumen of the PAC and abutting against the endocardium of the right ventricle.

The output in milliamps (mA) is increased to achieve capture; up to 20–140 mA may be required to achieve capture. Factors that increase the threshold for capture include well-developed musculature, obesity, chronic obstructive pulmonary disease (COPD), hypoxaemia, myocardial infarction and positive pressure ventilation. This mode of temporary pacing is painful. Analgesic and anxiolytic medications increase tolerability. Transcutaneous pacing is a temporary emergency intervention.

Clinical case
A 64-year old patient with a biventricular pacemaker is in the ICU with pneumonia. He is sedated, there is a tracheal tube in place, and mechanical ventilation is being provided. The heart rate is 35/min, and the 12-lead ECG shows a complete heart block. The blood pressure is low. What should be done?

Clinical pearl
Pacing threshold = the minimum output amplitude required to initiate pacing.
Sense = the ability of the pacemaker to sense the heart's electrical activity.
Capture = a pacemaker spike/output successfully initiates cardiac conduction.

Summary points

- Cardiac pacing may improve heart function.
- A magnet may convert a pacemaker to a 'VOO' mode and may disable the cardioverter/defibrillator function.
- Sensing and capture thresholds as well as intrinsic heart rhythms may change during critical illness.
- When a pacemaker fails, underlying causes such as metabolic and electrolyte derangements should be excluded.
- Emergency pacing may be a life-saving intervention.

Cardiac surgery

The recent experience of cardiac surgery has been humbling for thousands of surgeons who have seen their livelihoods eroded by interventional cardiologists. This is illustrative of the vagaries of the modern world; with rampant technology, apparently essential practitioners may wake up to find that their roles have been superseded. Cardiac surgeons are attempting to redefine a niche for themselves. They are operating on sicker and older patients, and are promoting new procedures, such as placement of ventricular assist devices. A patient's risk of mortality following cardiac surgery may be approximated from validated risk scoring systems, such as the Euroscore (www.euroscore.org). With modern cardiac surgery, postoperative intensive care is challenging and may impact significantly on survival.

Pandora's box of complications

An array of complications may occur following cardiac surgery. With cardiopulmonary bypass (CPB), there is exposure to artificial surfaces, which may result in systemic inflammatory response syndrome (SIRS), inflammation and activation of coagulation. Cross-clamping of the aorta may lead to plaque displacement or aortic damage. Embolisation of plaques may manifest as stroke or damage to other organs. When flow during CPB is low, damage to the kidneys and brain may occur. Some myocardial damage is inevitable. Conduction abnormalities such as complete heart block are common, especially following aortic valve surgery. Atrial fibrillation complicates 20–30% of cardiac surgeries. Some degree of coagulopathy often occurs following CPB. Factors contributing include surgical bleeding, consumptive coagulopathy, platelet dysfunction, haemodilution, hyperfibrinolyis, hypothermia, acidaemia and heparin or protamine effects. Heparin, apart from causing bleeding, may trigger life-threatening heparin-induced thrombocytopenia (p. 134). Patients are at risk for fluid, electrolyte, acid–base and glucose abnormalities following CPB.

Cardiogenic shock and haemorrhagic shock (p. 132) are important causes of instability following heart surgery. However, there are other key diagnoses, which are easily overlooked (Table 1).

Concealed bleeding

The mediastinal drains may be clotted or the bleeding may be into the posterior mediastinum or pleural spaces. This diagnosis may be suggested by a falling haemoglobin or by radiological features; there may be mediastinal widening or a layering opacification of lung fields representing haemothoraces. Treatment is surgical.

Systolic anterior motion of the mitral valve leaflet (SAM)

SAM most commonly occurs following mitral valve repair or when there is an underlying hypertrophic cardiomyopathy. The anterior leaflet of the mitral valve may be long and floppy, and may be pulled into the ventricular outflow tract during systole. This results in obstruction to flow and to mitral regurgitation. Echocardiography is useful for corroboration. SAM is aggravated by inotropes, hypovolaemia and vasodilatation. Treatment is with fluid, vasoconstrictors and beta-blockers.

Right heart failure (p. 94)

The right heart is vulnerable during CPB. Echocardiography reveals a dilated, poorly contractile right ventricle and an empty left ventricle with preserved function.

Diastolic dysfunction

Ventricular relaxation is energy dependent. Myocardial stunning, especially with pre-existing left ventricular hypertrophy, often manifests as diastolic dysfunction. Patients are exquisitely sensitive to hypovolaemia. Treatment may include low-dose inotropes, fluid resuscitation and atrioventricular (AV) pacing at a rate of 70–90/min with a short PR interval to allow maximal time for ventricular relaxation prior to atrial contraction.

Table 1 **Differential diagnosis of haemodynamic instability following heart surgery**										
	BP	CVP	PCWP	PAP	CI/SVO$_2$	SVR	S$_a$O$_2$	Peak pressure	CXR	Echo
Tamponade	↓	↑	↑	↑	↓	↔/↑	↔/↓	↔	↔	Chamber compression
Haemorrhage	↓	↓	↓	↓	↓	↔/↑	↔/↓	↔	Opacification	Empty LV
Cardiogenic shock	↓	↑	↑	↑	↓	↔/↑	↔/↓	↔	Enlarged heart, pulmonary congestion	↓ Ejection fraction
Diastolic dysfunction	↓/↔/↑	↑	↑	↑	↓	↔/↑	↔/↓	↔	↔	LVH, normal EF, diastolic dysfunction
SAM	↓	↓	↔/↑	↔/↑	↓	↓/↔	↔/↓	↔	↔	SAM, MR, gradient across LVOT
Pneumothorax	↓	↑	↓	↔/↑	↓	↔	↓	↑	Decreased unilateral lung markings	Empty LV
Right heart failure	↓	↑	↓	↔/↑	↓	↔	↔/↓	↔	Prominent pulmonary vasculature	Empty LV, dilated RV, TR
Vasoplegia	↓	↓	↓	↓	↔/↑	↓	↔	↔	↔	Empty LV, normal EF

BP, blood pressure; CI, cardiac index; CVP, central venous pressure; CXR, chest radiograph; echo, echocardiography; EF, ejection fraction; LV, left ventricle; LVH, left ventricular hypertrophy; LVOT, left ventricle outflow tract; MR, mitral regurgitation; PAP, pulmonary artery pressure; PCWP, pulmonary capillary wedge pressure; RV, right ventricle; SAM, systolic anterior motion; SVO$_2$, mixed venous oxygen saturation; TR, tricuspid regurgitation; peak pressure = ventilator peak pressure; ↓, decrease; ↔, no change; , increase.

Tamponade

This is a tricky diagnosis as the features are seldom classical. The only chamber compressed is often the left atrium, which is posterior. This can easily be missed even with echocardiography. Whenever there is unexplained hypotension and decreased urine output, tamponade should be considered. Pulsus paradoxus and elevated jugular venous pulsation may be evident. Surgical exploration is warranted.

Tension pneumothorax

If the pleural spaces are entered during surgery, there is increased risk of tension pneumothorax. The diagnosis and decision to treat are clinical. Features include increased resonance to percussion, diminished unilateral breath sounds, tracheal shift, pulsus paradoxus, hypotension, increased peak and plateau ventilator pressures and decreased oxygen saturation. If the patient is stable and there is diagnostic doubt, an urgent chest radiograph is indicated.

Vasoplegia

Refractory hypotension with vasodilatation may occur. Anaphylaxis and protamine reactions may present in this manner. Angiotensin-converting enzyme (ACE) inhibitors on the morning of surgery increase susceptibility. The underlying mechanism may be a SIRS-type response. A dose of steroids, such as 8 mg of dexamethasone, may be helpful. Treatment is typically with noradrenaline (norepinephrine) and vasopressin infusions. Methylene blue (1–2 mg/kg) has been described when hypotension persists.

ICU management

Output from chest drains should be monitored. Haemoglobin, platelet count, coagulation tests, electrolytes and blood gases are usually checked. A 12-lead ECG and a chest radiograph (p. 106) should be obtained on admission.

Respiratory

A plan to wean mechanical ventilation and wake and extubate patients should be instituted when there is no contraindication. Pulmonary oedema and atelectasis occur commonly. Positive end-expiratory pressure and diuretics may be beneficial.

Cardiovascular

When heart function is poor, inotropes should be weaned slowly over days. A balloon pump should be discontinued when there is haemodynamic stability. Epicardial pacing wires allow temporary postoperative pacing. Occasionally, a permanent pacemaker is required. Aspirin should be restarted.

Statins, ACE inhibitors and beta-blockers may have long-term benefit. Beta-blockers or amiodarone may decrease the likelihood of atrial fibrillation. Potassium and magnesium supplementation decreases the likelihood of arrhythmias.

Kidneys/fluid/electrolytes

Electrolyte and acid–base abnormalities should be corrected. Tight glucose control improves outcome. Renal dysfunction may occur secondary to hypovolaemia, hypotension or acute tubular necrosis (p. 110), and renal replacement therapy may be needed (p. 34).

Infections

Infection with *Staphylococcus aureus*, including community-acquired methicillin-resistant S. *aureus*, or other organisms may complicate heart surgery. Antibiotic prophylaxis frequently includes vancomycin and may be administered for up to 48 h. Mediastinitis and osteomyelitis are devastating complications.

Echocardiography

Echocardiography may provide useful information following heart surgery about regional wall motion, volume status, heart function, valvular function, pericardial effusions, cardiac clots, aortic dissections and shunts. Echocardiography can help to differentiate among the various causes of shock.

> ### Clinical case
> A 75-year-old patient presents 6 h following coronary artery bypass surgery. Mechanical ventilation is ongoing. The blood pressure (BP) is decreasing despite noradrenaline (norepinephrine) infusion. The systolic BP varies by 15 mmHg during the respiratory cycle. The heart rate is 110/min. Jugular venous distension is noted. What is the most likely diagnosis?

> ### Summary points
> - An array of complications may occur following cardiac surgery.
> - Cardiogenic and haemorrhagic shock are common.
> - Tamponade and concealed bleeding may be overlooked.
> - Beta-blockers, aspirin, ACE inhibitors and statins may improve outcome.

Pulmonary hypertension

The pulmonary circulation receives the entire cardiac output. Normally, the pulmonary circulation is a low-pressure, low-resistance, high-capacity and thin-walled circuit. There is a large vascular reservoir that may be recruited to accommodate an increase in flow, maintaining the mean pulmonary artery pressure at approximately 12–16 mmHg. Pulmonary hypertension (PHT) is defined by mean pulmonary artery pressure >25 mmHg at rest or 30 mmHg during exercise. The right ventricle (RV) is a thin-walled pump. When the pressure increases in the pulmonary circuit, the RV may be unable to cope with the increased load, and right-sided heart failure may result.

Aetiologies of PHT

- Primary and secondary causes
- Intrinsic (from disease in lung itself) and extrinsic causes (e.g. cardiac disease)
- Acute and chronic causes.

Acute and chronic pulmonary hypertension are compared in Table 1.

$$\text{Pressure} = \text{flow} \times \text{resistance}$$

PHT may result from an increase in pulmonary blood flow or resistance to flow. Three important mechanisms resulting in PHT are, therefore, an increase in left atrial pressure (e.g. mitral stenosis), a left-to-right heart shunt (e.g. ventricular septal defect) and an increase in pulmonary vascular resistance (i.e. vasoconstrictive, obstructive or obliterative) (see Table 2).

Consequences/diagnosis

PHT can lead to a decrease in cardiac output and mean arterial pressure, RV and left ventricle (LV) failure, and hypoxaemia (Fig. 1).

Symptoms include dyspnoea, angina, fatigue, syncope and abdominal distension.

Physical examination may reveal a left parasternal heave, a loud pulmonary component of the second heart sound (S2) and a systolic murmur of tricuspid regurgitation. Peripheral signs of RV failure (e.g. cyanosis, hepatomegaly, jugular venous distension) may also be apparent.

Possible *electrocardiogram (ECG) findings* include RV hypertrophy and right atrial enlargement. With a pulmonary embolism (PE), the ECG is likely to show normal sinus rhythm or sinus tachycardia. Occasionally, the ECG may show right axis deviation and signs of right heart strain (S1Q3T3): S wave in lead I, Q wave in lead III and an inverted T wave in lead III.

The typical *chest radiograph* or CT scan (Fig. 2) may show enlarged right and left pulmonary arteries, prominence of the RV and the hilar pulmonary artery trunk, rapid tapering of vascular markings or hyperlucent lung periphery.

Table 1 **Features of acute and chronic pulmonary hypertension**
Acute PHT
Severe and sudden: increase in right ventricular (RV) afterload→increased end-diastolic volume, decreased ejection fraction, decreased stroke volume→decreased cardiac index
Can develop acute right heart failure
RV can generate limited mean pulmonary artery pressure (up to 40 mmHg)
RV ischaemia can develop
Acute pulmonary embolism is a common cause
Chronic PHT
Progressive so that the RV dilates and hypertrophies from chronic pressure and volume overload
Gradual RV dysfunction
Tricuspid regurgitation may occur
RV failure may result
RV can generate higher pressures than with acute PHT
RV ischaemia can develop
Chronic obstructive pulmonary disease is a common cause

Table 2 **Differential diagnosis of PHT on the ICU**
Causes of acute PHT
H: hypothermia/hypoxaemia
A: acidosis
M: mitral valve flail
P: pain, PEEP, pneumothorax
E: embolism
R: respiratory diseases (e.g. asthma, pneumonia)
Causes of chronic PHT
Cardiac disease (e.g. left heart failure, mitral valve disease)
Chronic thromboemboli
Collagen vascular disease
Hypertrophy of small artery walls
Left-to-right shunts
Polycythaemia
Portal hypertension

PEEP, positive end-expiratory pressure.

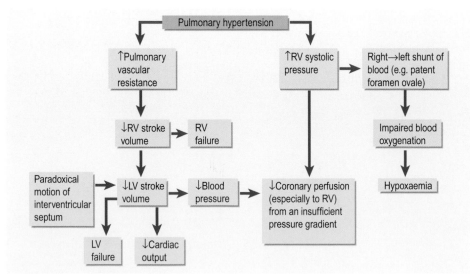

Fig. 1 **The pathogenesis of clinical deterioration with PHT.**

Table 3 **Drugs for PHT**	
Drug	**Mechanism**
Calcium channel blockers	Decrease intracellular calcium→vasodilation
Nitric oxide	Stimulates soluble guanylate cyclase→increases cGMP→vasodilation
Prostacyclin	Stimulates adenylate cyclase→increases cAMP→vasodilation
Sildenafil	Inhibits phosphodiesterase in the lung to inhibit breakdown of cAMP→vasodilation
Bosentan	Blocks endothelin-1 receptors to block vasoconstriction and smooth muscle cell proliferation

cAMP, cyclic adenosine monophosphate; cGMP, cyclic guanosine monophosphate

Echocardiography is useful in clarifying diagnoses. Left and right heart function as well as the heart valves may be assessed. Doppler measurements allow quantification of pulmonary pressures and cardiac output. For suspected PE, lung perfusion scans, pulmonary angiography and spiral computerised tomography scans are useful for diagnosis. Cardiac catheterisation is the gold standard for diagnosis of PHT. This enables evaluation of pulmonary pressure, cardiac output, response to vasodilators (such as nitric oxide and prostacyclin), intracardiac shunts and coronary circulation. A pulmonary artery catheter may be useful in tracking patient progress and efficacy of therapy.

Treatment

The priority is to treat any underlying cause of PHT (Fig. 3, Table 3). Oxygen is the easiest effective intervention. Most treatments are geared towards decreasing RV afterload and treating RV failure.

Nitric oxide can be administered via inhalation, resulting in pulmonary vasodilation that occurs selectively in ventilated areas. It has a greater effect on the pulmonary circulation than the systemic because of its short half-life. However, it is expensive. Inhaled prostacyclin is a suitable and cheap alternative to inhaled nitric oxide.

Fig. 2 **CT scan with features of pulmonary hypertension.**

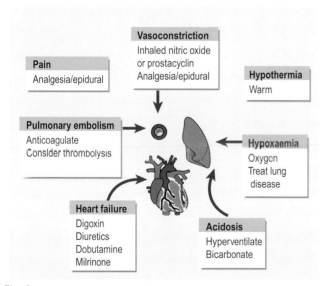

Fig. 3 **Emergency treatment of PHT.**

Clinical case

A 45-year-old man underwent an open fixation of a fractured tibia 2 days ago. There were no complications during surgery, and the patient was doing well until he suddenly felt short of breath. On examination, he is distressed, obtunded, diaphoretic and has petechiae on his chest and in his axillae. The heart rate is 115/min, blood pressure is 150/80 mmHg, respiratory rate is 28/min, tympanic temperature is 37.9°C, and peripheral oxygen saturation is 92% on a high-concentration oxygen mask. Cardiac examination reveals a parasternal heave and a loud pulmonary component of the second heart sound. What is the most likely diagnosis and how may this be established?

Summary points

- Pulmonary embolism is an important cause of acute PHT on the ICU.
- PHT can cause RV failure, especially if it is acute.
- Treatment should be aimed at underlying causes and at promoting pulmonary vasodilation.
- Oxygen is a safe and effective treatment for PHT.

Valvular and congenital heart disease

Pressure–volume loops

A plot of the relationship between ventricular volume and simultaneous ventricular pressure is a basis for understanding mechanical events during the cardiac cycle and the adaptation to both pressure and volume overload lesions that may occur with valvular heart disease. In Figure 1, line 'A' demonstrates the diastolic pressure–volume relationship, and point 'EDV' describes the *preload* of the left ventricle, i.e. the volume in the ventricle that contributes to the stretch of the sarcomere immediately before contraction. The slope of line 'A' describes the *compliance* of the ventricle, i.e. the change in volume for a given change in pressure. Ventricular hypertrophy or wall thickening leads to a decrease in compliance and thus ventricular filling requires higher filling pressures.

During isovolumic contraction, 'B', developed pressure builds in the ventricle until it exceeds pressure at the aortic valve (or left ventricular outflow tract if an obstructive lesion is present) and ejection occurs, 'C'. Following ejection and aortic valve closure, isovolumic relaxation occurs, 'D'. *Stroke volume* is defined as the difference between end systolic volume 'ESV' and EDV. The *afterload* of the ventricle is defined by the wall tension, i.e. force per unit of cross-sectional area, against which it must contract, and is described by Laplace's law, which states that wall tension is equal to Pr/2h where P = peak intraventricular pressure, r = ventricular chamber radius and h = wall thickness.

Oxygen consumption

Most of the energy utilized by the heart is expended for cardiac contraction. Oxygen consumption for mechanical work is proportional to the area within the pressure – volume loop, with the greatest amount consumed for pressure development during isovolumic contraction. Lesions producing increased ventricular pressure demands, such as aortic stenosis for example, not only lead to increase in oxygen consumption but also stimulate ventricular hypertrophy. From Laplace's law it follows that increased wall thickness

helps normalise wall tension and preserve ejection fraction despite the increases in developed pressure necessary for forward flow to occur. Valvular heart lesions leading to increases in ventricular volume, including aortic and mitral regurgitation, also produce an increase in myocardial oxygen consumption, but this increase in volume work is far less costly than increases in pressure work. Haemodynamic management goals for the most common valvular lesions are listed in Table 1.

Postoperative considerations

Left ventricular dysfunction most often occurs as a consequence of longstanding preoperative pressure or volume overload, but may be a result of inadequate intraoperative myocardial protection or valve dysfunction. Right ventricular performance may not only be compromised as a result of the factors above, but may result from pulmonary hypertension or uncorrected tricuspid regurgitation and volume overload. Pharmacological and/or mechanical support of ventricular function may be required. Pulmonary hypertension, commonly seen in

patients with left-sided valve disease and elevated left atrial pressure (LAP), may persist following surgery because of pulmonary vascular changes that occur with longstanding disease. In addition to careful management of oxygenation, acid–base balance, temperature and analgesia/sedation, inhaled pulmonary vasodilators may be administered to minimise right ventricular afterload. Conduction disturbances and dysrhythmias are common and may require temporary pacing for several days immediately postoperatively. Occasionally, a permanent pacemaker will be necessary. All patients with mechanical valve prostheses and patients with bioprostheses and thrombosis risk factors (e.g. atrial fibrillation, severe left ventricular dysfunction, hypercoagulable state or prior thromboembolism) require anticoagulation. Current anticoagulation guidelines are listed in Table 2. Aspirin is recommended in addition to anticoagulation to reduce the risk of thromboembolism. All patients with prosthetic valves require antibiotic prophylaxis for the prevention of endocarditis (www.americanheart.org).

Congenital heart disease (CHD)

Normal fetal and neonatal circulation

In utero, pulmonary and systemic circulations exist in parallel, with mixing

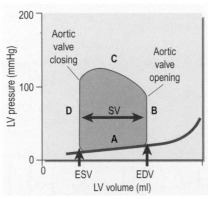

Fig. 1 **Pressure–volume loop.**

Table 2 **Anticoagulation guidelines**	
	INR
First 3 months all valves	2.5–3.5
Mechanical aortic	2.0–3.0
Mechanical mitral	2.5–3.5
Bioprosthetic + risk factors	2.0–3.0

INR, international normalised ratio.

Table 1 **Haemodynamic goals for valvular lesions**				
	Rhythm	**Rate**	**Afterload**	**Other**
AS	Sinus/AV pace	Avoid tachycardia	Maintain diastolic BP	Avoid wide pulse pressure Ensure adequate LVEDV
AR	Sinus not as important	Avoid bradycardia	Reduce/control afterload	Support contractility Avoid excessive LVEDV
MS	Sinus where possible ↑ Likelihood of AF	Heart rate 70–90	Maintain diastolic BP	↑ risk of pulmonary oedema Avoid ↑ in PVR
MR	Sinus where possible ↑ Likelihood of AF	Heart rate 80–100	Reduce/control afterload	Support contractility Avoid ↑ in PVR

AF, atrial fibrillation; AR, aortic regurgitation; AS, aortic stenosis; AV, atrioventricular; BP, blood pressure; LVEDV, left ventricular end-diastolic volume; MR, mitral regurgitation; MS, mitral stenosis; PVR, pulmonary vascular resistance.

occurring at the level of the patent foramen ovale (PFO) and patent ductus arteriosus (PDA). Increased vascular resistance in the pulmonary vascular bed shunts most of the blood flow away from the lungs into the systemic circulation. At birth, with the onset of spontaneous ventilation and increased oxygen tension, pulmonary vascular resistance decreases and pulmonary blood flow (PBF) increases. Loss of the low-resistance placental vascular bed increases systemic vascular resistance, decreasing flow through the PDA until it closes in response to the increased oxygen tension. Increased pulmonary venous return to the left atrium causes LAP to exceed right atrial pressure (RAP) with functional closure of the PFO (Fig. 2).

Classification

Congenital cardiac malformations are generally characterised by the direction of central cardiac shunting. *Complex shunts* are those with both shunting and obstructive lesions. The magnitude and direction of simple shunts are determined by the orifice size (restrictive versus non-restrictive) and relative differences in systemic and pulmonary vascular resistance.

Left-to-right shunts increase PBF and lead to right ventricular volume overload. If the shunt magnitude is great enough, excessive PBF may produce pulmonary oedema and lead to pulmonary vascular occlusive changes, pulmonary hypertension and reversal of shunt direction, a condition known as *Eisenmenger syndrome.*

Right-to-left shunts decrease PBF and lead to increased venous admixture, arterial desaturation and cyanosis. Erythrocytosis is the compensatory response to chronic hypoxaemia, and haematocrits may exceed 70%, increasing blood viscosity, reducing tissue perfusion and increasing cardiac workload.

Mixing lesions are characterised by mixing of the pulmonary and systemic circulations. The net effects on blood flow and arterial oxygen saturation are related to the relative differences in systemic and pulmonary vascular resistance. Factors that regulate vascular tone may be manipulated to affect the direction and magnitude of blood flow, although vascular changes may be relatively fixed in the adult.

Oxygen content data from blood samples obtained during cardiac catheterisation can be used to calculate pulmonary blood flow (Qp) and systemic blood flow (Qs) (Table 3).

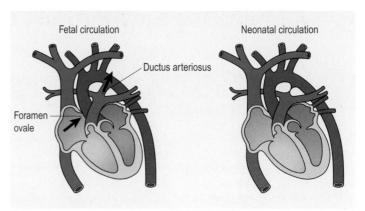

Fig. 2 **Fetal and neonatal circulation.**

Table 3 **Shunt classification**		
Shunt direction	**Qp/Qs ratio**	**Examples**
L to R	Qp/Qs > 1	ASD, VSD, PDA, AVSD (AV canal)
R to L	QP/Qs < 1	TOF, pulmonary atresia, Ebstein's anomaly
Complex		Truncus arteriosus, TGA, DORV, HLHS

ASD, atrial septal defect; AV, atrioventricular; AVSD, atrioventricular septal defect; DORV, double outlet right ventricle; HLHS, hypoplastic left heart syndrome; PDA, patent ductus arteriosus; TGA, transposition of the great arteries; TOF, tetralogy of Fallot; VSD, ventricular septal defect.

Cyanotic heart disease

Cyanotic congenital heart disease in adults is a multisystem disorder. Compensatory erythrocytosis leads to an increase in red cell mass with haematocrits reaching 70% or more. At these levels, symptoms related to hyperviscosity may occur (headache, visual disturbances, fatigue, myalgias, paraesthesias). Dehydration, when present, may contribute to symptomatic hyperviscosity and should be treated promptly with volume repletion. Phlebotomy, by depleting iron stores, may aggravate rather than alleviate symptoms because of the production of less deformable, microspherocytic red cells.

Haemostatic abnormalities related to cyanotic CHD include reduced platelet count, quantitative von Willebrand factor defects and increased tissue vascularity. Most bleeding is mild and mucocutaneous, although haemoptysis, menorrhagia and perioperative bleeding can occur. Paradoxically, these patients are predisposed to in situ thrombosis of the pulmonary vasculature and pulmonary infarction. Decisions regarding anticoagulation management in this population are extremely difficult.

Increased red cell turnover and haem breakdown lead to excessive levels of unconjugated bilirubin in the bile and a propensity for cholelithiasis. Biliary colic is relatively common, and an increased incidence of acute cholecystitis is a risk factor for Gram-negative bacteraemia and infective endocarditis. Renal function is generally preserved, although proteinuria and hyperuricaemia are common, and adults occasionally suffer from acute gouty arthritis. The presence of right-to-left shunting increases the risk of paradoxical emboli, and patients are at significant risk of cerebrovascular events. Extreme caution to avoid air bubbles and microparticle filters should be employed with intravenous access to avoid iatrogenic embolism.

Shunt equations

$$Qp \text{ (L/min)} = VO_2/CpvO_2 - CP_aO_2$$
$$Qs \text{ (L/min)} = VO_2/CaO_2 - CmvO_2$$
$$Qp/Qs = S_aO_2 - SmvO_2/SpvO_2 - Sp_aO_2$$

Summary points

- Physiological changes can be predicted based on whether lesions arise from volume or pressure overload.
- In patients with CHD, identify the source and nature of pulmonary blood flow.
- Always consider the need for subacute bacterial endocarditis prophylaxis.
- Cyanotic heart disease is a multisystemic disorder.

Respiratory system

Respiratory failure

Respiratory failure describes ineffective gas exchange across the lungs. It is frequently the primary reason for intensive care unit (ICU) admission. Respiratory failure represents a diverse group of disease processes, which manifest as abnormalities in the O_2 and CO_2 content of blood. Hypoxaemic (type 1) respiratory failure occurs when arterial P_aO_2 is <50–60 mmHg (6.5–8 kPa). Hypercarbic (type 2) respiratory failure is characterised by P_aCO_2 >49 mmHg (6.5 kPa).

Patients with respiratory failure may exhibit hypopnoea, tachypnoea, tachycardia, difficulty clearing secretions, ineffective breathing and increased work of breathing. Ineffective breathing or increased work of breathing may be accompanied by accessory respiratory muscle use, retractions or paradoxical abdominal motion. Respiratory failure results in tissue hypoxia and acid–base disturbances. Further disturbances may ensue, including circulatory arrest.

Control of ventilation

Ventilation normally varies in response to CO_2 production to maintain P_aCO_2 within a narrow range of 40 ± 4 mmHg (5.3 ± 0.53 kPa). The chief control of ventilation is via chemoreceptors in the medulla, which respond to changes in pH. Receptors in the central nervous system (CNS), vasculature, lungs and airways also contribute to the control of ventilation by responding to chemical and mechanical triggers. Responses are mediated by the nervous system (spinal cord, phrenic nerves and intercostal nerves) and respiratory musculature. The contraction of the respiratory muscles overcomes lung elastance, chest wall elastance and airway resistance, resulting in air movement.

Ventilation and perfusion relationships

Adequate exchange of O_2 and, to a lesser extent, CO_2 depends on maintaining both ventilation (V) and perfusion (Q) to lung units. When ventilation and perfusion are disparate, *V/Q mismatch* exists and gas exchange is compromised. Portions of the lung with a low V/Q ratio (relative shunt) will contribute blood to the left atrium with a high P_aCO_2 and low Po_2 (closer to systemic venous content). Some compensation is achieved by areas of the lung with high V/Q ratios (relative dead space), where the P_aO_2 of exiting blood is even higher than areas with a normal V/Q. However, the ability of high V/Q areas to compensate for low V/Q areas is limited because of the flat portion of the top of the haemoglobin–oxygen dissociation curve. CO_2 exchange does not have this limitation and, therefore, V/Q mismatch causes hypoxaemia much more readily than hypercapnia.

A *shunt* is present when blood flow from the right ventricle does not participate in gas exchange before returning to the heart. This is normally less than 10% of blood flow.

Dead space is that volume of the airways and lungs that receives ventilation but does not participate in gas exchange. *Anatomical dead space* represents portions of the respiratory tree that do not *normally* participate in gas exchange, such as the nasopharynx, trachea, bronchi and bronchioles. This is increased in intubated patients, when the conducting airways are artificially extended. *Physiological dead space* is larger, representing the sum of anatomical dead space and diseased lung areas not participating in gas exchange. Physiological dead space is usually 20–30% of tidal volume. Low cardiac output and pulmonary embolus are causes of increased dead space; blood flow does not get to ventilated lung regions (Fig. 1).

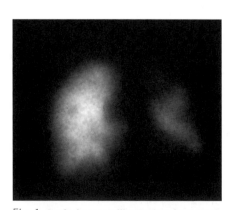

Fig. 1 **Perfusion scan illustrating decreased blood flow to lung regions on the left with high probability of pulmonary embolus.** The white areas (right lung) reflect good perfusion. The dark areas (left lung) reveal poor perfusion.

As dead space increases, CO_2 elimination is compromised. Increases in CO_2 content are usually mitigated by increases in minute ventilation in the spontaneously breathing patient. With marked increases in dead space, the respiratory system may not be able to increase ventilation enough to prevent hypercapnia.

Examples of respiratory failure in the ICU

The causes of hypoxaemia and hypercapnia can be categorised as low inspired O_2, hypoventilation, V/Q mismatch and increased O_2 utilisation, all of which have multiple pathological causes (Table 1). Increased shunt can be caused by cardiovascular abnormalities or pulmonary parenchymal disturbances, where ventilation has been compromised because alveoli are diseased, collapsed or filled with a non-air substance.

Hypoventilation is a decrease in alveolar ventilation, resulting in an increased P_ACO_2. This results in a lower P_AO_2 and therefore a lower P_aO_2. Hypoxaemia related to isolated hypoventilation improves readily with increased F_IO_2. Hypoventilation may result when there is a maladaptive decrease in the impetus to breathe, incompetence of the neuromuscular ventilatory apparatus or an increased load on the respiratory system.

Respiratory failure may be precipitated when the load on the respiratory system is increased by increases in airway resistance, decreases in compliance or V/Q mismatch. Therefore, many aetiologies of respiratory failure culminate with hypoventilation when a fatigued patient is unable to cope with the increased demands on the respiratory system.

The acute respiratory distress syndrome (ARDS) is a cause of respiratory failure characterised by bilateral pulmonary infiltrates, decreased lung compliance and a P_aO_2– F_IO_2 ratio <200 mmHg (26.7 kPa) in the absence of atrial hypertension. Aetiologies of ARDS are diverse and include sepsis, pneumonia, aspiration, trauma and many others. Transfusion-related acute lung injury (TRALI) is an

Table 1 Causes of respiratory failure with examples

Central failure	Ineffective breathing	Decreased compliance	Increased resistance to breathing	Increased dead space	Increased shunt	Increased oxygen consumption
Respiratory depressants (e.g. opiates)	ICU neuropathy/ myopathy	ARDS	Asthma	COPD	Pneumonia	Sepsis
Stroke	Flail chest	Restrictive lung diseases	COPD	Asthma	ARDS	Hyperthermia/fever
Central sleep apnoea	Drug-induced myopathy	Pneumothorax	Secretions	Pulmonary embolus	Pulmonary oedema	Burns
Ondine's curse	Spinal cord injury	Increased intra-abdominal pressure	Laryngospasm	Low cardiac output	Pneumothorax	Hyperthyroidism
Hypothyroidism	Guillain–Barré syndrome	Obesity	Tracheal stenosis	Excessive PEEP	Congenital cardiac disease	Neuroleptic malignant syndrome
Brainstem infarct	Motor neurone disease	Kyphoscoliosis	Epiglottitis		Pulmonary embolus	Malignant hyperthermia
	Myasthenia gravis	Pleural effusions	Airway tumour		COPD	Status epilepticus
		Sleep apnoea	Sleep apnoea		Asthma	

example of ARDS, which usually occurs within 4 h of a blood component transfusion and is characterised by hypoxaemia and dyspnoea secondary to non-cardiogenic pulmonary oedema.

Therapies

Along with treatment of the underlying aetiology, management of respiratory failure may include supplementary O_2, bronchodilator therapy and assisted ventilation. Invasive positive pressure ventilation is provided via a tracheal or tracheostomy tube.

Non-invasive positive pressure ventilation (NIPPV) is an alternative to conventional invasive ventilation and has been utilised in the therapy of multiple types of acute respiratory failure. NIPPV is provided by a nose or face mask and can encompass multiple modes of ventilation. Advantages of NIPPV include patient comfort, natural airway defences are maintained, patients retain the ability to eat and speak, and complications of intubation may be avoided (e.g. ventilator-associated pneumonia). Disadvantages include retention and inspissation of lung secretions, facial ulcers and gastric distension. NIPPV requires the participation of a cooperative patient.

When NIPPV is effective, patients usually experience benefit within the first 2 h of therapy. The respiratory rate and accessory muscle use decreases, and gas exchange improves. There is evidence in favour of NIPPV or *continuous positive airway pressure* (CPAP) in chronic obstructive pulmonary disease (COPD), for cardiogenic pulmonary oedema, following major thoracic and abdominal surgery or in patients with *Pneumocystis jiroveci* pneumonia (PCP).

It is important to diagnose failure of NIPPV and CPAP early and to institute invasive ventilation prior to

complications such as cardiorespiratory arrest or aspiration of gastric contents. If weaning from mechanical ventilation is unlikely in view of established respiratory failure, patients may decide that invasive ventilation should not be initiated or that it should be discontinued.

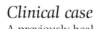

Clinical case

A previously healthy 45-year-old male is receiving postoperative analgesia with a morphine patient-controlled anaesthetic (PCA) following open reduction and internal fixation of an isolated femur fracture. The patient is transferred to the ICU after becoming very drowsy. An arterial blood gas reveals pH of 7.23, P_aO_2 of 90 mmHg and P_aCO_2 of 65 mmHg with the patient receiving 60% supplemental O_2. Is the patient's respiratory failure explained by opioid-induced respiratory depression? What investigations are indicated?

Summary points

■ The respiratory system includes the brainstem, the phrenic nerve, the respiratory muscles, the pulmonary vasculature, the heart, the lungs and the conducting airways.
■ Compromise of any of these may result in respiratory failure.
■ ICU patients frequently have several coexisting causes of respiratory failure.
■ Non-invasive ventilation, if initiated early, may improve respiratory function and stave off invasive mechanical ventilation.
■ Copious secretions and uncooperative patients do not augur well for non-invasive ventilation.

Asthma

Airway inflammation and hyper-responsiveness are the hallmarks of asthma; multiple cytokines and inflammatory mediators have been implicated in its pathogenesis. Hypertrophied smooth muscle and mucous glands, bronchial oedema and mucus plugging all contribute to airway narrowing and air trapping in asthma. Hypoxaemia is common in severe asthma, but can usually be treated with supplementary oxygen. A more alarming feature of asthma is progressive dynamic lung hyperinflation. High airway resistance hampers expiratory flow, leading to incomplete alveolar emptying and increasing alveolar pressure, a condition known as intrinsic positive end-expiratory pressure (PEEP). Hyperinflated lungs have poor compliance; they are difficult to inflate further (Fig. 1). This results in increased work of breathing and exhaustion. Severe hyperinflation may lead to haemodynamic collapse and obstructive shock (Fig. 2). The mechanism for this is similar to that in tension pneumothorax where increased intrathoracic pressure limits blood return to the heart.

Signs and symptoms of a severe asthma attack

The predominant symptom of asthma is dyspnoea. Severe attacks are refractory to patients' home bronchodilators. Signs include tachypnoea, tachycardia, diaphoresis, wheezing throughout the respiratory cycle and accessory muscle use. Pulsus paradoxus >20–25 often occurs with marked intrinsic PEEP. Severity of wheezing is not a reliable marker of airway obstruction as disappearance of wheezing could indicate total obstruction of the airway and impending respiratory collapse. Other signs of life-threatening respiratory failure include cyanosis, confusion, hypotension and bradycardia. Pneumothorax and pneumomediastinum are complications of severe asthma attack, and unilateral decreased breath sounds or crepitus may be present. Serial measurement of peak expiratory flow may reveal progressive worsening.

Laboratory findings

Initially, arterial blood gases show respiratory alkalosis and mild hypoxaemia. CO_2 retention begins to occur once the forced expiratory volume in 1 s (FEV_1) has fallen to approximately 25% of normal. An unexpectedly calm patient having a severe attack is suggestive of CO_2 narcosis. Lactic acidosis may also be present. Steroids cause eosinophilic leucocytosis. Steroids and bronchodilators can produce a mild hypokalaemia.

Imaging

Chest radiographs are indicated in acute asthma attacks to rule out co-morbidity such as pneumothorax, pneumo-pericardium, pneumomediastinum or other lung pathology.

Management of a severe asthma attack

All patients should receive high concentrations of supplementary oxygen. Inhaled beta-agonists should be administered immediately. A common starting regimen is four puffs of albuterol via a metered dose inhaler or 2.5 mg of nebulised albuterol (0.5 mL of a 0.5% solution in 2.5 mL of normal saline) every 20 min for 1 h, then hourly depending on

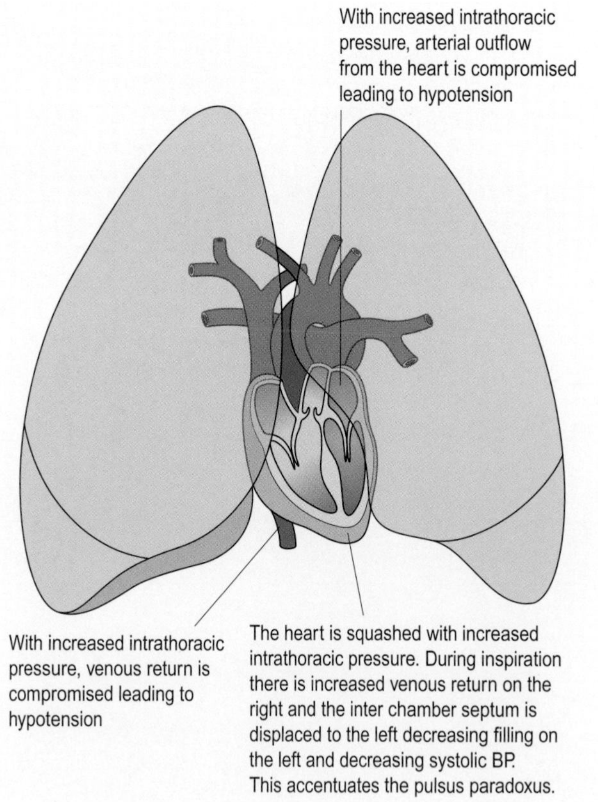

With increased intrathoracic pressure, arterial outflow from the heart is compromised leading to hypotension

With increased intrathoracic pressure, venous return is compromised leading to hypotension

The heart is squashed with increased intrathoracic pressure. During inspiration there is increased venous return on the right and the inter chamber septum is displaced to the left decreasing filling on the left and decreasing systolic BP. This accentuates the pulsus paradoxus.

Fig. 1 **The haemodynamic problems associated with intrinsic PEEP and hyperinflation.**

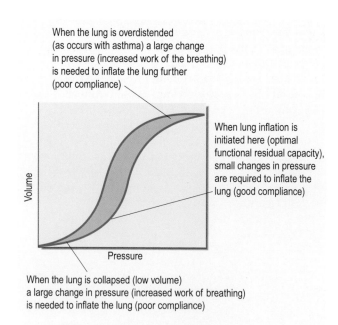

When the lung is overdistended (as occurs with asthma) a large change in pressure (increased work of the breathing) is needed to inflate the lung further (poor compliance)

When lung inflation is initiated here (optimal functional residual capacity), small changes in pressure are required to inflate the lung (good compliance)

Volume

Pressure

When the lung is collapsed (low volume) a large change in pressure (increased work of breathing) is needed to inflate the lung (poor compliance)

Fig. 2 **Diagram illustrating poor lung compliance in severe asthma.**

clinical response. With refractory asthma, the dosage and frequency may be increased, and should be limited only by side-effects such as tachyarrhythmias. Subcutaneous adrenaline (epinephrine) or terbutaline may be given if the patient is breathing so poorly that an inhaled drug is ineffective.

Systemic steroids are effective only after 6–12 h and should be given early. A common starting regimen is oral prednisone 60–80 mg every 6–8 h. Intravenous methylprednisolone 40 mg every 6 h can also be used, but has not been shown to be superior to oral prednisone. Once improvement has occurred, the prednisone dosing can be decreased to 60–80 mg/day. Steroids should be continued until the patient's pulmonary function has returned to baseline, which may be as long as 10–14 days.

Tracheal intubation

The decision to intubate is a complicated one, based on clinical judgement of impending respiratory failure in spite of optimal medical management. Assisted ventilation may be life saving, but a tracheal tube is a major irritant that may worsen bronchospasm and make asthma even more resistant to treatment. In general, worsening dyspnoea, decreased ability to speak, respiratory acidosis and somnolence are indications that assisted ventilation may be needed. Non-invasive ventilatory support has shown some promise as a temporising measure in status asthmaticus, but the benefit of this approach is unproven and controversial.

Sedation prior to intubation is often accomplished with a short-acting benzodiazepine, such as midazolam, combined with succinylcholine. Ketamine is sometimes used for patients with status asthmaticus as it causes bronchodilation. Paralysis using non-depolarising muscle relaxants allows ventilation with lower mean airway pressures in patients who would otherwise require extremely high inflation pressures to ventilate adequately. Vecuronium and other steroid muscle relaxants may be preferable to atracurium, which causes histamine release and may worsen bronchospasm. Caution is warranted as all non-depolarising muscle relaxants have increased potential to cause an ICU myopathy when combined with systemic steroids, making it more difficult to wean mechanical ventilation. Muscle relaxant use should be limited and, if deemed necessary, a nerve stimulator should be used to ensure that the doses administered are kept to a minimum. Sedation and paralysis may worsen the hypotension and haemodynamic instability that occurs with intrinsic PEEP. Prophylactic fluid administration and drawing up an intravenous vasoconstrictor, such as phenylephrine, are prudent measures prior to giving sedative medications. Oxygen desaturation may occur rapidly, and intubation should be undertaken only by an experienced practitioner.

Mechanical ventilation

The principles of mechanical ventilation can be summarised as follows: avoid high inflation pressure, allow time for expiration, avoid PEEP, tolerate hypercapnia (up to P_aCO_2 of 90 mmHg) and try to synchronise mechanical ventilation with breathing. Ventilation for the first 24 h should be controlled to allow for recovery from exhaustion. Thereafter, it is reasonable to wean to assisted modes. Plateau pressure is the best predictor of hyperinflation (intrinsic PEEP) and should be kept below 35 cmH$_2$O. This can be achieved by limiting tidal volumes (6 mL/kg), increasing inspiratory flow rate (80–100 L/min) and increasing expiratory time (inspiratory–expiratory ratio <1:3).

> ### Clinical case
>
> A 43-year-old female is admitted for an asthma attack. She is given oxygen, beta-agonists and oral steroids. She has a peak expiratory flow rate (PEFR) of 60% of her predicted value and signs in keeping with acute asthma. Thirty minutes later, the lung examination reveals decreased wheezing and a slow heart rate. She is calm and moderately drowsy. A repeat PEFR is 15% of her predicted value. What should be the next step in her treatment?

> ### Summary points
>
> - Give oxygen, beta-agonists and steroids early.
> - Dynamic hyperinflation and intrinsic PEEP cause severe haemodynamic compromise.
> - A calm patient who has stopped wheezing may be on the brink of cardiorespiratory arrest.
> - Mechanical ventilation should be with low tidal volumes, no PEEP, high inspiratory flow rate and long expiratory time.

Chronic obstructive pulmonary disease

Intensive care units (ICUs) should not be dumping grounds for people with endstage chronic obstructive pulmonary disease (COPD) who have little prospect of recovery. To many people, death is preferable to lifelong dependence on a mechanical ventilator. ICU admission is warranted when there are reversible complications, which should be identified and treated expeditiously.

Epidemiology

COPD is traditionally separated into emphysema and chronic bronchitis, although many patients exhibit traits of both. The overwhelming risk factor for COPD is tobacco smoking, with a relative risk between 9:1 and 25:1. Approximately 5% of cases occur with alpha-1 antitrypsin deficiency, which is present in 1:3000 and is responsible for a disproportionate share of emphysema in young patients.

Pathophysiology

Emphysema is characterised by enlargement of the air spaces and destruction of capillary beds owing to loss of alveolar walls. This is thought to occur through the actions of lysosomal elastase released by neutrophils. Cigarette smoke is a chemoattractant for neutrophils and represses physiological elastase inhibitors. Patients with alpha-1 antitrypsin deficiency lack this inhibitor altogether. The distribution of alveolar destruction varies depending on the cause: centri-acinar in smokers and panacinar in patients with alpha-1 antitrypsin deficiency.

Chronic bronchitis is defined as a chronic, productive cough for 3 months in two consecutive years. Histologically, it is associated with bronchial mucous gland hypertrophy (measured by the Reid index), bronchial smooth muscle hyperplasia and small airway inflammation with neutrophilic infiltrates (Fig. 1).

Patients with obstructive lung disease have decreased forced expiratory volume in 1s (FEV_1), forced vital capacity (FVC) and FEV_1/FVC ratio and increased residual volume (RV) and total lung capacity (TLC) (Figs 2 and 3).

Emphysema is associated with moderate hypoxaemia, usually with normal P_{CO_2}. Destruction of alveoli increases physiologic dead space, but hypoxic vasoconstriction limits V/Q mismatch. In patients with chronic bronchitis, hypoxaemia is often severe with elevated P_{CO_2}. Pulmonary artery pressures are elevated in both conditions, but cor pulmonale is more common with chronic bronchitis with more severe hypoxaemia.

Traditionally, the stereotyped 'pink puffer' and 'blue bloater' have helped to define the opposite ends of the clinical spectrum manifested by COPD patients. Emphysematous pink puffers are barrel-chested individuals who breathe with pursed lips using accessory muscles. They are not cyanotic, do not have a prominent cough, and their symptoms do not tend to vary from day to day. Blue bloaters are patients with chronic bronchitis who are overweight, oedematous and cyanotic, with mottled skin and a prominent intermittent interminable cough. It is unclear

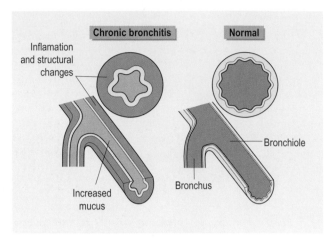

Fig. 1 **Airway changes in chronic bronchitis.**

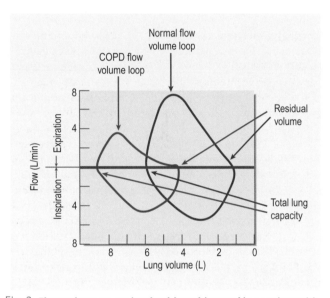

Fig. 2 **Flow volume traces in a healthy subject and in a patient with COPD.**

why some patients go down the path to pink puffer or blue bloater. There may be a genetic predisposition to one or the other based on tolerance of elevated CO_2 levels in order to decrease the work of breathing.

Chest radiograph

Chest radiograph typically shows hyperinflation, hyperlucency and hilar prominence if pulmonary hypertension is present.

Management

Management of the chronically ill COPD patient should focus on reversible complications and coexisting diseases. These include infection, cor pulmonale, atrial fibrillation, pulmonary embolism, bronchospasm, polycythaemia and hypoxaemia.

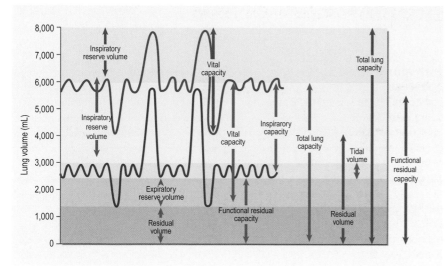

Fig. 3 **Pulmonary function tests: healthy patient (red) and a patient with COPD (blue).** IRV, inspiratory reserve volume; ERV, expiratory reserve volume; RV, residual volume; VC, vital capacity; FRC, functional residual capacity; TLC, total lung capacity; TV, tidal volume.

It is important to allow sufficient time for exhalation by limiting the inspiratory to expiratory ratio. Tidal volumes and minute ventilation should be limited to avoid pneumothorax, decreased cardiac output or mediastinal or subcutaneous emphysema. Moderate hypercapnia is well tolerated. The use of positive end-expiratory pressure (PEEP) is controversial. Traditionally, PEEP was kept to a bare minimum to avoid further hyperinflation. In emphysematous patients, it is becoming increasingly common to provide a small amount of external PEEP to stent open the small airways that would otherwise close with the loss of radial traction in the emphysematous lung. Sedation should be minimised and, following initial progress, a weaning protocol should be instituted. A tracheostomy may be considered if there are copious secretions and the patient has a poor cough.

Medical management

1 During exacerbations, scheduled nebulised treatment as often as hourly with ipratropium and a beta2-agonist such as albuterol is indicated.

2 Short courses of systemic steroids are effective treatments for COPD exacerbations. Intravenous methylprednisolone 1–2 mg/kg every 6–12 h is typical. After 2–3 days, this may be converted to oral prednisone 60 mg for 2 weeks, and then tapered over 2 weeks.

3 For severe exacerbations, intravenous antibiotics are indicated. The most common bacteria are those that cause community-acquired pneumonia, such as *Streptococcus pneumoniae* and *Haemophilus influenzae*. Other organisms may be present such as *Pseudomonas aeruginosa* and *Klebsiella pneumoniae*. Empiric treatment is typically a third-generation cephalosporin or antipseudomonal penicillin, plus a fluoroquinolone or aminoglycosides for synergy.

4 Methylxanthines such as aminophylline and theophylline are controversial, and should be used only when other treatment modalities are contraindicated or ineffective.

5 Hydration may help with the mobilisation of secretions. On the other hand, diuretics may improve oxygenation and right heart failure. With atrial fibrillation, restoration of sinus rhythm may improve symptoms. Venesection may be indicated for severe polycythaemia.

Non-invasive ventilation or continuous positive airway pressure (CPAP) may be alternatives to intubation and mechanical ventilation. Contraindications to non-invasive ventilation are impaired consciousness, an uncooperative patient, vomiting risk, significant arrhythmia or hypotension, and excessive secretions. When patients are responding to therapy, heart rate and respiratory rate should decrease, and respiratory acidosis should resolve.

The decision to intubate should not be taken lightly. End-of-life issues and the possibility of failure to wean off the ventilator should be discussed. In general, reasons to intubate include signs of cardiovascular collapse, hypotension, altered mental status, overt pneumonia, upper airway obstruction, copious sputum and poor cough reflex.

Ventilation

Patients with COPD develop dynamic hyperinflation secondary to airway obstruction. This hyperinflation reduces venous return, which can lead to haemodynamic instability. The main ventilatory strategy is to treat hypoxaemia and severe respiratory acidosis while avoiding excessive pressures in already hyperinflated lungs.

Clinical case

A 64-year-old female has been intubated for 5 days in the ICU following her COPD exacerbation. Efforts to wean her off the ventilator have repeatedly failed. Prior to this exacerbation, the patient was functioning fairly well at home. She was properly treated on admission to the ICU with beta2-agonists, steroids and antibiotics, and was initially paralysed with a vecuronium infusion for the first 12 h of intubation to minimise dyssynchrony with the ventilator. What may be the reason for failure to wean? How would you assess this, and what should be done?

Summary points

- COPD treatment in the ICU should focus on reversible problems: hypoxia, infection, bronchospasm, cor pulmonale.
- Consider other causes of respiratory failure, such as pulmonary embolism.
- Oxygen, beta-agonists, anticholinergics, antibiotics and steroids are the cornerstones of treatment.
- Ventilator strategy: treat hypoxaemia and severe acidosis. Limit inflation pressures and allow time for exhalation.

The ICU chest radiograph

The portable chest radiograph (pCXR) is the most common radiology study performed in the intensive care unit (ICU). It is useful in a broad spectrum of diagnostic and therapeutic situations. It is a fast, inexpensive and high-yield test. The pCXR often yields useful information when patients have cardiorespiratory pathology or when there are devices that are seen on the radiograph. These include tracheal tubes, tracheostomy tubes, feeding tubes, chest drains, pacemaker wires, central venous catheters and pulmonary artery catheters.

Most patients have a pCXR when they are admitted to the ICU. This is useful in several respects. It allows the ICU team to confirm that all the tubes and catheters are appropriately positioned. It provides a baseline study, which may be useful for retrospective comparison as a patient's condition changes with time. The pCXR may also be helpful in providing information about cardiac and respiratory diseases as well as a patient's state of hydration. The clinician should also examine every CXR for pleural effusions, pneumothoraces and mediastinal pathology.

A pCXR is indicated when there is a deterioration in a patient's cardiac or pulmonary function. Examples include pneumonia, acute respiratory distress syndrome (ARDS), congestive cardiac failure, fluid overload, bronchospasm, pulmonary embolism, pneumothorax, pleural effusion, atelectasis and aspiration. It is generally, but not universally, agreed that a pCXR is indicated following a procedure, such as intubation, tracheostomy, central line placement or passage of a feeding tube. While the pCXR undoubtedly yields valuable information, routine radiographs are wasteful and expose patients to unnecessary radiation.

Technique of the portable chest radiograph

The pCXR is useful in that it can be performed in the ICU. However, the pCXR also has shortfalls. The shorter focus–film distance results in misleading magnification of structures, especially the heart. A high kilovoltage technique cannot be used because portable machines are unable to deliver a sufficiently high kilovoltage and the maximum current is limited so that long exposure times are needed, increasing movement artefact. Both these limitations lead to decreased image quality. Portable lateral radiographs are even less likely to be successful because of extremely long exposure times. Positioning of patients for portable radiography is difficult, and the resulting radiographs are often of poor quality. Thus, the ICU physician should use the pCXR for broad diagnostic and confirmatory purposes, such as line positioning and effusions, and not for making subtle diagnoses that require a higher quality image found on a standard chest radiograph or computerised tomography scan.

Intrepretation of the portable chest radiograph

An ICU clinician often has to interpret a pCXR in emergency circumstances, frequently without a radiologist's expertise. Accurate interpretation necessitates a thorough and systematic approach that can be applied to all studies. A typical pCXR from an ICU patient is shown in Fig. 1 and will be used as an example interpretation. The first step is to identify the type of study, patient information, date and time of the pCXR and quality of the film. A good-quality pCXR should not be rotated, should include all the anatomical structures of interest and should allow some visualisation of the vertebral bodies behind the cardiac silhouette. The next step is to identify foreign material, such as tubes, catheters, valves and wires, and determine if they are different from a prior study. Fig. 1 demonstrates typical lines and tubes that may be present in ICU patients.

A systematic approach to identifying all lines, tubes and hardware is to focus on the area of the carina: the majority of central venous lines, tracheal tubes, nasogastric or small bowel feeding tubes and mediastinal thoracostomy tubes end close to this anatomical landmark or pass beyond it. The proper positioning of these items is listed in Table 1.

Based on the information in Table 1, the astute observer will note that, in Fig. 1, the pulmonary artery catheter (B) is advanced approximately 3 cm too distal in the right inferior pulmonary artery, and the tracheal tube (F) is perilously close to the right mainstem bronchus and should be pulled back. Thoracostomy tubes or intercostal drains are typically located laterally or superiorly.

The cardiac silhouette and lung fields should be inspected for abnormalities, including pneumothorax, possible

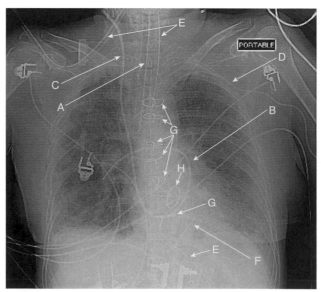

Fig. 1 **Typical pCXR in an ICU patient.** A, endotracheal tube; B, pulmonary artery catheter; C, right internal jugular central venous catheter; D, left subcutaneous central venous catheter; E, nasogastric tube; F, mediastinal thoracostomy tube; G, sternal wires; H, mitral valve ring.

Table 1	**Proper positioning of tubes and catheters**
Central venous catheter	Tip just above the right atrium (to the right of the carina)
Pulmonary artery catheter	Tip in main pulmonary artery (at the hilum)
Endotracheal tube	Tip 3–4 cm above the carina
Thoracostomy tube	Along the pleural space without kinks
Nasogastric/small bowel tubes	Directed behind the heart with a slight distal bend to the left tracking below the diaphragm

Table 2	**Abnormalities in cardiac silhouette and lung fields**
Pneumothorax	Radiolucent lung field with collapsed lung. Mediastinum shifts away in tension pneumothorax
Pulmonary infiltrate	Radio-opaque segment of lung. Air bronchograms may be present
Atelectasis	Radio-opaque dependent portions of lung with loss of volume
Effusion/hydro-/ haemothorax	Blunting of costophrenic angles Radio-opaque lung field
Pulmonary oedema	Perihilar fullness, upper lobe blood diversion or cephalisation of pulmonary vasculature

infiltrates, atelectasis, effusion or suggestion of pulmonary oedema. Descriptions of these findings are given in Table 2.

In Fig. 1, the astute observer may note a probable small right apical pneumothorax (a sliver of increased lucency and loss of lung markings at the apex) and probable bilateral basal atelectasis or small effusions (increased basal opacification with blunting of costophrenic angles).

Clinical case

A 61-year-old man is in the ICU recovering after thoraco-abdominal aneurysm repair with prolonged respiratory failure and is unable to eat. Placement of a small bowel feeding tube is attempted. The tube is secured at 54 cm from the tip. The patient tolerates the procedure well. Secretions cannot be withdrawn from the tube. An abdominal radiograph is obtained, but the tube is not visualised. A pCXR is obtained (Fig. 3). What is the correct next step in the management of this patient?

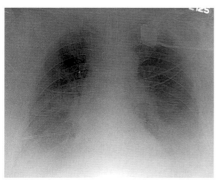

Fig. 3 **Clinical case pCXR.**

An unsuspected finding on a pCXR may occasionally be attributable to an iatrogenic misadventure. For example, see Fig. 2.

The final step in inspecting the pCXR is to evaluate the bony structures for any abnormalities. In the ICU setting, this includes evaluation of the ribs, clavicles and any part of the shoulder joint visualised for any abnormalities. The use of the pCXR to evaluate bony structures is limited. Should an abnormality be suspected, dedicated films of the area should be obtained.

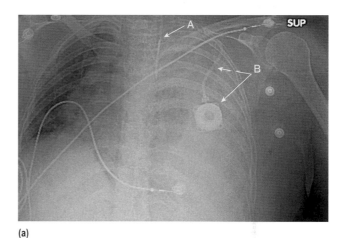
(a)
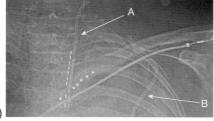
(b)

Fig. 2 **(a) A large left (probable) effusion is seen after placement of a new left internal jugular central venous catheter (A) in a patient with an existing left subclavian subcutaneous reservoir port (B). Upon close inspection (b), it can be appreciated that the new internal jugular line takes a straight course perpendicular (dashed arrow) to the subclavian port (asterisks), representing probable perforation of the left subclavian vein with the tip of the new line infusing intravenous fluids into the pleural space, resulting in the large effusion.**

Summary points

- The pCXR is a high-yield and convenient examination for ICU patients.
- The pCXR may provide valuable information when there is a change in pulmonary or cardiac function.
- A pCXR may be useful in confirming the correct position of a catheter or breathing tube and may reveal complications associated with the procedure.
- Examination of the pCXR should be systematic to prevent missed findings.

Gastrointestinal/ renal system

Renal failure

Twenty per cent of the cardiac output is delivered to the kidneys, emphasising the crucial role played by these organs. The kidneys are essential for the elimination of toxins and wastes, the regulation of electrolytes and pH, and for fluid homeostasis. They also have an important role in the production of the hormone erythropoietin. Acute renal failure (ARF) in the intensive care unit (ICU) is associated with a mortality of 50–80%. Up to 15% of ICU patients are at risk for ARF. It is important to prevent ARF where possible, to address the causes of ARF, to treat the complications of ARF (Fig. 1) and to institute renal replacement therapy when indicated. The only intervention proven to protect the kidneys against insults is the administration of fluid.

Definitions and complications

ARF is the rapid loss of kidney function over hours to days (Box 1). This is in contrast to chronic renal failure which occurs over months to years. ARF may occur with normal, increased or diminished urine output. Anuria is urine output <100 mL/24 h, oliguria is between 100 and 400 mL/24 h, and non-oliguria is ≥400 mL/24 h. Prognosis tends to be better for non-oliguric renal failure. Normal urine output is considered to be 0.5–1 mL/kg/h. Complications associated with ARF are shown in Fig. 1.

Causes

Prerenal renal failure is the mechanism of injury in 35% of cases of ARF. With timely identification, rapid restoration of renal blood flow may prevent acute tubular damage. Causes of prerenal ARF include *intravascular* hypovolaemia, septic shock, drugs [e.g. non-steroidal anti-inflammatory drugs (NSAIDs) and angiotensin-converting enzyme (ACE) inhibitors], heart failure and liver failure or the hepatorenal syndrome. Patients who have underlying renal disease with borderline blood flow are especially vulnerable to prerenal insults. People

Box 1. Acute renal failure

Acute renal failure may be defined as:

- Increase in serum creatinine level by ≥44 μmol/L over baseline
- Increase in serum creatinine level over 50% of baseline
- Reduction in creatinine clearance >50%.

with chronic hypertension may require higher than 'normal' blood pressure to maintain adequate renal perfusion.

Intrinsic renal failure is associated with a direct injury to the kidneys. Acute tubular necrosis (ATN) carries 70–80% mortality in the ICU. Fifty per cent of cases of ARF are secondary to ischaemic ATN. This can occur in association with a progressive prerenal process, surgery (especially cardiac, aortic and hepatobiliary) and increased intra-abdominal pressure. Measurement of bladder pressure is an indirect way of measuring abdominal pressure and is useful when an abdominal compartment syndrome is suspected. ATN occurs with toxic insults such as aminoglycosides, radiocontrast dye, cisplatin, amphotericin B, ciclosporin, haemoglobin and myoglobin pigment and crystals (e.g. uric acid).

Acute interstitial nephritis (AIN) is an intrinsic process most commonly due to an allergic reaction to a drug (e.g. beta-lactam antibiotics, sulpha drugs, NSAIDs, furosemide). Other possible aetiologies include autoimmune diseases (e.g. systemic lupus erythematosus), infections (e.g. Legionnaire's disease) and infiltrative diseases (e.g. sarcoid, lymphoma). AIN is often reversible with resolution of the underlying aetiology.

Vascular renal failure occurs with bilateral renal artery stenosis, renal artery thrombosis, hypertensive crises, haemolytic uraemic syndrome, thrombotic thrombocytopenic purpura and disseminated intravascular coagulation.

Glomerulonephritis is inflammation of the glomerulus for which serological and immunopathological assays are needed to identify the cause and to guide appropriate therapy.

Post-renal renal failure is associated with obstruction of urine flow, which occurs in approximately 10% of ARF cases. Common aetiologies include benign prostatic hypertrophy, prostate or cervical cancer, retroperitoneal disorders (e.g. retroperitoneal fibrosis), malignancy, lymphadenopathy and intratubular crystals (e.g. sulphonamide, uric acid).

Prerenal ARF and ATN may be difficult to distinguish. Blood urea and creatinine concentrations do not always accurately reflect renal function. For example, urea is increased with gastrointestinal bleeding and creatinine is increased following seizures. Urine sodium provides additional useful information. It is elevated in ATN because the injured tubules are unable to reabsorb sodium. FENA (the fractional excretion of sodium) is a useful equation (Fig. 2), except if the patient is receiving diuretics. The fractional excretion of urea (FEurea) may be more accurate. Replace urea for sodium in the FENA equation and use the cutoffs of <35 and >50 instead of the 1%. If

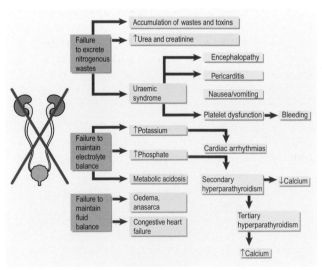

Fig. 1 **Complications associated with ARF.**

History: renal disease, hypertension, diabetes, nephrotoxic drugs or contrast dye, recent surgery
Examination: end organ damage (diabetes, hypertension), dehydration, heart failure, renal artery bruits, peripheral pulses
Urine: urinalysis, FENA*, sediment, electrolytes, osmolality, output, passage of urine catheter (may be difficult with post-renal ARF)

Type of ARF	Sediment	Proteinuria	Osmolality (mOsm/kg)	FENA*	Specific gravity	Urine Na	Urea to Cr ratio
Pre-renal	Bland, possibly hyaline caste	Trace/none	> 500	< 1%	> 1.025	< 20 mEq/L	> 70
Acute tubular necrosis	'Muddy brown' pigmented casts**	Mild/moderate	< 350	> 1%	< 1.015	> 20 mEq/L	< 70
Acute interstitial nephritis	WBCs and WBC casts, eosinophils, RBCs	Mild/moderate	< 350	> 1%	< 1.015	> 20 mEq/L	
Vascular	Bland, RBCs (if necrosis)						
Glomerulonephritis	Dysmorphic RBCs and RBC casts	Moderate/severe	> 500	< 1%	> 1.025	< 20 mEq/L	
Post-renal	WBCs, crystals, possibly RBCs	Trace/none	< 350	> 1%	< 1.015	> 20 mEq/L	

*Fractional excretion of sodium (FENA)= $\dfrac{\text{Urine Na/plasma Na}}{\text{Urine Cr/plasma Cr}}$

**Contrast and pigment nephrotoxins may result in urine osmolality of > 500 mOsm/kg, FENA < 1%, specific gravity of > 1.025, urine Na < 20 mEq/L.

Fig. 2 **Algorithm to determine the aetiology of ARF.** WBC, white blood cell; RBC, red blood cell; Cr, creatinine; Na, sodium.

FENA or FEurea is high, the concentrating ability of the kidneys is preserved. Renal stones are frequently seen on plain radiograph. A renal ultrasound may provide information on renal blood flow and may be useful for the diagnosis of hydronephrosis when there is obstruction to urine flow. When the kidneys are shrunken, this may suggest a chronic element to the renal dysfunction. Computerised tomography scans and angiography may provide further information. Renal biopsy is crucial for determining the cause of glomerulonephritis. Other specialised studies include serum calcium and uric acid for malignancy, creatinine kinase for rhabdomyolysis, serum protein electrophoresis and urine protein electrophoresis for multiple myeloma, and eosinophilia for allergic interstitial nephritis.

Prevention/treatment

When there is a reversible cause, this should be identified and treated expeditiously. Restore renal perfusion, typically with volume, when prerenal ARF is suspected. Treat the associated pathology when AIN is diagnosed. Obstruction to urine flow with urethral or suprapubic catheterisation is often curative for post-renal ARF. The treatment of ATN is usually supportive, including maintenance of sufficiently high blood pressure. The complications of ARF may be life threatening. They include hyperkalaemia, acidaemia, hyperphosphataemia, fluid overload, pericardial effusion and encephalopathy. These should be identified and treated. If they are refractory to conventional therapy, renal replacement (i.e. dialysis) should not be delayed (p. 34). Further renal insults, such as nephrotoxic drugs, should be avoided, and the dosages of drugs that are dependent on renal excretion should be modified according to the creatinine clearance.

Renal protection

Various interventions have been attempted to provide renal protection. These include dopamine, dopexamine, diuretics, diltiazem, bicarbonate, N-acetylcysteine and natriuretic peptide analogues. Generally, they do not work and may do more harm than good. The only useful intervention is intravascular fluid administration. There may be a role for low-osmolality contrast media and prophylactic bicarbonate or N-acetylcysteine to decrease the risk of radiocontrast-induced ARF.

Clinical case

A 60-year-old male with non-Hodgkin's lymphoma has a severe urinary tract infection complicated by bacteraemia. Gentamicin is administered when blood cultures reveal a Gram-negative organism with sensitivity to gentamicin. Over 3 days, the creatinine increases from 120 to 350 μmol/L. The urea increases from 5 to 26 mmol/L. The serum sodium is 140 mEq/L, urine sodium is 14 mEq/L, and urine creatinine is 70 μmol/L. What is the most likely diagnosis and why?

Summary points

■ Ischaemic insult to the kidneys and prerenal renal failure are the most common causes of ARF.
■ Early identification of the aetiology of ARF may allow for successful intervention (Fig. 2).
■ Many elderly patients are at risk of ARF because of pre-existing problems that predispose to renal failure.
■ NSAIDs may cause renal failure by inducing acute interstitial nephritis or prerenal renal failure.

Gastrointestinal bleeding

The most common gastrointestinal (GI) disorder in the intensive care unit (ICU) is acute GI bleeding, with upper GI bleeds being more common than lower GI bleeds. Efforts to prevent this complication should be prioritised because the mortality of GI bleeds is 8–10%. There is a frequent association of GI bleeding with myocardial ischaemia or infarction; elderly patients are especially vulnerable to the resultant hypovolaemic and anaemic shock. About 14% of those with a major GI haemorrhage develop myocardial infarction.

Causes

The differentiation of upper from lower GI bleeding is by the location of the bleed relative to the ligament of Treitz.

Stress-related erosive syndrome (SRES) is the most common cause of an upper GI bleed in the ICU. Virtually all ICU patients have stress-related mucosal disease within 1 day of admission, with 1–4% developing clinically important bleeding. SRES consists of discrete gastric mucosal lesions secondary to stress associated with critical illness. These lesions may worsen, extend, haemorrhage and become diffuse in the upper GI tract. Although most bleeding is self-limiting, it is associated with increased morbidity and mortality. *SRES haemorrhage* is SRES that progresses to frank haemorrhage and hypovolaemia, with a decrease in haemoglobin $\geq 2\,g/dL$, typically necessitating at least 2 units of packed red blood cells within 24 h or surgical intervention.

Mesenteric vasculopathy usually occurs at lower GI sites and results in a small proportion of GI bleeds. Two subtypes are occlusive disease from thromboembolism and non-occlusive disease from vasospasm. Symptoms include abdominal pain and post-prandial pain, which may progress to an acute abdomen. Vasoconstricting drugs, diffuse vascular or atherosclerotic disease, and thrombophilia all increase patients' susceptibility to mesenteric vasculopathy.

Variceal bleeding carries a high mortality of approximately 40% even with treatment. It typically occurs with portal hypertension, often secondary to liver cirrhosis.

Peptic ulcer disease may occur in the stomach, duodenum and/or oesophagus. A history of dyspepsia and epigastric pain may be reflective of pre-existing peptic ulcer disease.

Less common causes of GI bleeding include Mallory–Weiss tear, oesophagitis, duodenitis and malignancy. *Medications* that may exacerbate or cause GI bleeds include non-steroidal anti-inflammatory drugs (NSAIDs), corticosteroids and anticoagulants.

Diagnosis and management

Figure 1 is an algorithm for the initial diagnosis and management of GI bleeds. A detailed history and physical examination are important with an emphasis on pre-existing disease, such as peptic ulcer disease or liver disease, and use of medications such as NSAIDs (Boxes 1 and 2). Haemoglobin and haematocrit may not initially reflect the severity of the bleed for up to 72 h, so serial checks are advisable. A type and screen is warranted in case blood transfusion is required. Tests of coagulation and platelet function may yield valuable information.

Consider an electrocardiogram and blood for troponin if myocardial ischaemia is suspected. Faecal occult blood testing may reveal blood in the patient's stool even if it is not grossly visible. A gastric tube insertion and lavage revealing coffee ground material or frank blood indicates an upper GI bleed.

An oesophagogastroduodenoscopy (OGD) allows visualisation of the upper GI tract; SRES may be diagnosed and lesions such as ulcers may be biopsied. Diagnostic accuracy is high. In addition to diagnosing sources of upper GI bleeds, OGD provides the means of stopping the bleeds with various methods, such as thermocoagulation, clips and sclerosing injection.

Colonoscopy is indicated for lower GI tract visualisation. Radionuclide scanning uses labelled red blood cells to find the source of a GI bleed if OGD and colonoscopy are inconclusive. Angiography may be resorted to if non-invasive techniques are unsuccessful in localising a bleed. A specific bleeding site may be targeted for embolisation or vasopressin administration to halt bleeding. Angiography is the gold standard for diagnosing mesenteric vasculopathy. Abdominal computerised tomography (CT) may also be useful in diagnosing mesenteric vasculopathy.

Surgery is usually indicated if there is profuse bleeding despite interventional OGD or angiography. It may include vagotomy, excision or oversewing of bleeding sites, gastric devascularisation or gastrectomy. For variceal bleeds, shunt surgery or transjugular intrahepatic portosystemic shunt (TIPS) may be needed. Vasopressin is a potent splanchnic and systemic vasoconstrictor. It may help with variceal bleeds. There are multiple systemic side-effects including coronary spasm. Octreotide is a somatostatin analogue causing splanchnic vasoconstriction and a decrease in portal pressure. It is an alternative to vasopressin for the treatment of variceal bleeding. Balloon tamponade may be used temporarily to control variceal bleeding for up to 24 h, but there is a 75% rebleed rate when the balloon is removed.

Proton pump inhibitors and histamine-2 receptor blockers inhibit gastric acid secretion and are useful for both prophylaxis and treatment. Prevention of SRES may be achieved when the gastric pH is maintained above 4. The downside to this approach is that overgrowth of bacteria may render patients more susceptible to nosocomial pneumonia.

Marshall and Warren were awarded the 2005 Nobel Prize in Physiology or Medicine for their discovery of 'the bacterium *Helicobacter pylori* and its role in gastritis and peptic ulcer disease'. *H. pylori* causes inflammation of the gastric and duodenal mucosa. For peptic ulcer disease, attempts should be made to diagnose *H. pylori* infection, and the addition of antibiotics, such as clarythromycin and metronidazole, and bismuth to a proton pump inhibitor or histamine-2 receptor blocker is usually indicated.

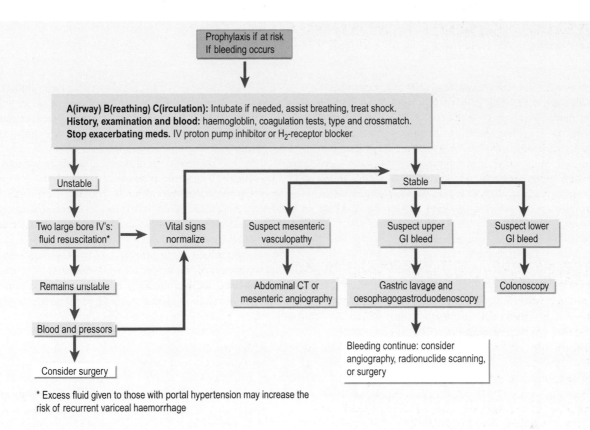

Fig. 1 **Initial diagnosis and management of GI bleeds.**

Box 1. Risk factors for GI bleeding in the ICU

*Coagulopathy**
*Respiratory failure with mechanical ventilation >48 h**
*Shock or hypotension
*Sepsis or multiple system organ failure
*Multiple or severe trauma
*Burns >35% of total body surface area
*Severe central nervous system injury
*Hepatic or renal failure
*Acute coronary syndrome
*Aspiration pneumonia
*Post organ transplant
*Post surgery
*Prolonged ICU admission
Anticoagulation
Portal hypertension
Peptic ulcer disease

*Risk factor specific for SRES
**Most significant risk factors for SRES

Box 2. Symptoms and signs of GI bleeding

Haematemesis: blood-stained vomitus
Melaena: dark-coloured or tarry stools, owing to mixing of blood with intestinal contents
Haematochezia: bloody stools
Coffee ground emesis or nasogastric tube aspiration
Bloody gastric aspirate
Unexplained decreased in haematocrit
Unexplained haemodynamic instability and signs of hypovolaemia
Abdominal pain and acute abdomen

Practice point

GI bleeding may result in severe blood loss and haemorrhagic shock. Initial treatment may include protection of the airway with a tracheal tube, intravenous volume resuscitation and blood transfusion. Only if a patient is stable should an OGD be attempted for diagnosis and treatment. Torrential bleeding is usually an indication for surgery.

Clinical case

A 64-year-old male with coronary artery disease is admitted to the ICU after a motor vehicle accident. On his third day in the ICU, he is noted to have two bouts of melaena. A gastric lavage reveals a bloody aspirate. In addition, his haematocrit has trended down. Two units of packed red blood cells are administered. What is the most likely cause of his GI bleed and why? What test is crucial for diagnosis?

Summary points

- In the ICU upper GI bleeds are more common than lower GI bleeds.
- Remember your ABCs in managing patients with GI bleeds.
- Consider prophylactic therapy in critically ill patients at risk of SRES.
- OGD is an effective diagnostic and management tool in upper GI bleeds.

Gastrointestinal motility disorders

Gastrointestinal (GI) hypermotility and hypomotility may result from primary pathological processes or may occur as a consequence of severe systemic illness.

Bowel obstruction

Bowel obstruction can be classified anatomically. (i) The problem may be in the lumen, such as foreign bodies, gallstones or faecal impaction. (ii) There may be lesions in the wall, such as tumours, diverticular disease, inflammatory bowel disease or strictures. (iii) The problem may be outside the bowel wall, such as adhesions, hernias, tumours or abscesses. (iv) There may be a torsion (volvulus).

For small bowel obstruction (SBO), the most common aetiologies are adhesions and hernias. For large bowel obstruction (LBO), neoplasia, diverticulitis and sigmoid volvulus are most common.

Small bowel obstruction

History
The four cardinal symptoms are colicky pain, distension, nausea and vomiting, and constipation. Pertinent history includes operations and co-morbidities.

Physical examination
Signs include distension and a tympanitic abdomen. Hernias and scars provide clues. Rectal examination may exclude constipation and faecal impaction. Skin overlying a hernia containing ischaemic bowel may be warm, erythematous and oedematous. With peritoneal signs – board-like rigidity, guarding or rebound tenderness – emergency laparotomy is indicated.

Leucocytosis may suggest strangulation, alkalaemia may occur with vomiting, and acidaemia with diarrhoea. Hypernatraemia and elevated urea are suggestive of hypovolaemia. Lactic acidosis occurs with bowel ischaemia and liver dysfunction.

Investigations
Radiograph features of SBO (Fig. 1) include dilated small intestine with air–fluid levels and paucity of gas in the colon and rectum. Features of

strangulation include pneumatosis and portal venous gas. An upright chest radiograph is useful to detect bowel perforation.

Computerised tomography (CT) has a sensitivity of 90–100% for SBO (Fig. 2). CT may reveal features mandating immediate surgery, such as a closed loop obstruction or signs of bowel ischaemia – wall thickening, pneumatosis and portal venous gas.

Initial therapy for SBO includes preventing oral intake, intravenous fluid (IVF), decompression using a nasogastric tube (NGT) and serial abdominal examinations.

Early postoperative SBO
This is SBO within 1 month of abdominal or pelvic surgery. Re-exploration is difficult owing to adhesions, and is associated with a high risk of complications. Strangulation is rare; conservative management is recommended. If there is no resolution within 5–7 days, parenteral nutrition and a gastrostomy tube for decompression should be considered.

Intussusception
This is an uncommon cause of SBO in adults. The most common predisposing factor is an intraluminal neoplasm, which acts as a 'lead point' for the proximal intestine or 'intussusceptum' to telescope inside the distal intestine or 'intussuscepiens'. Patients may report recurrent episodes of obstruction, accompanied by passage of bloody stools mixed with mucus, so-called 'redcurrant jelly'. Investigations include contrast study and CT scan. Management is operative.

Large bowel obstruction

The workup of LBO is very similar to that of SBO. Management is *always* operative.

Volvulus

Sigmoid volvulus occurs when there is a redundant loop of sigmoid with a narrow base of attachment of the mesosigmoid. This allows the redundant bowel to twist and obstruct. *Caecal* volvulus occurs in the setting of recent

surgery and left colonic obstruction. Plain abdominal films are diagnostic of volvulus in 50% of cases. Endoscopy is the gold standard for diagnosis – in addition, it may be therapeutic for sigmoid volvulus (successful in 75–90% of cases).

If endoscopic detorsion is successful, and there is no ischaemia, elective colon resection must be performed because there is a recurrence rate of up to 50%. Urgent surgery is indicated for sigmoid volvulus if there is colonic ischaemia, or if endoscopic detorsion fails. Surgery is indicated for caecal volvulus.

Colonic pseudo-obstruction

Also known as Ogilvie's syndrome this is non-mechanical, functional obstruction of the large intestine thought to be an

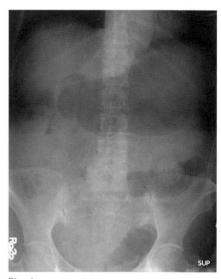

Fig. 1 **Supine plain abdominal radiograph demonstrating the multiple dilated small bowel loops of small bowel obstruction.** The valvulae conniventes are visible across the whole width of the dilated bowel. There is a paucity of gas in the large bowel. Note the left lower quadrant colostomy.

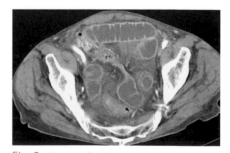

Fig. 2 **CT scan showing small bowel obstruction with adhesive band.**

imbalance of GI autonomic tone. On plain films, there is a dilated proximal colon with preservation of haustral markings, a normal calibre small intestine unless there is an incompetent ileocaecal valve, and a transition point may be seen (most commonly at the splenic flexure). Colonoscopy or gastrografin enema may exclude a mechanical defect. Management is conservative. Intravenous neostigmine or epidural local anaesthesia to promote motility have been described. Intestinal decompression is indicated when the caecal diameter is >12 cm or the patient fails to improve within 48–72 h. This is accomplished by colonoscopy and air insufflation. It is successful in 80% of cases; in the remaining 20%, repeat colonoscopy is successful in 85%. A decompressive tube may decrease recurrence. Mucosal ischaemia warrants surgery.

Ileus

Ileus denotes dysmotility in the absence of mechanical obstruction. It follows loss of coordinated peristaltic intestinal contractions, usually lasting 3–5 days after abdominal operations. Ileus may also be the result of local or systemic inflammation or infection. The classic features of ileus include:

- abdominal distension;
- failure to pass flatus;
- high nasogastric outputs; and
- nausea and vomiting, dehydration, electrolyte abnormalities.

Investigations
Plain abdominal films show gas distending the small and large bowel, including the rectum. CT scan may exclude mechanical obstruction.

Treatment
Keep the patient NPO (nil by mouth), decompress with a NGT, minimise opiates and correct fluid and electrolyte derangements.

Constipation

There are myriad causes of constipation. Chief among these are (over)medication and not maintaining a healthy bowel regimen. Drugs associated include opiates, anticholinergics, antihypertensives (calcium channel blockers), antispasmodics, anticonvulsants and antipsychotics (phenothiazines). Constipation may progress to faecal impaction.

Colitis

Clostridium difficile, a Gram-positive, anaerobic, spore-forming bacterium, is the most common cause of infectious diarrhoea in hospital. There is a spectrum of disease, from asymptomatic carriage to self-limited colitis to pseudomembranous colitis to toxic megacolon and, finally, to fulminant colitis. The predominant risk factor for overgrowth of toxigenic strains is the use of antibiotics. Restriction of antibiotic duration is crucial for prevention.

There may be crampy abdominal pain, distension and tenderness. Paradoxically, in the postoperative patient who develops toxic megacolon, there may be a reflex ileus and constipation, rather than diarrhoea. Fever, leucocytosis, dehydration and acidosis accompany severe cases. If unrecognised, the condition may progress to colonic perforation, peritonitis and septic shock (Fig. 3). Stop antibiotics and start oral metronidazole. Do not administer antimotility agents until *C. difficile* is excluded.

Diagnosis is with enzyme-linked immunosorbent assay (ELISA) for toxins in stool. ELISA should be repeated at least twice if negative. Abdominal radiographs are useful for perforation and to monitor colonic diameter. If initial response (<48 h) is poor, switch to intravenous metronidazole and oral vancomycin. Worsening of symptoms, sepsis, toxic megacolon, fulminant colitis or perforation require colonic resection.

Ischaemic colitis is difficult to diagnose. The diagnosis may be made at the time of laparotomy. The symptoms are pain and diarrhoea, classically 'redcurrant jelly' stools owing to the mixing of blood with mucus. The pain is sudden, crampy, often in the lower abdomen and more on the left. A reflex ileus may be triggered, leading to abdominal distension, nausea and vomiting. Rectal examination is positive for blood. Leucocytosis with a left shift may be found. Gangrene, sepsis and shock may develop.

Abdominal films may show intraperitoneal air and mucosal 'thumbprinting', which reflects oedema of the colonic mucosa. Colonoscopy is the study of choice, revealing discoloured mucosa, haemorrhagic nodules and frank ulceration. Patients with perforation, septic shock or who are deteriorating require urgent laparotomy. Conservative treatment includes NPO, IVF, analgesia and broad-spectrum antibiotics; most patients improve within 24–48 h.

Diarrhoea in patients receiving enteral feeding

Modifiable factors include high feed osmolarity, lactose intolerance, bacterial contamination, bolus (as opposed to continuous) feeding and lack of dietary fibre.

Clinical case
A woman was admitted with SBO, probably resulting from adhesions. Conservative management failed, and she was taken for laparotomy. She had a postoperative ileus complicated by aspiration pneumonia. After 7 days of cefepime for pneumonia, she has developed diarrhoea. Her vital signs are stable, her white blood cell count, having normalised, starts to rise again. Abdominal examination is benign. What is the likely diagnosis?

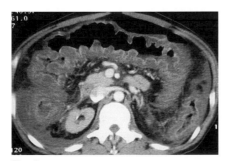

Fig. 3 **CT scan showing pseudomembranous colitis with frank perforation.**

Summary points

- Bowel obstruction is characterised by pain, distension, nausea and vomiting, and obstipation.
- Examine the abdomen and *always* do a rectal examination.
- There is a role for conservative management of small bowel obstruction but not large bowel obstruction.
- The complications of obstruction and colitis include ischaemia, perforation and sepsis.
- Always consider *C. difficile* colitis.

Cholecystitis and pancreatitis

Cholecystitis

Acute cholecystitis can occur with or without gallstones. Calculous gallbladder disease can be complicated by gangrene, perforation and sepsis. Acalculous cholecystitis predominates in the intensive care unit (ICU). Patients undergoing cardiac and aortic surgical procedures, trauma patients, septic patients and burn patients are at higher risk.

The pathophysiology of acalculous cholecystitis involves ischaemia of the gallbladder wall (Fig. 1). Inadequate perfusion may result from shock or limited hepatic venous outflow, as with mechanical ventilation with high positive end-expiratory pressure (PEEP). Increased gallbladder intraluminal pressure also limits perfusion. Fasting, total parenteral nutrition and biliary sludge are thought to be associated with acalculous cholecystitis for this reason.

The usual presentation of acute cholecystitis includes right upper quadrant pain, nausea, vomiting and fever. However, these symptoms and signs are difficult to assess in critically ill patients. A high index of suspicion is necessary in ICU patients with signs of systemic inflammation, especially if risk factors for gallbladder hypoperfusion exist.

The diagnosis is confirmed with ultrasound examination, which is done at the bedside. Gallbladder wall thickening and pericholecystic fluid are diagnostic. Additional findings include gallstones, sludge and intramural air. Biliary nuclear scintigraphy can be used in equivocal cases, but there is a significant false-positive rate owing to the frequency of biliary stasis in ICU patients. In addition, this requires transport to the nuclear medicine area. Similarly, computerised tomography (CT) scan requires transport out of the ICU. CT is insensitive for gallstones but can show signs of cholecystitis. The main advantage of CT imaging is the ability to identify other intra-abdominal pathology such as pancreatitis, intra-abdominal abscess, bowel obstruction and mass lesions of solid organs (Fig. 2).

The optimal therapy is cholecystectomy. Laparoscopic cholecystectomy may be technically difficult owing to the high incidence of gallbladder gangrene or perforation. Critically ill patients often require

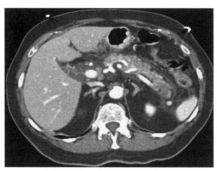

Fig. 2 **This CT slice of the abdomen shows evidence of pancreatitis, choledocholithiasis and choledocholithiasis.** The overall picture is consistent with gallstone pancreatitis.

aggressive resuscitation and antibiotic therapy. Those patients who remain too unstable to undergo operation may better tolerate percutaneous cholecystostomy, which drains the septic focus and decreases intraluminal pressure. Interval cholecystectomy can be performed when the patient improves.

Acute acalculous cholecystitis has a mortality rate as high as 50% attributable largely to the underlying predisposing illness.

Pancreatitis

Pancreatitis is divided into acute and chronic processes. Acute pancreatitis can be a patient's ICU admission diagnosis, or it can complicate a patient's ICU course. Chronic pancreatitis rarely warrants ICU admission unless complicated by an acute exacerbation or if treatment is required for an associated problem such as delirium tremens. The majority of cases of acute pancreatitis are the result of either biliary stone disease or alcohol consumption. These are typically implicated when pancreatitis is the admission diagnosis. Less common aetiologies of acute pancreatitis are more frequently implicated when the diagnosis is made during an ICU stay.

The pathophysiology of acute pancreatitis has been debated for decades. The result is release of lytic enzymes that cause varying degrees of autodigestion and therefore glandular destruction (Fig. 1). There is often a profound inflammatory response that is the basis for much of the systemic effects. This response has a tremendous variability. The majority (approximately 80%) of cases are self-limiting with fluid and nutritional support. The clinical course of the remainder is far more severe. This group can develop pancreatic pseudocysts, pancreatic necrosis and multiple organ system failure. The more fulminant cases are frequently fatal.

Typically, a history of acute, severe, epigastric abdominal pain, often with nausea and vomiting, is elicited. Elevated serum levels of pancreatic enzymes amylase and lipase are usually suggestive, but are neither sensitive nor specific. Perforated or ischaemic bowel can give a false-positive result, and pancreatic insufficiency may lead to false-negative enzyme levels. CT is

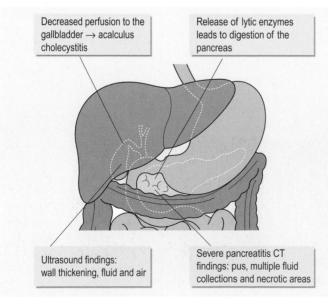

Decreased perfusion to the gallbladder → acalculus cholecystitis

Release of lytic enzymes leads to digestion of the pancreas

Ultrasound findings: wall thickening, fluid and air

Severe pancreatitis CT findings: pus, multiple fluid collections and necrotic areas

Fig. 1 **Cholecystitis and pancreatitis.**

frequently used in cases of severe pancreatitis. CT can define areas of necrosis or pseudocyst formation (Table 1, Fig. 3). Ultrasound commonly misses these findings.

One of the most important distinctions in severe pancreatitis is between sterile and infected necrosis. Although CT may show retroperitoneal gas or a clearly defined abscess, it is often necessary to perform an image-directed fine needle biopsy of the pancreas to diagnosis infection.

ICU management of acute pancreatitis can be required for a variety of reasons, but close monitoring of vigorous volume resuscitation and support of dysfunctional vital organs are the usual indications. Early involvement of a multidisciplinary team consisting of intensivists, surgeons, gastroenterologists and interventional radiologists is ideal.

Airway protection and mechanical ventilatory support are frequently required. Acute respiratory distress syndrome (ARDS) can complicate severe episodes of acute pancreatitis. Aggressive volume resuscitation is instituted; intravascular volume depletion secondary to third space loss is usually present. Vasopressor and inotropic support can be necessary with shock resulting from infected necrosis. These patients have a poor prognosis. Invasive haemodynamic monitoring provides information about tissue perfusion and may help to guide resuscitation.

Nutritional support is essential for patients with pancreatitis. Historically,

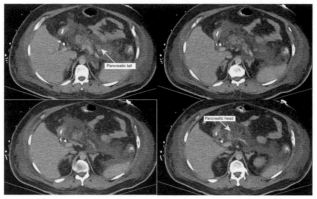

Fig. 3 **These CT slices of the abdomen show evidence of pancreatitis with necrosis.** The pancreatic tail enhances normally and is surrounded by fluid. This is consistent with pancreatitis. The head and neck have tissue that does not enhance, consistent with necrosis.

bowel rest has been prescribed, but more recent data suggest that enteral nutrition is desirable if tolerated. Post-pyloric feeding may be the preferred route, although this remains controversial. Patients who cannot tolerate enteral nutrition for 5–7 days should receive parenteral nutrition. Tight glucose control is important.

The use of broad-spectrum antimicrobials is debated. The basis for their use in pancreatic necrosis arises from the fact that mortality rises when necrotic pancreatic tissue becomes infected. There are data to support the use of imipenem in acute pancreatitis complicated by necrosis.

Infected pancreatic necrosis is an indication for laparotomy, necresectomy and drainage. These patients often require prolonged ICU care with periodic reoperation for ongoing debridement of non-viable pancreatic tissue. Rarely, operation is performed after several weeks of severe pancreatitis without evidence of improvement or when there is rapid clinical deterioration. Cholecystectomy is indicated when the aetiology of

pancreatitis is biliary stone disease. Surgery is usually delayed until recovery from acute pancreatitis. If biliary drainage is indicated for biliary obstruction, either percutaneous or endoscopic techniques are employed in the setting of acute pancreatitis.

The Acute Physiology and Chronic Health Evaluation (APACHE) scoring systems and other prognosticators have been employed with limited success to predict outcome of acute pancreatitis (Table 2).

Table 1 **Computerised tomography grading of severity of pancreatitis**	
(A) Normal pancreas	0
(B) Oedematous pancreatitis	1
(C) B plus mild extrapancreatic changes	2
(D) Severe extrapancreatic changes including one fluid collection	3
(E) Multiple or extensive extrapancreatic collections	4
Necrosis	
None	0
< One-third	2
> One-third, < one-half	4
> Half	6
CT severity index = CT grade + necrosis score	
	Complications:
0–3	8%
4–6	35%
7–10	92%
	Deaths:
0–3	3%
4–6	6%
7–10	17%

<table>
<tr><td colspan="2">Table 2 Clinical and laboratory correlates of poor outcome with pancreatitis</td></tr>
<tr><td>Initial assessment:</td><td>Clinical impression of severity
Body mass index > 30
Pleural effusion on chest radiograph
APACHE II score > 8</td></tr>
<tr><td>24 h after admission:</td><td>Clinical impression of severity
APACHE II score > 8
Glasgow score 3 or more
Persisting organ failure, especially if multiple
C-reactive protein > 150 mg/L</td></tr>
<tr><td>48 h after admission:</td><td>Clinical impression of severity
Glasgow score 3 or more
C-reactive protein > 150 mg/L
Persisting organ failure for 48 h
Multiple or progressive organ failure</td></tr>
</table>

Clinical case

A patient is being treated on the ICU for aspiration pneumonia complicated by respiratory failure and shock. He has a background history of daily alcohol abuse. The patient is sedated with a tracheal tube in place. Treatment includes antibiotics, fluid resuscitation and pressor agents. Three days after ICU admission, he develops abdominal distension, jaundice, hypotension and abdominal tenderness. What is the diagnosis?

Summary points

- Acalculous cholecystitis predominates in the ICU.
- Ultrasound is useful to diagnose cholecystitis.
- CT scan is important in diagnosing pancreatitis and for providing information about prognosis.
- Pancreatitis may be associated with cytokine release, systemic inflammatory response syndrome (SIRS) and multiorgan dysfunction.

Liver failure

The liver plays crucial roles in metabolism, detoxification and synthesis; liver disease (Table 1) in critically ill patients is associated with increased mortality. With acute liver failure, transplantation may be the only hope of survival.

Fulminant hepatic failure is defined as acute liver failure in patients without a history of chronic liver disease with the hallmarks of hepatic encephalopathy and coagulopathy (Fig. 1). The symptoms and signs may be abrupt and non-specific: nausea/vomiting, malaise, headache, dehydration, abdominal pain, fever, anorexia, dark urine, jaundice.

Hepatic encephalopathy is altered mentation secondary to liver dysfunction. Asterixis – flapping motion of hands when outstretched and dorsiflexed – is a feature of hepatic encephalopathy. Grade I is the least severe and carries the best prognosis. The patient will be mildly confused. A patient with grade IV encephalopathy is comatose and unrousable.

Paracentesis of ascitic fluid allows evaluation of the serum-to-ascites albumin gradient (Table 2). This may shed light on the aetiology of the ascites and liver failure.

The coagulopathy, hypotension and heart failure that may result from liver failure may be difficult to distinguish from sepsis with disseminated intravascular coagulopathy (DIC). Hypotension resulting from sepsis may cause 'shock liver', resulting in an elevation of transaminase proteins, lactate levels and, possibly, hypoglycaemia and hyperbilirubinaemia. Sepsis with DIC should be suspected if there is a worsening thrombocytopenia.

The consequences of liver failure are detailed in Fig. 1.

Severity and treatment

Targeting treatment for different aetiologies is important. Examples include high-dose penicillin G for *Amanita* mushroom poisoning, delivery of the baby for acute fatty liver of pregnancy, and zinc or trientine therapy for Wilson's disease. The Child–Turcotte–Pugh scoring system is used to assess the severity and emergency of acute liver failure (Table 3).

Monitor for and treat complications

Nutritional and metabolic

Provision of nutrition and frequent glucose monitoring are essential. Enteral nutrition may be preferable to maintain gut integrity and decrease bacterial translocation. Metabolic acidosis may reflect worsening hepatic function. High lactate has been associated with poor prognosis.

Cardiovascular

With oedema and ascites, judging adequate intravascular volume status may be challenging. Invasive

Table 1 **Causes of liver failure**		
Drug/toxin	**Infection**	**Other**
Paracetamol/acetaminophen (see p. 154)	Hepatitis A	Idiopathic: pregnancy [e.g. acute fatty liver of pregnancy, HELLP syndrome (**h**aemolysis, **e**levated **l**iver enzymes, **l**ow **p**latelets) during pregnancy]
Alcohol	Hepatitis B (most common cause worldwide)	
Idiosyncratic drug reaction (e.g. halothane, isoniazid)	Hepatitis C	Metabolic disorders (e.g. Wilson's disease)
Amanita mushroom poisoning	Rarely hepatitis D or E	Sepsis
		Shock
		Hypercoagulable states causing thrombosis
		Malignancy

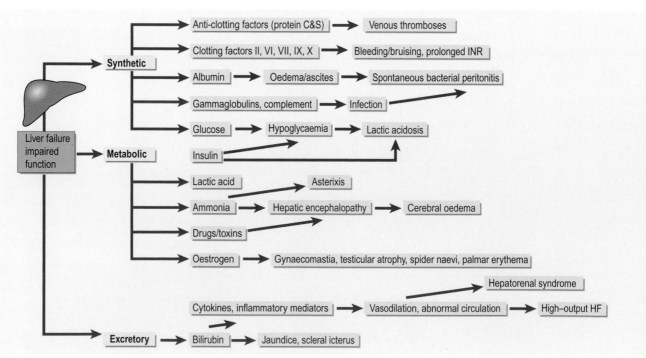

Fig. 1 **Consequences of liver failure.**

haemodynamic monitoring is usual practice. This includes an arterial line, a central venous catheter and cardiac output measuring technology (e.g. oesophageal Doppler, pulmonary artery catheter). Fluid resuscitation is frequently needed.

Haematological

Factor VII has a short half-life. The international normalised ratio (INR), which measures the so-called extrinsic coagulation pathway, is therefore a sensitive tracker of changes in liver function. Fresh frozen plasma or vitamin K may be needed to treat bleeding or to cover an invasive procedure or surgery. The downside is that these interventions decrease the utility of the INR as an index of liver function. Bleeding from piles and oesophageal varices may occur with portal hypertension. Counterintuitively, liver failure may increase the likelihood of thrombosis secondary to protein C and S deficiency. Thrombosis prophylaxis may be appropriate.

Neurological

Hepatic encephalopathy may occur in the setting of gastrointestinal bleeding, infection, alkalosis, hypokalaemia, sedatives/tranquillisers, high dietary proteins, azotaemia/uraemia and progressive hepatic dysfunction. Precipitating factors should be treated. Ammonia may be measured, although the levels do not correlate with the severity of encephalopathy. A low-protein diet and alteration of the gut flora with lactulose and/or antibiotics (e.g. metronidazole, neomycin) may decrease encephalopathy.

Patients with grade III or IV encephalopathy are at a high risk of cerebral oedema. Intracranial pressure (ICP) monitoring may be useful; goals are to maintain ICP <20 mmHg and cerebral perfusion pressure (CPP) >60 mmHg. Jugular venous saturation provides information about global cerebral perfusion. Simple measures such as elevating the head of the bed and preventing head turning may facilitate venous drainage and decreased ICP. Mannitol may be administered to decrease ICP with the proviso that plasma osmolality is monitored. Noradrenaline (norepinephrine), vasopressin and phenylephrine may be used to maintain CPP. A head scan may provide additional information (e.g. uncal herniation). Ventilation to normocapnia and maintenance of normal body temperature may improve neurological outcome.

Respiratory

Patients may complain of exertional dyspnoea or platypnoea (easier breathing when recumbent rather than erect) owing to hepatopulmonary syndrome. This occurs in the setting of liver disease and is accompanied by hypoxaemia, intrapulmonary vascular dilatations and right-to-left intrapulmonary shunting. The diagnosis may be confirmed with a lung perfusion scan or contrast-enhanced echocardiography.

Infectious

Gram-positive infections are most common. Daily cultures should be obtained because patients may not have an elevated white cell count or a fever. Empiric broad-spectrum antibiotics may be reasonable if there is clinical deterioration, and antifungal agents may be added if a patient does not respond. Typical sites of infection include peritoneum (spontaneous bacterial peritonitis), blood and lungs. Ascitic fluid is a good culture medium for bacteria; paracentesis typically shows ≥ 250 neutrophils/mm^3. Organisms may be grown from the fluid.

Renal

Hepatorenal syndrome refers to decreased renal function secondary to abnormal arterial circulation and increased activity of the endogenous vasoactive system from liver failure. Replenish electrolytes and perform dialysis as needed. The most effective treatment of hepatorenal syndrome is liver transplantation.

Clinical case

A 30-year-old male presents with acute non-paracetamol (acetaminophen)-induced hepatic failure. He has grade II encephalopathy and no clinical evidence of ascites on physical examination. Is close observation on the medical ward appropriate management?

Table 2 Serum-to-ascites albumin gradient (SAAG)

SAAG >1.1	SAAG <1.1
Portal hypertension	No portal hypertension
Causes: cirrhosis, Budd–Chiari syndrome, cardiac disease, portal vein thrombosis, myxoedema, massive liver metastases	*Causes:* malignancy (e.g. massive hepatic metastases, hepatocellular carcinoma, primary mesothelioma), pancreatic disease, bile leak, infections (e.g. bacterial peritonitis), hypoalbuminaemia (e.g. nephrotic syndrome)

Summary points

- Liver failure affects the whole body.
- The INR is useful for tracking changes in liver function.
- Severe lactate elevation may be a marker of poor prognosis.
- Early admission to an ICU is essential.
- Transplantation may be life saving.

Table 3 The Child–Turcotte–Pugh scoring system

Points	1	2	3
Grade of encephalopathy	No encephalopathy	I–II	III–IV
Presence of ascites	Absent	Slight or controlled by diuretics	Moderate or worse, despite diuretics
Serum bilirubin (μmol/L)	<34.2	34.2–51.3	>51.3
Bilirubin (μmol/L) for those with primary biliary cirrhosis, primary sclerosing cholangitis or other cholestatic liver diseases	<68.4	68.4–171	>171
Serum albumin (g/L)	>35	28–35	<28
INR	<1.7	1.7–2.3	>2.3

5–7 points, mild or class A; 8–10 points, moderate or class B; 11–15 points, severe or class C.

Endocrine system

Endocrine function in the ICU

The role of the hypothalamic–pituitary axis for homeostasis during stress is critical. The initial response to stress from injury, infection, inflammation and starvation is an increase in the release of anterior pituitary hormones. This early hormonal stimulation promotes a catabolic state to provide efficient metabolic substrates for the vital organs such as the brain and heart and to support host defence responses. Prolonged critical illness generally leads to depressed hypothalamic stimulation of pituitary function with a loss of the normal pulsatility in hormone secretion coupled with peripheral tissue unresponsiveness.

Adrenal function and glucocorticoids

Stress activates the hypothalamus–pituitary–adrenal (HPA) axis to cause release of corticotropin-releasing hormone (CRH) from the hypothalamus and increased release of corticotropin (ACTH) from the anterior pituitary (Fig. 1). This acute stress response shifts adrenal production from mineralocorticoids (aldosterone) and adrenal androgens (dehydroepiandrosterone, DHEA) to glucocorticoids with an increase in cortisol secretion. Prolonged stress and illness lead to an uncoupling of normal feedback mechanisms. This imbalance between immunostimulant (DHEA) and immunosuppressant (cortisol) hormones has important implications for infection susceptibility in chronic illness. Glucocorticoids are responsible for increased production of glucose, free fatty acids and amino acids, maintenance of cardiac contractility and vasomotor tone, and anti-inflammatory effects.

Cortisol circulates primarily bound to cortisol-binding globulin (CBG), while approximately 10% circulates as biologically active free cortisol. CBG is decreased in critical illness with an increase in free cortisol levels. Normal diurnal secretion is abolished in critical illness, and random cortisol levels are typically measured. While it is difficult to define 'normal' cortisol levels in critical illness, levels $<18\,\mu g/dL$, and many would suggest even levels $<25\,\mu g/dL$, are inappropriately low. Provocative testing may be helpful to assess adrenal function and reserve. Corticotropin is administered intravenously, and cortisol levels are measured at 30- and 60-min intervals.

Adrenal insufficiency is associated with increased morbidity and mortality during critical illness, and clinicians must have a high index of suspicion. Clinical features are non-specific and may include fatigue, depression, fever, hypotension, hyponatraemia, hypoglycaemia or eosinophilia.

Thyroid function

In non-thyroidal illness (NTI), there is a fall in circulating triiodothyronine (T3) levels, primarily due to a decrease in peripheral conversion of thyroxine (T4) into T3 and a concomitant increase in the production of reverse T3 (rT3) (Fig. 2). Typically, levels of T4 and thyroid-stimulating hormone (TSH) remain within a low–normal range, although there is a reduction in TSH response to thyrotropin-releasing hormone (TRH) and a loss of normal pulsatile TSH secretion.

Critically ill patients with overt primary hypothyroidism will demonstrate markedly elevated TSH levels and may have clinical features of hypothyroidism, including hypothermia, bradycardia, hypotension, depressed mental status or dry skin. The decision to treat these individuals must be based on clinical context and other medical factors, including possible cardiac disease or pituitary disorder with concomitant subclinical adrenal insufficiency.

Significantly decreased TSH levels are generally found in patients with primary hyperthyroidism, although critically ill patients receiving dopamine or glucocorticoids may have low TSH levels due to direct inhibition of TSH release. Treatment with methimazole or propylthiouracil should only be considered in patients with extremely low or undetectable TSH if they also have elevated T3 or T4 levels.

Somatotropic axis

Growth hormone (GH) is secreted from the anterior pituitary in a pulsatile fashion in response to hypothalamic growth

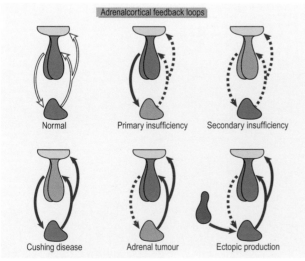

Fig. 1 **Adrenocortical feedback loops.**

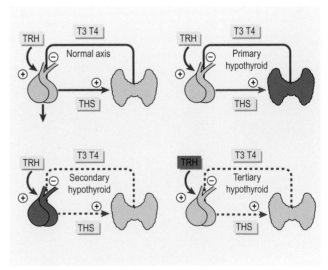

Fig. 2 **Thyroid feedback mechanisms.**

hormone-releasing hormone (GHRH) and a novel class of peptides including ghrelin. GH has a number of direct metabolic effects, including lipolysis, insulin antagonism, amino acid transport and immune cell stimulation. Indirectly, GH promotes anabolism and growth. During stress, GH pulse frequency is increased and GH levels are elevated. With prolonged critical illness, the pulsatile secretory pattern of GH release becomes irregular, and peak GH levels are reduced, contributing to a chronic wasting condition.

In an attempt to prevent muscle loss and promote positive nitrogen balance, it is tempting to consider GH supplementation in critically ill patients. Trials in children with hypermetabolic conditions related to burn injury have shown improved outcomes, whereas trials in critically ill adults have generally been unfavourable.

Hyperglycaemia and insulin resistance

Stress-induced hyperglycaemia is relatively common, occurring in up to half of critically ill patients, with a higher prevalence in the elderly. Hyperglycaemia in the intensive care unit (ICU) may be due to multiple factors including the gluconeogenic and glycogenolytic effects of neurohormonal responses to illness or injury, cytokine-induced insulin resistance, drug administration (catecholamines, glucocorticoids), dextrose-containing solutions, excessive feeding, diabetes mellitus, pancreatitis, obesity and the metabolic syndrome. Studies have demonstrated worse outcomes in patients with hyperglycaemia and improved outcomes in patients in whom glucose levels were controlled with insulin administration.

Androgens

Testosterone is the most important endogenous anabolic steroid, and its depressed levels during critical illness may have important implications for wound healing and muscle wasting. Androgen replacement therapy in men has been associated with increased muscle mass and strength, improvements in ventilator weaning and increased mobilisation and ability to participate in physical therapy. Replacement therapy may be considered in both men and women with chronic critical illness wasting, although androgen replacement therapy is contraindicated in breast or prostate carcinoma, and may cause hepatotoxicity, polycythaemia, oedema and female virilisation.

Prolactin

Prolactin has important immunoregulatory functions with receptors on human B and T lymphocytes. Factors leading to increased prolactin levels in response to acute stress or injury are not entirely characterised, although dopaminergic pathways are likely to be involved. Reduced levels of prolactin with prolonged stress may play a role in the compromised immune function and susceptibility to infection of chronically ill patients.

Practice point

Is dopamine a good idea?
↓ GH secretion
↓ TSH secretion
↓ Prolactin secretion

Summary points

- Tight and consistent glycaemic control for both diabetic and non-diabetic patients decreases morbidity and mortality.
- Adrenal insufficiency should be considered when there is hypotension refractory to pressor treatment.
- Euthyroid sick syndrome should be differentiated from a true thyroid illness.
- There is no indication to check or administer growth hormone or its derivatives to ICU patients.

Diabetes mellitus in the ICU

Diabetes mellitus is becoming increasingly common in westernised populations as we become more idle and obese. Diabetes is of major economic significance as it accounts for over 10% of health care expenditure in some populations (Hogan et al 2003). Box 1 lists reasons why diabetics might end up in the intensive care unit (ICU). Type I diabetics often have a normal body mass, but type II diabetics often show features of the so-called 'metabolic syndrome X' – they are centrally obese, hypertensive, hyperlipidaemic and relatively resistant to the effects of insulin.

Diabetic ketoacidosis and its mechanisms

Starved patients normally become ketotic as they shift to fat metabolism (see p. 52). Fatty acids are exported from fat tissue to the liver, where they are broken down into acetate and exported as ketone bodies (acetoacetate and beta-hydroxybutyrate). In the presence of acidosis, the predominant ketoacid produced is beta-hydroxybutyrate.

In the absence of insulin, cells 'starve in the midst of plenty' – despite high blood glucose levels, cells cannot take up the sugar because of lack of insulin. Ketones are poured out as a result of this perceived 'starvation'. Sugar leaks into the urine causing an osmotic diuresis, with dehydration. Ketoacidosis causes vomiting, which worsens the dehydration.

In pregnant diabetic women, marked acidosis may be present without substantial hyperglycaemia. In other patients with ketoacidosis and a blood glucose that is not markedly elevated (under ~ 14 mmol/L), you should suspect that the ketoacidosis has another cause, e.g. alcoholic ketosis.

Managing ketotic coma

Initial attention should be paid to the basic ABC – airway, respiration and circulatory management. Careful assessment is vital, paying attention to what precipitated the ketosis, associated diseases and fluid and electrolyte deficits (Box 2). All management should ideally be documented on a single large flowchart, so that every participant in management can see what is happening!

Box 1. Factors associated with ICU admission

1. *Hyperglycaemic, ketotic coma* in type I diabetics (with absolute insulin deficiency due to autoimmune destruction of beta cells in the pancreas).
2. *Hyperglycaemic 'non-ketotic' coma* with markedly elevated sugar levels in type II diabetics. Type II diabetics often have a degree of resistance to the effects of insulin, as well as abnormal patterns of insulin release. Careful testing reveals that a significant number of such patients have some degree of ketosis.
3. *Hypoglycaemic coma*, often related to failure to take food with hypoglycaemic medication or other accidents of administration of such drugs. Severe 'neuroglycopenia' of even a few minutes duration may result in irreversible neurological injury.
4. *Complications of diabetes* or of other intercurrent diseases. Diabetics often end up as critically ill patients owing to complications shown in Fig. 1.
5. *Insulin resistance*. A patient not previously identified as 'diabetic' may be admitted to the ICU for a reason unrelated to diabetes (commonly following trauma or major surgery), and the diabetes may become manifest, as the underlying condition causes insulin resistance. Recent evidence suggests that such insulin resistance is not only related to the 'trauma' of surgery, but also to the patient being in a starved state! (see p. 52).

Box 2. Key management points

1. *Fluid replacement* is the cornerstone. A common deficit is 100 mL/kg. A reasonable best guess fluid replacement regimen in someone with a baseline mass of 70 kg is 1 L over 30 min, 1 L over 1 h, 1 L over 2 h and then 1 L every 4 h until euvolaemia, but caution may be needed, especially in those with other disease such as pre-existing heart failure. There is controversy about which fluid should be given, but commonly used fluids are Ringer's lactate/Plasmalyte® and normal saline. The disadvantage of normal saline is that, because its strong ion difference (SID) is zero, it replaces ketoacidosis with a 'dilutional' hyperchloraemic acidosis, which may take days to settle (see p. 44).
2. *Provision of insulin* is vital. This should ideally be as a continuous infusion of insulin. About 0.1 U/kg/h will commonly be required, remembering that there is some adsorption of insulin to plastic. With marked insulin resistance, vast amounts of insulin may occasionally be required, up to many hundreds of units per day.

   In suboptimal circumstances, intramuscular insulin may be effective, but subcutaneous insulin should not be given. Recent studies show that 'uncomplicated' diabetic ketoacidosis can be managed with the newer ultrashort-acting insulin analogues – Insulin Aspart, Lispro – given subcutaneously! Intermittent intravenous (IV) boluses of insulin are a *poor* option, as the half-life of insulin in the circulation is tiny, and even the biological effect of IV insulin is short-lived. Complications of therapy may be more common with large IV boluses of insulin.

3. *Potassium replacement* will be needed, and should be started when the serum potassium declines to under 5.5 mmol/L. Initially start at 15 mmol/L of replacement fluid, but larger amounts may be required, given with due caution. Phosphate levels should be watched and severe hypophosphataemia addressed, but routine replacement is thought to be harmful. Avoid mixing calcium-containing and phosphate-containing solutions.
4. *Antibiotics* should be given where there is any likelihood of infection. If pus is present, it *must* be drained as soon as possible. Diabetic ketoacidosis masks features of infection by causing both hypothermia and leucocytosis.
5. It is seldom, if ever, necessary to administer alkalinising agents such as bicarbonate or tris-hydroxymethyl aminomethane (THAM). However, with severe acidosis, such agents may be of value under carefully controlled conditions, including careful observation and management of respiration.

If serum sodium is normal in the presence of marked hyperglycaemia, the incautious clinician may get a surprise – as hyperglycaemia is controlled, the sodium will rise (Box 3)!

Hyperosmolar states without ketosis

Small amounts of insulin are sufficient to turn off ketone formation but, with insulin deficiency and severe intercurrent illness, extreme hyperglycaemia can occur, ultimately resulting in coma. Glucose levels may reach 60 mmol/L or more. Onset is often over a longer period of time than is the case with ketotic coma, and the patients are correspondingly sicker.

Because of the extreme dehydration and marked hyperglycaemia encountered, hyperviscosity is common, and may have devastating consequences including cerebral vascular occlusion. Most authorities recommend more gradual correction of fluid deficits in hyperosmolar coma, and there is again controversy about which fluid should be used. Whatever approach is taken, morbidity and mortality are high. Meticulous fluid balance, slow rehydration and anticoagulation using low-molecular-weight heparin are thought to be important components of management.

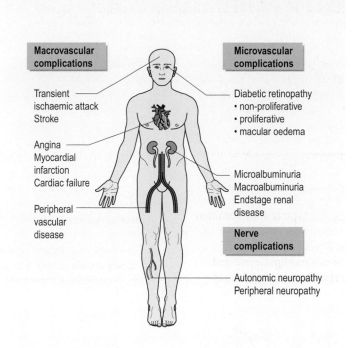

Fig. 1 **Complications of diabetes mellitus.**

Box 3. 'Correcting' sodium according to glucose level

Astute clinicians have observed how, as high glucose levels are corrected, due to osmotic shifts, serum sodium rises. Effectively, for every 10 mmol/L glucose above a value of 10, you can correct the serum sodium by +3 mmol. So, if the measured sodium is 130 mmol/L and the glucose is 50 mmol/L, when the glucose is corrected, you can expect the sodium to rise to about 142 mmol/L. This is *not* a form of pseudohyponatraemia, but reflects the fluid deficit!

Other diabetic problems

Many patients in the ICU will have either diabetes or impaired glucose tolerance. Recent evidence suggests that tight glucose control is important, particularly in preventing infective complications during their ICU admission (see Clinical case). Every diabetic should also be scrutinised for complications of diabetes (Fig. 1). These include macrovascular complications (cerebrovascular disease and stroke, ischaemic heart disease and peripheral vascular disease), microvascular complications (retinopathy leading to blindness, renal disease causing proteinuria and, ultimately, renal failure) and nerve complications including peripheral neuropathy and autonomic neuropathy.

Most diabetics in the ICU will require insulin infusion, with glucose and potassium as appropriate. 'Sliding scales' are an anachronism and should not be used.

Clinical case

A 50-year-old woman with a history of impaired glucose tolerance is admitted to the ICU with pancreatitis and acute respiratory distress syndrome requiring ventilatory support. How would you manage her blood sugar, and what targets would you set?

Summary points

■ Diabetics commonly end up in the ICU.
■ Meticulous glycaemic control in the ICU is vitally important.
■ Appropriate fluid replacement is the cornerstone of management of ketoacidotic and hyperosmolar states.
■ Most diabetics in the ICU require insulin infusion.
■ Be on the lookout for complications of diabetes in your diabetic patients!

Endocrine emergencies

Endocrine emergencies arise from hyperfunction or hypofunction of an endocrine organ (Table 1). Often, barely compensated conditions are perturbed by a stressful event, leading to decompensation and clinical sequelae.

Diabetic ketoacidosis (DKA)

DKA is a life-threatening deficiency of insulin that leads to excess glycogenolysis, gluconeogenesis, lipolysis and generation of ketone bodies. Hyperglycaemia causes an osmotic diuresis with spillage of electrolytes, glucose and free water in the urine. This leads to marked hypovolaemia and electrolyte abnormalities. The most common precipitants include infection, missed insulin doses, myocardial infarction and stroke.

Clinical features include polyuria, polydipsia, abdominal pain, nausea, fatigue, altered mental status, Kussmaul breathing, tachycardia, hypotension and acetone breath odour. Laboratory findings include hyperglycaemia (usually 20–40 mmol/L) and elevated anion gap metabolic acidosis (due to ketones). Serum potassium levels may be elevated as a result of acidosis, but total body potassium stores are markedly depleted by urinary losses. Other electrolytes (magnesium, phosphate) are often depleted as well.

Treatment is aggressive volume resuscitation with normal saline, coupled with an insulin infusion. Dextrose saline should be used when blood glucose decreases below 15 mmol/L. Potassium and other electrolytes must be added to replace urinary losses.

Hyperosmolar non-ketotic coma (HONK)

HONK syndrome is a condition related to DKA that results from a relative lack of insulin, but not a complete absence. It is often seen in type II diabetes, when insulin production is adequate to prevent ketoacidosis but not hyperglycaemia. Extreme hyperglycaemia (typically worse than DKA) causes severe hypovolaemia, electrolyte abnormalities and altered central nervous system (CNS) function.

Signs and symptoms of HONK are similar to those of DKA. Laboratory findings include hyperglycaemia (often 30–40 mmol/L), a normal pH and hyperosmolality (>320 mOsm/kg). Treatment is similar to DKA.

Thyroid storm

Thyroid storm is a life-threatening hypermetabolic disorder caused by abnormally high levels of T4 or T3. Patients usually have pre-existing compensated hyperthyroidism (most commonly Graves' disease or toxic nodular goitre), although it can be iatrogenic (from exogenous T4, iodine, amiodarone or lithium). Thyroid storm usually evolves in response to a stressor such as surgery, illness or trauma. Differential diagnoses include malignant hyperthermia, neuroleptic malignant syndrome, phaeochromocytoma and the serotonin syndrome.

Signs and symptoms include cardiovascular (tachyarrhythmias, high-output heart failure, hypertension, angina), neurological (nervousness, tremors, increased reflexes) and constitutional (weakness, anorexia, fever, nausea, diarrhoea). Levels of free T3 and/or T4 are elevated, while TSH levels are suppressed by feedback inhibition.

Pharmacological therapy involves beta blockade (e.g. propranolol) followed by antithyroid medications (propylthiouracil, methimazole or sodium iodide) to render the patient euthyroid. After stabilisation, definitive therapy consists of thyroidectomy or radioactive ablation of the thyroid gland. Adjunctive therapy involves temperature management, intravenous fluids and corticosteroids (accelerated metabolism may cause relative adrenal insufficiency).

Myxoedema coma

Myxoedema coma is an extreme form of decompensated hypothyroidism resulting from insufficient T4 or T3 levels, generally due to failure of the thyroid gland (primary hypothyroidism). As with thyroid storm, myxoedema coma usually develops in response to a stressful event, such as surgery, infection, trauma, myocardial infarction or burn. Differential diagnoses include CNS event (stroke, meningitis), metabolic abnormalities (electrolytes, hypoglycaemia, diabetic ketoacidosis, adrenal insufficiency), infectious (urinary tract infection most common in the elderly), myocardial infarction, hypoxaemia and depression, among others.

Signs and symptoms include cardiovascular (bradycardia, hypotension or hypertension), neurological (lethargy, delayed reflex

Table 1 **Major features of hyperfunction and hypofunction of organs**		
Syndrome	**Clinical features**	**Treatment**
Thyroid storm	Arrhythmias, fever, anxiety, hypertension, hyperreflexia	Antithyroid drugs, beta blockade, ablative surgery or radiation, ± corticosteroids
	History of hyperthyroidism	
	Elevated T3/T4, low TSH	Search for inciting event (surgery, infection, myocardial infarction)
Myxoedema coma	Bradycardia, lethargy, hypothermia	Warming, intravenous fluids, thyroid hormone replacement
	History of hypothyroidism	
	Low T3 and/or T4	Search for inciting event
DKA/HONK	Polydipsia, polyuria, lethargy, hypotension	Fluid resuscitation, electrolyte repletion, insulin therapy
	Hyperglycaemia ± anion-gap acidosis	Search for inciting event
Adrenal insufficiency	Fatigue, nausea, hypotension, fever	Intravenous fluids, dextrose, corticosteroid (± mineralocorticoid) replacement
	Hyperkalaemia, hyponatraemia	
	Abnormal ACTH stimulation test	Search for inciting event
Phaeochromocytoma	Anxiety, flushing, tachycardia, hypertension	Blood pressure control with alpha-adrenergic blockade and subsequent beta blockade
	Elevated catecholamine levels	Intravenous fluids

ACTH, adrenocorticotropic hormone; DKA, diabetic ketoacidosis; HONK, hyperosmolar non-ketotic dehydration syndrome; TSH, thyroid-stimulating hormone.

relaxation, altered mentation) and constitutional (hypothermia, alopecia, constipation). Non-specific laboratory findings include anaemia, elevated creatine kinase, elevated creatinine, hyperlipidaemia, hypoglycaemia, hyponatraemia and respiratory acidosis.

Initial treatment consists of correction of hypovolaemia and electrolyte abnormalities, treatment of hypothermia and careful monitoring of cardiovascular status. Empiric antibiotics are often warranted. Blood and urine cultures should be obtained and a chest radiograph examined. Lumbar puncture may be appropriate as well. Supplemental glucocorticoids (e.g. hydrocortisone 100 mg every 8 h) should be given until adrenal insufficiency is ruled out in the case of pituitary failure.

Definitive therapy is treatment with intravenous thyroid hormone. Both T3 and T4 are available, but T4 is recommended. A typical regimen consists of 100–500 μg intravenously (IV), then 75–100 μg IV per day until the patient is able to take oral T4.

Adrenal insufficiency

Adrenal insufficiency is an absolute or relative deficiency of cortisol (and perhaps aldosterone) production by the adrenal cortex. It can result from primary adrenal failure or secondary adrenal insufficiency [inadequate adrenocorticotropic hormone (ACTH) production]. As with other endocrine emergencies, patients often have compensated adrenal insufficiency with an acute crisis precipitated by some stressor (e.g. infection, trauma, surgery). A controversy exists in critically ill patients with 'relative adrenal insufficiency'. Patients in shock states with refractory hypotension will sometimes improve with the administration of glucocorticoids, even with normal cortisol levels.

Signs and symptoms include fatigue, lightheadedness, nausea and vomiting, abdominal pain, fever, tachycardia, hypotension and confusion. Patients in shock may show hypotension refractory to multiple vasopressors. Laboratory findings include hyponatraemia, hyperkalaemia, hypoglycaemia, prerenal azotaemia, anaemia, lymphocytosis and eosinophilia.

Once clinically suspected, the diagnosis of adrenal insufficiency is confirmed by an ACTH stimulation test. A baseline cortisol level is drawn, synthetic ACTH is administered, and cortisol levels are measured at 30 and 60 min. A failure of serum cortisol to increase beyond a threshold level (usually 500 nmol/L or more than 250 nmol/L above baseline) indicates true adrenal insufficiency.

Definitive treatment consists of replacing both glucocorticoids (e.g. hydrocortisone) and mineralocorticoids (e.g. fludrocortisone). Adjunctive therapy includes aggressive volume repletion and treatment of hypoglycaemia with intravenous dextrose.

Phaeochromocytoma

Phaeochromocytomas are tumours (usually benign) of catecholamine-producing chromaffin cells. Some 90% arise in the adrenal medulla. Some cases are associated with the multiple endocrine neoplasia (MEN) type II syndromes. Excess catecholamines produce signs and symptoms including

anxiety, flushing, palpitations, headaches, nausea, dyspnoea, chest pain, paroxysmal hypertension, tachydysrhythmias, diaphoresis and tremors.

Diagnosis is made by elevated 24-h urinary excretion of catecholamines – adrenaline (epinephrine) and noradrenaline (norepinephrine) – and their metabolites (vanillylmandelic acid and metanephrines), as well as elevated plasma catecholamines. After biochemical tests confirm the tumour, localisation is performed by imaging (magnetic resonance imaging and nuclear medicine studies).

Definitive therapy is surgical removal, but initial stabilisation is necessary, as intraoperative manipulation of the tumour can cause large amounts of catecholamines to be released. Medical therapy includes adrenergic blockade, blood pressure control and ensuring normal volume status. Adrenergic blockade is achieved first using alpha-adrenergic antagonists (usually phentolamine or phenoxybenzamine). Beta blockade is instituted only once alpha-blockers are used, as unopposed alpha-adrenergic tone can cause hypertensive crisis.

> ### Clinical pearls
>
> 1. Phaeochromocytomas follow the 'rule of 10s': 10% are extra-adrenal, 10% are bilateral and 10% are malignant.
> 2. The classic findings of paroxysmal hypertension, flushing and headache, suggest phaeochromocytoma as a diagnosis.

> ### Clinical case
>
> A 44-year-old woman recently underwent an open reduction and internal fixation of a tibial fracture sustained in a motor vehicle accident. She was otherwise uninjured. She claims no prior medical history except having taken 'some sort of thyroid pill' in the past, but had stopped when she moved recently. Twelve hours postoperatively, she is found to be in some distress on the surgical ward. Her heart rate is 140 bpm and irregularly irregular, respirations 26/min, blood pressure is 150/95 mmHg, temperature is 39°C, and oxygen saturation is 99% on 2 L of oxygen by nasal cannula. She is anxious and diaphoretic. Physical examination is remarkable for a diffuse goitre and proptosis. She is transferred to the surgical ICU for further care.
>
> What is the differential diagnosis of this patient's condition? What further studies would you order?

> ### Summary points
>
> - Endocrine emergencies often arise from barely compensated conditions perturbed by stressful inciting events.
> - The treatment for both HONK and DKA is fluids (lots) electrolyte repletion and insulin.
> - First-line therapy for thyroid storm is beta blockade and antithyroid medication, followed by ablative therapies.
> - Replacement therapy for hypothyroidism may unmask concurrent adrenal insufficiency.
> - Patients in shock with refractory hypotension may imrove with glucocorticoids, even with normal baseline cortisol.

Haematological
system

Clotting and bleeding: a delicate balance

Through veins and vessels the life
blood pours
While battle rages with fierce and
constant pitch
Twixt choleric furies striving to
stem the sanguine flow
And surgeons' scalpels slicing
faster than they can sew.
Anonymous medieval poet

The mechanisms underlying many
intensive care unit (ICU) deaths involve
diametrically opposing pathological
processes: thrombosis and haemorrhage.
Patients may be at risk of major
bleeding following trauma, surgery,
anticoagulant medicines, disseminated
intravascular coagulopathy and various
infections such as viral haemorrhagic
fevers. On the other hand, intravascular
clotting is responsible for strokes, heart
attacks, venous thromboses and
pulmonary emboli. The typical ICU
patient may alternately be at risk of both
major haemorrhagic and thrombotic
complications during their ICU stay. A
working knowledge of physiological
mechanisms of clotting and bleeding
helps clinicians to identify patients at
risk and to intervene appropriately to
treat excessive bleeding and to prevent
inappropriate clotting. We look here at
the normal physiology surrounding
coagulation. Subsequent pages deal with
mechanisms of coagulation
derangements as well as their
prevention and treatment.

The clot war (see Figs 1 and 2)

Figure 1 shows the key physiological
clotting mechanisms. Fig. 2 shows the
key physiological anti-clotting
mechanisms. Inactivated clotting agents
are blue, activated clotting agents are
pink and anti-clotting agents are green.
The intact endothelium is essential for
anti-clotting activity. The activated
platelet and the tissue factor-bearing cell
are the initiators of clotting.

Clotting agents

Headquarters
- Tissue factor-bearing cell
- Activated platelets.

Key clotting agents
- The activator – tissue factor
- The initiator – factor VIIa

- The messengers – factors IXa and Xa
- The conductor - thrombin (factor IIa)
- The amplifiers – factors Va and VIIIa
- The binder - fibrin (factor Ia)
- The stabiliser – factor XIIIa

- Platelet activators [thrombin, platelet-activating factor (PAF), adenosine diphosphate (ADP), thromboxane (TXA$_2$), von Willebrand factor (vWF), adrenaline (epinephrine), collagen, arachidonic acid].

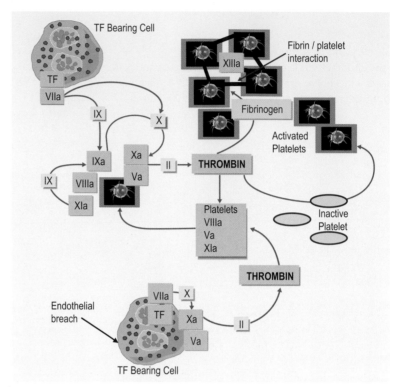

Fig. 1 **Key physiological clotting mechanisms.**

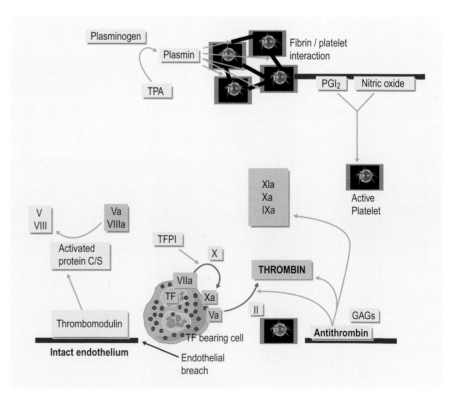

Fig. 2 **Key physiological anti-clotting mechanisms.**

Anti-clotting agents

Headquarters:
- Endothelium.

Key anti-clotting agents:
- The inhibitor – tissue factor pathway inhibitor
- The opposers – antithrombin and glycosaminoglycans (GAGs)
- The interceptor – thrombomodulin
- The inactivators – protein C and protein S
- The repulsers – nitric oxide (NO) and prostacyclin (PGI$_2$)
- The cleaver - plasmin.

Normal clotting mechanisms (Fig. 1)

When the endothelium is denuded, cells bearing tissue factor (the activator – TF) are exposed. TF binds avidly to factor VII. This complex activates factors X and IX. Factor Xa enlists factor V, and they bring thrombin into play. The small amount of thrombin (the conductor) produced sends out an array of activating signals, most notably to platelets, FVIII and FV (the amplifiers), fibrinogen/fibrin (the binder), FXIII (the stabiliser) and FXI. Activated platelets swarm to the signal, exude sticky pseudopods, extrude granules (e.g. ADP, TXA$_2$, PAF) to attract more platelets to plug the breech by combining with fibrin (the binder). FXIIIa (the stabiliser) stabilises the fibrin–platelet clot. FVa and FVIIIa (the amplifiers) complex with FXa and FIXa, respectively, and bind to activated platelets. On the activated platelet surface, a massive thrombin burst occurs, which sends out its signals and accelerates clotting.

Normal anti-clotting mechanisms (Fig. 2)

The intact endothelium usually prevents clotting. Nitric oxide and prostacyclin (PGI$_2$) (the repulsers) are constitutively produced and prevent platelet aggregation and adhesion. Tissue factor pathway inhibitor (TFPI, the inhibitor) opposes the TF/VIIa/Xa complex. In areas where the endothelium has not been breeched, thrombomudulin (the interceptor) receives a signal from thrombin (the conductor) and dispatches protein C and protein S (the inactivators) to inactivate factors VIIIa and Va. Antithrombin (AT) and glycosaminoglycans (GAGs) are also dispatched by intact endothelium to oppose clotting agents. Plasmin, a proteolytic enzyme, is activated by tissue plasminogen activator (TPA). Plasmin prevents rampant clot extension and promotes clot lysis or cleavage.

Bleeding and clotting tendencies

These regulatory and counter-regulatory mechanisms ensure that, under normal circumstances, clotting occurs only at sites of injury and that blood flows freely in the intact vessels. When the balance shifts, pathological bleeding or clotting can occur. The reasons for such shifts include congenital abnormalities, disease processes and drugs that interfere with clotting and bleeding. Patients on ICUs frequently have bleeding and clotting problems as part of multiorgan dysfunction or secondary to drugs or sepsis.

Coagulopathy on the ICU

Bleeding tendencies present on the ICU for a variety of reasons. Acquired causes are common. Thrombocytopenia occurs with severe sepsis, and coagulopathy, or haematological failure, may be a component of multiorgan failure. Liver failure, kidney failure, bone marrow failure and metabolic derangement all contribute to bleeding diatheses.

Thrombophilia on the ICU

A tendency to clot is an underappreciated problem on the ICU. Patients are bedridden and may have undergone surgery. They are sitters for major thrombotic episodes. Patients on heparin who have a precipitous decrease in platelet count may, apparently paradoxically, be at risk for thrombosis. Importantly, ICU patients frequently have acquired decreased concentrations of antithrombin, protein C and S. Tissue factor, an important initiator of clotting, is usually exposed with endothelial injury. In certain pathological states, such as severe sepsis, soluble tissue factor may be detected in plasma.

Bleeding, when unabated, usually leads to slow protracted death, during which time the clinician has many opportunities to stem the flow. A major clot, such as a pulmonary embolus, may kill in an instant. Thrombosis prophylaxis is a priority for most ICU patients.

> ### Clinical case
>
> A 22-year-old woman is admitted to the ICU with a diagnosis of bacterial meningitis. She has bruises and petechiae over her body. Laboratory results reveal a mild anaemia (Hb=11 g/dL), a low platelet count (platelets=110×10^9/L), and a mild coagulopathy [international normalised ratio (INR)=1.4 and partial thromboplastin time (PTT)=43 s]. The haematologist recommends that activated protein C and antithrombin should be administered. The ICU fellow wants to treat with platelet and plasma transfusions. Who is correct?

> ### Summary points
>
> - There is a delicate balance between clotting and anti-clotting mechanisms.
> - This balance is frequently disturbed in critically ill patients.
> - Thrombin and activated platelets are central in coordinating and promoting clotting.
> - The intact endothelium is essential for preventing pathological clotting.
> - Thrombosis is a frequent cause of in-hospital mortality.

Bleeding in the ICU

Causes of bleeding

Congenital

von Willebrand's disease (vWD) is the most common inherited bleeding diathesis (Table 1), with an estimated 1% of the population having a form of the disorder. The defect is in von Willebrand factor (vWF), required for platelet adhesiveness and as a carrier for factor VIII. There are three types of vWD. Desmopressin (DDAVP), a drug that mobilises endogenous vWF, may prevent or treat bleeding with mild forms of vWD, but is not indicated for type 2B or type 3 vWD. Blood products, including cryoprecipitate, fresh frozen plasma (FFP) and platelets, may be used to treat vWD. Factor VIII/vWF concentrates provide definitive treatment. Platelet aggregometry and near-patient platelet function testing, such as the PFA-100, may yield information about severity. Automated vWF ristocetin cofactor (vWF:RCo) assay allows both quantitative (types 1 and 3) and qualitative (type 2) diagnosis of vWD.

Haemophilia A, a lack of factor VIII (FVIII), is the most common clotting factor deficiency. It is an X-linked condition, so males are typically affected. Females may carry the gene and be mildly affected. The relative lack of FVIII varies from patient to patient. Serious bleeding is rare when FVIII levels are above 5% of normal but, for surgical purposes, more than 50% is desirable. Recombinant FVIII is given at the time of surgery to achieve adequate levels. Christmas disease (FIX deficiency) is also X-linked, and is treated with once-daily FIX infusions to maintain normal levels after surgery. Deficiencies in other clotting factors can also cause significant bleeding, and treatment is usually by replacement of the relevant factor. Patients who receive multiple courses of coagulation factors, typically FVIII, may develop antibodies or inhibitors. In such instances, recombinant activated FVII (rFVIIa) may stimulate coagulation through thrombin generation despite the clotting factor deficiency.

Acquired coagulopathies

Acquired bleeding tendencies are far more common than hereditary disorders (Fig. 1).

Drugs

Aspirin, heparin and warfarin are the most common anticoagulants. Aspirin is not typically associated with bleeding. Heparin-induced bleeding may be reversed with protamine, and warfarin may be neutralised with vitamin K or with FFP. Herbal remedies, especially Ginkgo biloba, may exacerbate bleeding. Low-molecular-weight heparins have a long half-life and have been implicated in increasing bleeding. Antiplatelet agents, such as clopidogrel, tirofiban, eptifibatide and abciximab, cause marked platelet inhibition. Platelet transfusion may partially reverse their effects. Newer anticoagulants, such as direct thrombin inhibitors – bivalirudin, hirudin, desirudin and argatroban – and fondaparinux, have long half-lives and no antidotes. Partial clearance may be achieved with dialysis.

Organ dysfunction

Apart from FVIII, the liver produces all the clotting factors. Liver failure results in profound coagulopathy. FVII has a short half-life, and its decline is mirrored by an increasing international normalised ratio (INR), the laboratory test that crudely reflects the extrinsic coagulation pathway. FFP, cryoprecipitate and recombinant FVII may be used to treat bleeding with liver failure. Renal failure results in platelet abnormalities. There may be some improvement with DDAVP, but platelet transfusion may be required. Bone marrow failure may occur with critical illness, especially with sepsis. Chemotherapeutic agents are also powerful antimetabolites and bone marrow suppressants. Severe thrombocytopenia may occur, and platelet transfusion is indicated when there is bleeding.

Disseminated intravascular coagulation

DIC occurs frequently with sepsis, meningitis, malaria and viral haemorrhagic fevers. Patients may have catastrophic bleeding and severe thrombocytopenia, but the underlying pathology is rampant activation of the

---

Table 1 Bleeding tendencies in the ICU

Category and mechanism	Examples	Mechanism
Congenital		
Platelet dysfunction	Von Willebrand disease, Glanzmann's thrombasthenia	vWF deficiency Abnormal platelet function
Factor deficiency	Haemophilia A, Christmas disease	Factor VIII deficiency Factor IX deficiency
Organ system dysfunction		
Liver failure	Paracetamol overdose	Low clotting factors
Renal failure	Acute tubular necrosis	Platelet dysfunction
Malignancy		
Haematological malignancies	Leukaemia	Thrombocytopenia with bone marrow failure
Physiological derangement		
Hypothermia	Heat loss during surgery	Impaired clotting factors function
Acidaemia	Lactic acidosis	
Drugs		
Thrombocytopenia	Chemotherapy drugs	Bone marrow suppression
Decreased clotting factors	Warfarin	Inhibition of vitamin K-dependent factors
Potentiation of antithrombin	Heparin, low-molecular-weight heparin	Inhibition of thrombin and other factors (e.g. FXa)
Factor Xa inhibition	Fondaparinux	Clotting FXa inhibition
Calcium binding	Citrate	Calcium inactivation
Thrombin antagonism	Argatroban, hirudin, bivalirudin, desirudin	Thrombin inhibition
Platelet inhibition	Aspirin, clopidogrel, abciximab, tirofiban	Decreased platelet activation or binding
Infections	Meningitis, malaria, sepsis, haemorrhagic fevers	Disseminated intravascular coagulation
Massive haemorrhage	Polytrauma	Dilutional coagulopathy
Foreign surface	Cardiopulmonary bypass	Consumptive coagulopathy Hyperfibrinolysis

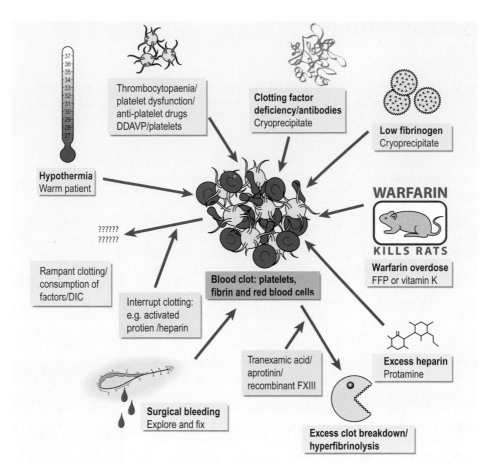

Fig. 1 **Causes (blue) and treatment (red) of bleeding in the ICU.**

coagulation system, leading to consumption of platelets and clotting factors. Treatment of DIC with blood components may worsen the DIC. Counterintuitively, the treatment for DIC may be with anticoagulant agents, such as heparin, recombinant activated protein C or tissue factor pathway inhibitor, in an attempt to decrease clotting activation. The best treatment of DIC is to treat the underlying disorder.

Surgical bleeding

The minority of patients who have undergone major surgery and are bleeding on the ICU have identifiable surgical sources of bleeding. Nonetheless, when the bleeding is unrelenting, a surgical source should always be suspected and excluded through re-exploration. Patients who lose a lot of blood also lose clotting factors and platelets. They become cold and acidaemic. And they have fresh wounds, which can easily bleed. It is important to keep patients warm and avoid excessive resuscitation with fluids known to exacerbate coagulopathy, including starches and albumin.

Pharmacological treatment of bleeding

DDAVP (e.g. 0.3 µg/kg IV) mobilises vWF and may be useful in treating bleeding where there is platelet dysfunction. Antifibrinolytic drugs – aprotinin, tranexamic acid (e.g. 50–100 mg/kg) and epsilon aminocaproic acid – stabilise clots and have been shown to decrease blood loss in several settings. Questions have been raised about the safety, efficacy and cost-effectiveness of aprotinin compared with tranexamic

acid. Recombinant clotting factors such as rFVIIa and rFXIIIa have shown promise in staunching bleeding when conventional measures, including blood components, have failed. Pharmacological treatment of bleeding is contraindicated for DIC and sepsis. The concern with all these agents is that they may tilt the delicate balance back towards thrombosis with devastating results.

Clinical case

A 76-year-old man is on the ICU following surgical replacement of the aortic arch with deep hypothermic arrest. There is bleeding at a rate is 250 mL/min. Blood pressure is 190/110, his heart rate is 110/min, temperature is 35.2°C, and there is metabolic acidosis. How should his bleeding be treated?

Summary points

- Acquired bleeding is more common than congenital.
- Drugs and blood components that promote clotting should generally not be administered when there is sepsis or DIC.
- Recombinant FVIIa may be useful for treating both congenital and acquired coagulopathies

Thrombosis in the ICU

Derangement in the delicate equilibrium between clotting and anti-clotting mechanisms occurs in virtually all intensive care unit (ICU) patients. As patients linger, bedridden, the risk of life-threatening thrombosis escalates. Identification of those at risk, early mobilisation and appropriate preventive strategies are priorities for the ICU team. Most ICU patients require thrombosis prophylaxis. Many are at increased risk and require therapeutic anticoagulation. When there is suspicion of venous thrombosis, bedside Doppler scanning may detect venous clots.

Virchow's triad

Virchow's triad describes the risk of blood clotting. Disruption to endothelial integrity, stasis of blood and shift in the clotting balance towards a procoagulant milieu frequently occur in ICU patients.

Thrombophilia is an abnormal tendency for the blood to clot. The cause may be congenital or acquired (see Table 1). Critically ill patients frequently have low concentrations of important endogenous anticoagulants, including antithrombin, tissue factor pathway inhibitor and the protein C/S complex. Arterial clots may result in strokes, bowel infarction, renal artery thrombosis and myocardial infarction. Venous thromboses (VTs) are more common. When venous clots break off and embolise, fatal pulmonary embolism may result. If there is a patent foramen ovale (PFO) in the heart, emboli may cross and embolise systemically, resulting in similar complications to arterial thromboses. The incidence of VTs in the ICU is >10%. Clots forming in the heart may also embolise systemically. Such clots typically occur in the settings of atrial fibrillation, ventricular aneurysms and mechanical heart valves. Transoesophageal echocardiography (TOE/TEE) is useful in detecting clots in the heart (see Fig. 1) and determining whether there is a PFO, implying increased risk of systemic embolisation.

Anticoagulant strategies

The most simple interventions to prevent clots are non-invasive, and include early mobilisation, calf compression devices, elastic stockings and physiotherapy.

Pharmacological anticoagulants act either by mimicking or promoting the actions of endogenous anticoagulants or by opposing the actions of procoagulant processes. The most important classes of drugs include platelet antagonists, thrombin inhibitors, agents that prevent factor synthesis, thrombolytics and recombinant anti-clotting factors (see Fig. 2 and Table 2).

Warfarin prevents the carboxylation of factors '1972' (IX, X, VII and II) as well as proteins C and S. Warfarin can therefore cause a procoagulant state before its anticoagulant actions kick in; it is advisable to continue intravenous anticoagulation until the international normalised ratio (INR) indicates a

Table 1 **Risk factors for thrombosis**		
Congenital	**Acquired**	**Precipitating**
Protein C or S deficiency	Malignancy	Immobility and bedrest
Activated protein C resistance (factor V Leiden)	Heparin-induced thrombocytopenia	Pregnancy/oral contraceptive pill
Abnormality of fibrinogen	Antiphospholipid syndrome	Obesity (body mass index > 30 kg/m²)
Abnormality or deficiency of antithrombin	Antithrombin deficiency	Smoking
Prothrombin 20210		Surgery, especially pelvic and orthopaedic
Increased factor XI, IX, VIII		
Hyperhomocysteinaemia		

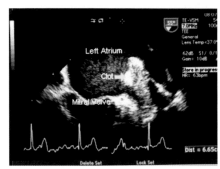

Fig. 1 Transoesophageal echocardiography: clot in left atrial appendage.

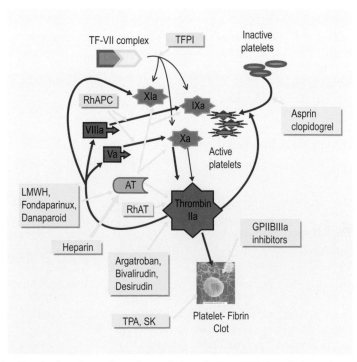

Fig. 2 The sites of action of some key anticoagulant medications. TFPI, tissue factor pathway inhibitor; RhAPC, recombinant human activated protein C; RhAT, recombinant human antithrombin; GPIIbIIIa, glycoprotein IIbIIIa; TPA, tissue plasminogen activator; SK, streptokinase; LWH, low molecular weight heparin. Activated clotting factors are shown with Roman numerals.

Table 2 Anticoagulant medications						
Drug	Mechanism	Metabolism	Dose for DVT prophylaxis	Dose for therapeutic anticoagulation	Therapeutic target	Reversal agent
Heparin	Potentiates antithrombin	Hepatic, RES and 50% renal excretion	5000 U SC twice to thrice daily	Bolus = 80 u/kg Infusion = 18 u/kg/h; adjust to target PTT	PTT = 60–80 s	Protamine: start with 25–50 mg
LMWH (e.g. enoxaparin)	Potentiates antithrombin: Xa inhibition	Mainly renal excretion twice daily	40 mg SC once to	1 mg/kg SC twice daily		None
Fondaparinux	Factor Xa inhibition	Renal	2.5 mg SC once daily			None
Warfarin	Prevents carboxylation of X, IX, VII, II	Hepatic		2–10 mg PO daily; adjust to target INR.	INR = 2–4	Vitamin K 1 mg or plasma; start with 2–4 units
Desirudin	Thrombin inhibition	Renal	10–15 mg SC twice daily			None
Bivalirudin	Thrombin inhibition	Renal		Bolus = 1 mg/kg Infusion = 0.2 mg/kg/h; adjust to target PTT	PT = 2–3 times control	None
Argatroban	Thrombin inhibition	Hepatic		Infusion = 2 mg/kg/min; adjust to target PTT	PTT = 60–80 s; may prolong INR	None

DVT, deep vein thrombosis; INR, international normalised ratio; PO, by mouth; PT, prothrombin time; PTT, partial thromboplastin time; RES, reticuloendothelial system; SC, subcutaneously.

therapeutic warfarin effect. Aspirin prevents platelet thromboxane production and is a weak platelet inhibitor. Clopidogrel blocks the platelet adenosine diphosphate (ADP) receptor and is a stronger inhibitor. Abciximab, tirofiban and eptifibatide are potent antiplatelet agents; they block the glycoprotein IIbIIIa receptor, thereby preventing platelet binding with fibrinogen. Tissue plasminogen activator and streptokinase promote clot breakdown and may be used in such situations as myocardial infarction or pulmonary embolism.

Unless they are at risk of bleeding, ICU patients should receive pharmacological thrombosis prophylaxis (Table 2). Indications for therapeutic anticoagulation include recent venous thrombosis or pulmonary embolism, atrial or ventricular thrombus, paroxysmal or chronic atrial fibrillation, mechanical heart valve, diagnosed thrombophilia and heparin-induced thrombocytopenia (HIT).

Heparin-induced thrombocytopenia

HIT typically presents 4–10 days after the onset of heparin therapy. If heparin has just been started and none has previously been administered for >100 days, HIT is unlikely. Most commonly, type I HIT occurs, which is a benign and transient thrombocytopenia. Type II HIT is mediated by immunoglobulin (Ig)M and IgG antibodies to the heparin–platelet factor 4 complex. Platelet aggregation, skin necrosis and both venous and arterial thrombosis result. Platelet count usually decreases by 50% from baseline, but is typically not $<20 \times 10^9$/L. Laboratory tests include enzyme-linked immunosorbent assay (ELISA) for antibodies, which is sensitive but non-specific. The laboratory standard for diagnosis is the serotonin release assay. The likelihood of HIT occurring is lower with LMWH. When HIT does occur, all forms of heparin *must* be stopped. Anticoagulation with argatroban or bivalirudin is appropriate, and consultation with a haematologist is advisable.

Inferior vena cava filters

When anticoagulation is contraindicated and there is a high risk of venous thrombosis, an ultrasound-guided inferior vena cava (IVC) filter may be inserted at the bedside. An IVC filter may be considered as an adjunct to anticoagulation therapy for those patients with pulmonary embolism. CO_2 is a non-nephrotoxic contrast agent and provides accurate determination of IVC anatomy. IVC filters should not be inserted in the setting of HIT.

Clinical case

A 64-year-old man with a history of hypertension and renal dysfunction had coronary angiography and placement of a coronary stent 6 weeks ago. He presented 2 days ago with atrial fibrillation and unstable angina, was admitted and a new stent was placed. Heparin has been infused since admission for a target partial thromboplastin time (PTT) of 60–80 s. Over the last couple of hours, the patient has developed localising neurological signs. The platelet count since admission has decreased from 160×10^9/L to 80×10^9/L.

Summary points

- Venous thrombosis occurs commonly in critically ill patients.
- Thrombosis prophylaxis is indicated for most ICU patients.
- HIT should be considered in any patient who has a decrease in platelet count following heparin.
- Argatroban or bivalirudin should be used for anticoagulation when a patient develops HIT.
- An IVC filter may be placed to decrease the likelihood of pulmonary embolism.

Infection

Prevention and treatment of infections

Principles of infection control in hospitals

Hospital-acquired infections (HAIs) occur in approximately 8% of patients at a cost of £1000 million per annum in the UK National Health Service. The basic principles of infection control include keeping wards and clinics clean, ensuring that staff act appropriately to prevent cross-infection, disposing of hospital waste in a safe manner and adequately decontaminating medical equipment.

Hand hygiene in health care workers is a highly effective way of preventing infection spreading between patients. Isolation of a case may be appropriate, particularly for highly transmissible infections, such as pulmonary tuberculosis or influenza, or when an infection with a resistant HAI, such as methicillin-resistant *Staphylococcus aureus* (MRSA) or vancomycin-resistant Enterococci (VRE), has been diagnosed (see p. 154).

Early recognition of infection in critically ill patients

Diagnosis of infection in critically ill patients can be very difficult as the normal markers of infection, such as fever and inflammatory markers, are often elevated as a result of the systemic inflammatory response in response to conditions such as hypovolaemia, bleeding and surgery as well as infection. The presence of multiple intravascular lines, endotracheal tubes and urinary tract catheters in combination with the immunocompromised condition of the critically ill patient promotes recurrent episodes of infection.

The major groups of infections seen in critically ill patients and suggested treatments are shown in Table 1. Regular examination of the patient for new signs is essential. Surveillance cultures, such as regular non-directed bronchial lavage, can be helpful in patients in critical care, and a complete septic screen (blood cultures, urinary cultures, line tip cultures and chest radiographs) should be carried out whenever fever or other signs of infection develop. Following diagnosis of infection, antibiotics should be given

for 5–7 days and then stopped, unless there is a good reason for their continuation (Box 1).

Selective decontamination of the digestive tract (SDD)

Infections in intensive care units (ICUs) are thought to follow oropharyngeal and intestinal colonisation with pathogenic microorganisms. SDD is based on the concept of colonisation resistance, the protective effect of the indigenous flora against secondary colonisation with Gram-negative aerobic bacteria. The aim of SDD is to eradicate carriage of potentially pathogenic bacteria from the oropharynx, stomach and gut. Topical, non-absorbed antibiotics, generally tobramycin, polymixin E and amphotericin B, are applied through a nasogastric tube, and treatment with parenteral antibiotics, most frequently cefotaxime, is added for the first 4 days.

Box 1. Principles of antibiotic treatment: 10 questions

- What are the likely causative organisms?
- Which agents are active against the likely pathogens?
- How can the microbiological diagnosis be made?
- What are the unwanted effects of the agent(s) chosen, including drug interactions?
- Which agent has the narrowest spectrum?
- How should the agent(s) be administered?
- What is the correct dose, taking into account renal and liver function and possible drug interactions?
- Should other treatment modalities (e.g. surgery, drainage of pus) be considered?
- Is therapy working?
- When should antibiotics be stopped?

Table 1 Infections associated with ICUs, with likely causative organisms and suggested treatment (NB. Policy may vary according to the local situation)

Condition	Likely organisms	Suggested*	Consider
Infections acquired on ICU			
VAP	Pseudomonas aeruginosa Staphylococcus aureus Escherichia coli Candida spp.	Piperacillin/tazobactam	Vancomycin Fluconazole
Line-associated sepsis/ fungaemia	Coagulase-negative staphylococci Enterococcus spp. Escherichia coli Candida spp.	Vancomycin	Piperacillin/ tazobactam Gentamicin Fluconazole
Occult bacteraemia fungaemia	Staphylococcus aureus Escherichia coli Candida spp.	Piperacillin/tazobactam	Vancomycin Gentamicin Fluconazole
Urinary tract infection	Escherichia coli Pseudomonas aeruginosa Candida spp.	Piperacillin/tazobactam	Gentamicin Fluconazole
Infective diarrhoea	Clostridium difficile	Metronidazole (by mouth)	Vancomycin (by mouth)
Infections requiring admission to the ICU			
Septic shock	Staphylococcus aureus Escherichia coli Streptococcus pneumoniae	Cefuroxime	Gentamicin Vancomycin[†]
Skin and soft tissue	Staphylococcus aureus Streptococcus pyogenes	Flucloxacillin	
CAP	Streptococcus pneumoniae Legionella pneumophila Respiratory viruses	Cefuroxime and macrolide	Vancomycin[†]
Urinary tract infection	Escherichia coli	Cefuroxime	Gentamicin
Abdominopelvic	Escherichia coli Bacteroides fragilis	Cefuroxime	Gentamicin Fluconazole
Meningitis	Neisseria meningitidis Streptococcus pneumoniae	Ceftriaxone 2 g q12 or Cefotaxime 2 g q8	Vancomycin

*Agents are administered intravenously unless indicated. Equivalent agents are indicated in Table 2 according to colour blocks.
[†]Consider addition of vancomycin or linezolid where patient is known to be colonised or at risk of MRSA or where C-MRSA is common.

The use of SDD is not universal in ICUs, and there is some controversy about its usefulness. It may be most effective in the subgroup of patients admitted to surgical ICUs following traumatic injuries (Box 2).

Box 2. Clinical learning point: crafty Candida can kill

Infections with Candida are common in critical care and should not be forgotten. The use of broad-spectrum antibiotics, the presence of prosthetic material and critical illness are factors that allow Candida to flourish in the body. Patients can become colonised in bowel flora, respiratory secretions, on skin and mucous membranes and along intravenous lines. Candida can then become invasive and result in pneumonia, fungaemia, endophthalmitis, urinary tract infection and endocarditis. Many Candida species, including *Candida albicans*, are susceptible to fluconazole. Other species, especially *C. krusei* and *C. glabrata*, can be resistant to fluconazole. Alternative agents such as amphotericin B or newer drugs such as voriconazole or caspofungin may be useful. *C. lusitania* can be resistant to amphotericin B. Susceptibility testing is helpful.

Table 2 Major groups of antibiotics (agents with broadly similar spectrum of activity are grouped according to colour)

Antibiotic group	Agent	Dosage	Spectrum of activity
Co-amoxiclav	Amoxicillin/clavulanate	1.2 g q8	GPC and GNR
Cephalosporins:			
First generation (FGC)	Cefazolin	0.25–1.5 g q6–8 h	GPC and GNR
Second generation (SGC)	Cefuroxime	0.75–1.5 g q8 h	GPC and GNR
Third generation (TGC)	Ceftriaxone	1–2 g q24 h	GPC and GNR
	Cefotaxime	1–2 g q8–12 h	GPC and GNR
Third generation (TGC) with antipseudomonal action	Ceftazidime	1–2 g q8–12 h	Extended GNR
Fourth generation (TGC)	Cefipime	1–2 g q12 h	Extended GNR, GPC
Antipseudomonal penicillins (APP)	Ticarcillin/clavulanate	3.1 g q4–6 h	Extended GNR, GPC
	Piperacillin/tazobactam	4.5 g q8 h	Extended GNR, GPC
Carbapenems	Imipenem/cilastatin	0.5–1 g q6 h	Extended GNR, GPC
	Meropenem	0.5–1 g q8 h	Extended GNR, GPC
Fluoroquinolones	Ciprofloxacin	0.2–0.4 g q12 h	Extended GNR
Aminoglycosides	Gentamicin	5–7 mg/kg q24 h*	Extended GNR
	Amikacin	15 mg/kg q24 h*	Extended GNR
Antistaphylococcal penicillins	Flucloxacillin	1–2 g q4–6 h	GPC
	Nafcillin	1–2 g q4 h	GPC
Glycopeptides	Vancomycin	15 mg/kg q12 h†	Extended GPC
	Teicoplanin	12 mg/kg q12 h‡	Extended GPC
	Oxazolidinone linezolid§	600 mg q12 h	Extended GPC
Macrolides	Erythromycin	15 mg/kg q6 h	GPC, *Legionella* spp.
Imidazoles	Fluconazole§	0.2–0.4 g q24 h	*Candida* spp.
Metronidazole	Metronidazole§	0.5 g q8 h	Anaerobes

*Trough serum levels should be kept below 1 μg/mL.
†Trough serum levels should be kept between 5 and 10 μg/mL.
‡Following loading with 12 mg/kg q12 h for three doses.
§Oral equivalent to intravenous dosing.
GPC, Gram-positive cocci (methicillin-susceptible *Staphylococcus aureus*, Streptococci); GNR, Gram-negative rods (*Escherichia coli*); Extended GNR (*Pseudomonas aeruginosa*); Extended GPC [methicillin-resistant *Staphylococcus aureus*, coagulase-negative staphylococci (CONS), Streptococci].

Clinical case

Diagnostic workup and treatment of a 'septic case':

A 54-year-old man is admitted with high fever and abdominal pain. He has tenderness and guarding in the right upper quadrant. He develops respiratory failure and hypotension. Blood count reveals neutrophilia. Inflammatory markers (C-reactive protein and erythrocyte sedimentation rate) are raised. Serum amylase and renal function tests are normal. Liver function tests show a cholestatic picture. The prothrombin time is lengthened by 5 s. Blood cultures grow *Escherichia coli* at 24 h. Urine microscopy and culture show no abnormalities. The chest radiograph suggests atelectasis in the right lower lobe. A computerised tomography scan of the abdomen is shown (Fig. 1). How should he be treated?

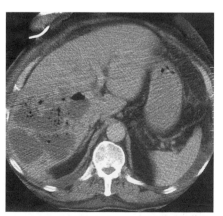

Fig. 1 **CT scan of the abdomen showing a large liver abscess.**

Summary points

- Basic principles of infection control, including hand hygiene and universal precautions, should be adhered to rigorously.
- Antibiotics should be used judiciously and according to local, national or international policy.
- Antibiotics with the narrowest spectrum should be given orally when possible and for short courses.

Sepsis and septic shock: aetiology and pathophysiology

Aetiology and pathophysiology

The sepsis syndrome occurs as a consequence of the complex interaction between host and invading pathogen. Sepsis is best regarded as a spectrum of disorders on a continuum, with localised inflammation at one end and severe generalised inflammatory response with multiorgan failure at the other end (Fig. 1). Increasing mortality rates are associated with progression along the continuum. Bacteria are commonly responsible for sepsis, particularly *Staphylococcus aureus*, *Escherichia coli* and *Streptococcus pneumoniae*. Other organisms, such as *Candida albicans*, are important in health care settings and, in areas of the world where malaria is prevalent, *Plasmodium falciparum* is frequently the aetiology. Typical syndromes associated with sepsis are pneumonia, urinary sepsis, intra-abdominal sepsis, and skin and soft tissue infection. See Boxes 1–4.

Bacterial components such as endotoxin and lipoteichoic acid, through their action on neutrophils and macrophages, induce a wide range of proinflammatory factors, including tumour necrosis factor (TNF)α and interleukin (IL)-1 and IL-6, and counter-regulatory host responses, IL-4 and IL-10, that turn off production of the proinflammatory cytokines. Recently, the pivotal roles of toll-like receptors on cell surfaces have been recognised in binding to bacterial components and in promoting cytokine production and cellular activation. Normally, there is a balance between pro- and anti-inflammatory responses. As a result of sepsis, the proinflammatory reaction (systemic inflammatory response syndrome or SIRS) can cascade out of control, with activation of complement, coagulation, widespread arterial vasodilatation and altered capillary permeability. A range of abnormalities may result, leading to multiorgan dysfunction and death. If there is a predominance of the compensatory anti-inflammatory response syndrome (CARS), which often occurs subsequently, patients become more vulnerable to infection, including opportunistic organisms (Fig. 2). SIRS and CARS are discussed more fully on p. 158. The complications of sepsis are shown in Figure 3.

Box 1. Ruminations on sepsis

'Sepsis is a classical example of a disease greater than the sum of its parts. It is a complex process in which intervention in one area might have only a modest effect in the overall outcome' (J . Cohen, 1992, *Mediators of Sepsis*).

'Septic shock leads to a state of metabolic anarchy in which the body can no longer control its own inflammatory response' (R.C. Bone, 1993, *Ann Intern Med*).

'Except on a few occasions the patient appears to die from the body's response to infection rather than from the infection itself' (William Osler, 1904, *The Evolution of Modern Medicine*).

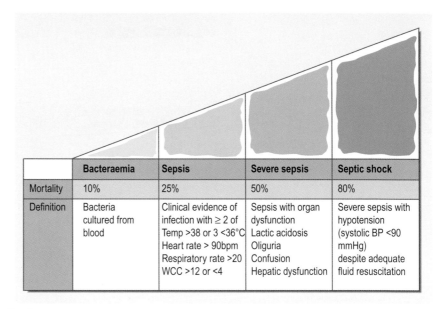

	Bacteraemia	Sepsis	Severe sepsis	Septic shock
Mortality	10%	25%	50%	80%
Definition	Bacteria cultured from blood	Clinical evidence of infection with ≥ 2 of Temp >38 or 3 <36°C Heart rate > 90bpm Respiratory rate >20 WCC >12 or <4	Sepsis with organ dysfunction Lactic acidosis Oliguria Confusion Hepatic dysfunction	Severe sepsis with hypotension (systolic BP <90 mmHg) despite adequate fluid resuscitation

Fig. 1 **Continuum of sepsis with definitions and approximate mortality rates** [adapted from Bone *et al*. (1992) *JAMA* 268: 3452–3455 with permission].

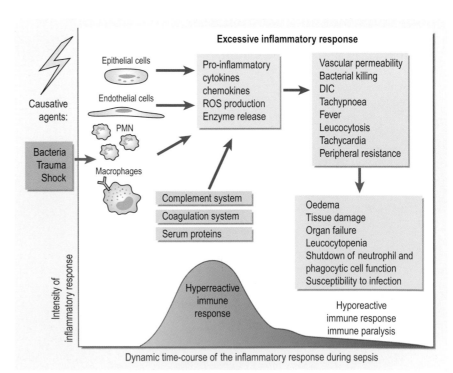

Fig. 2 **The time course of the inflammatory response during sepsis** [from Riedemann (2003) *Nature Med* 9: 517 with permission].

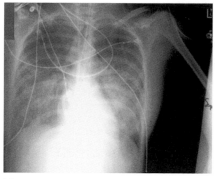

(a)

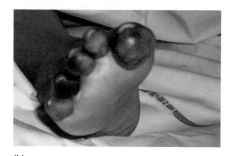

(b)

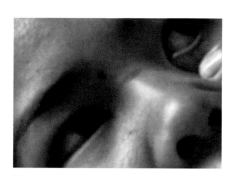

(c)

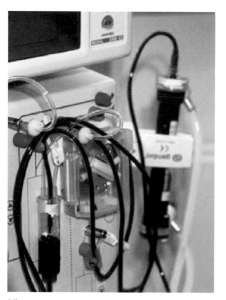

(d)

Fig. 3 Complications of sepsis: respiratory distress (a), hypoperfusion with gangrenous digits (b), jaundice (c) and renal failure (d).

Box 2. *Intensive insulin therapy in critical*

Hyperglycaemia and insulin resistance are common in critical illness and may predispose to infections, organ failure and death. A study of patients with critical illness showed that maintaining blood glucose between 80 and 110 mg/dL (4.4–6.1 mmol/L) using intravenous insulin resulted in fewer episodes of bacteraemia, reduction in rates of organ failure and reduced mortality. Keeping blood glucose below 150 mg/dl (8.3 mmol/L) may be as effective and associated with fewer episodes of hypoglycaemia.

Box 3. *What's new in sepsis?*

Recombinant human activated protein C (rhAPC)

Recent trials have shown that early administration of rhAPC may be associated with reduction in mortality (number needed to treat = 16) due to severe sepsis. RhAPC may have both anticoagulant and anti-inflammatory properties. This therapy is not without its detractors who point out that:

- It only seems to benefit the sicker patients (APACHE II score ≥25)
- It is not a benign therapy and increases the risk of dangerous bleeding
- Different batches of rhAPC may differ in their efficacy
- There are many cheap therapies of proven efficacy, which have been displaced from the limelight by rhAPC. An example is early administration of appropriate antimicrobial therapy
- It is an expensive treatment. Health care resources may be more sensibly allocated.

Vasopressin

Vasopressin, as its name suggests, has a direct vasoconstrictor effect. It has relatively little direct effect on either heart rate or cardiac output, unlike epinephrine, which is inotropic and is associated with tachycardia. However, a little goes a long way, and higher doses than those suggested have been associated with myocardial ischaemia and reduced cardiac output, especially in patients with cardiac disease. Vasopressin is usually reserved for refractory shock.

Sepsis and septic shock: treatment

Box 4. *Early goal-directed therapy for the treatment of sepsis and shock*

Rapid attention to the correction of metabolic and haemodynamic parameters has been shown to improve survival in patients with septic shock. Rapid recognition of septic shock is imperative, as is prompt administration of antibiotics. The initial goals of resuscitation using invasive monitoring, fluid resuscitation and vasopressor therapy are:

- Central venous pressure of between 8 and 12 cmH$_2$O
- Mean arterial pressure ≥65 mmHg
- Urine output ≥0.5 mL/kg/h
- Central venous or mixed venous oxygen saturation ≥ 70% (Fig. 4).

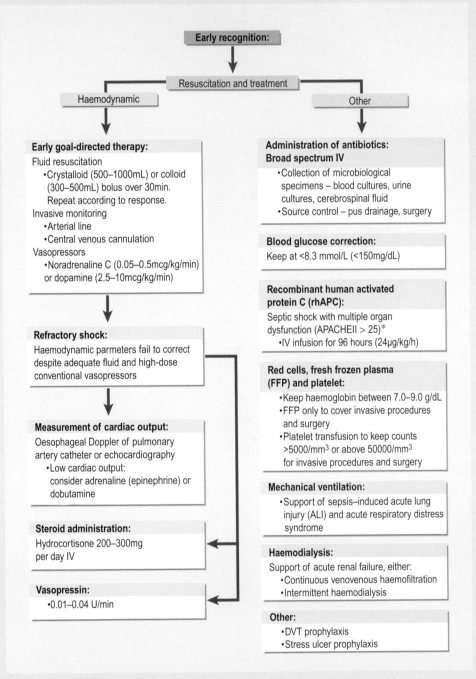

Fig. 4 **Flow chart outlining the treatment of sepsis and shock.** *The use of rhAPC for sepsis is controversial (http://content.nejm.org/cgi/content/full/355/16/1640).

Clinical case

An 18-year-old female college student was admitted with a history, given by her mother, of having been very unwell overnight. She had developed a flu-like illness with fever and shakes and had diarrhoea during the night. By morning, her mother had noticed a rash over the limbs and had brought her to hospital. On examination, she was unwell. There was a coalescing purpuric rash over the limbs, face and trunks (Fig. 5). She was drowsy, but could answer questions. She was febrile, 39°C, her pulse was 110/min and regular, respiratory rate was 30 breaths/min and her blood pressure was 86/33 units. A clinical diagnosis of meningococcal sepsis was made, and she was given 2.4 g of benzyl penicillin IV after blood cultures had been taken. Investigations revealed evidence of severe sepsis with multiorgan dysfunction and shock:

- Raised inflammatory markers: C-reactive protein (CRP) >285 mg/L; white cell count 18 000/mm³
- Renal impairment: urea 8.5 mmol/L (blood urea nitrogen=24 mg/dL); creatinine 186 Umol/L (2.1 mg/dL); urine output <10 mL/h
- Deranged liver function test: albumin 27 g/L; bilirubin 21 Umol/L; alanine aminotransferase (ALT) 75 IU/L; alkaline phosphate (ALP) 323 IU/L
- Disseminated intravascular coagulation: platelet count 82×10⁹/L; prothrombin time 22.5 s; activated partial thromboplastin time 189 s; elevated D-dimers
- Lactic acidosis: lactate 4.0 mmol/L; base excess – 6.5 mmol/L.
- Acute lung injury (ALI): chest radiograph. Arterial blood gas: pH 7.50; P_{CO_2}=2.8 kPa (21 mmHg); P_{O_2}=7.47 kPa (56 mmHg) on room air (P_aO_2/F_iO_2=267)
- Positive blood cultures: *Neisseria meningitidis* isolated after 24 h.
- How would you treat this patient?

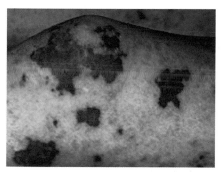

Fig. 5 **Purpuric rash of meningococcal septicaemia.**

Summary points

- Sepsis syndrome is the body's response to a number of diverse pathogens.
- Prompt recognition, early goal-directed resuscitation and administration of antibiotics are key to damage limitation.
- Close regulation of blood glucose with insulin and physiological steroid therapy may have a therapeutic role.
- Novel therapies such as rhAPC and vasopressin may be useful.

Central nervous system infection

Infections of the nervous system are devastating conditions that can progress rapidly and produce death or serious disability in a short period of time.

Sites where central nervous system (CNS) infection can occur are shown in Fig. 1. The more prevalent CNS infections are acute bacterial meningitis and viral meningoencephalitis. In some areas of the world, chronic tuberculous meningitis is a common condition. Intracerebral abscess and subdural empyema occur rarely, but are associated with serious neurological impairment.

Acute bacterial meningitis

Acute bacterial meningitis develops over hours or days. The common pathogens in adults are *Neisseria meningitidis* and *Streptococcus pneumoniae*. The combination of fever, headache, neck stiffness and photophobia should alert the clinician to a possible diagnosis of acute bacterial meningitis. Alterations in mental status may occur.

Bacterial pathogens causing meningitis normally gain access to the body by adherence to and colonisation of nasopharyngeal membranes. Entry to the bloodstream seems to occur at this site, with invasion of the meninges probably occurring through the choroid plexuses. Cerebrospinal fluid (CSF) examination is key to the diagnosis of bacterial meningitis, and typical findings are indicated in Table 1. It is important to exclude raised intracranial pressure (ICP) before undertaking lumbar puncture (LP) for CSF examination. This is best done by computerised tomography (CT) or magnetic resonance imaging (MRI) scanning. Clinical findings of impaired consciousness and focal neurological signs are indicators of raised ICP. In the absence of such findings, then a LP can be done without a scan.

Prompt implementation of therapy is essential. It is normal practice to collect a blood culture and then to administer antibiotics and steroids. The evidence for the use of steroids in the treatment of *Haemophilus* meningitis in children is fairly strong, and there is a growing body of evidence that steroids have a beneficial effect in adults with meningitis. Steroids (dexamethasone 0.15 mg/kg every 6 h intravenously), commenced with antibiotics or 15 min previously, are continued for 2–4 days. Antibiotic therapy is continued for 7 days for *N. meningitidis* and *H. influenzae* and for 10–14 days for *S. pneumoniae*. In most cases, benzyl penicillin 2.4 g given every 4 h is effective. Many areas of the world have high levels of resistance to penicillin in *S. pneumoniae*.

Carbapenem antibiotics or third-generation cephalosporins with vancomycin will be appropriate in such circumstances.

Neurological sequelae are common after acute bacterial meningitis. Sensorineural hearing loss may occur in up to one-third of cases. Hydrocephalus, cognitive impairment and cortical blindness are other adverse events. Mortality rates remain high; some 50% of patients presenting with coma will die despite intensive therapy.

Viral encephalitis

Invasion of the brain tissue by virus particles is termed viral encephalitis. This serious condition is rare but is associated with high mortality and, in survivors, with a high incidence of neurological sequelae. Numerous viruses can invade the brain, the commonest worldwide are arboviruses (such as West Nile virus), rabies, Japanese B encephalitis and Herpes simplex virus (HSV).

HSV encephalitis (HSE) causes haemorrhagic necrosis of the brain, with a predilection for the temporal lobes. Typical presentation involves a non-specific prodrome or flu-like illness. This is followed by headache and drowsiness. There may be behavioural change, visual hallucinations, seizures and coma.

Diagnosis is based upon clinical findings and examination of CSF. Typically, there is a lymphocytic proliferation, protein and red cells may be elevated. CSF glucose is usually normal, but is occasionally reduced. Imaging is best done

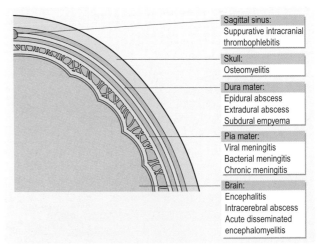

Sagittal sinus:
Suppurative intracranial thrombophlebitis

Skull:
Osteomyelitis

Dura mater:
Epidural abscess
Extradural abscess
Subdural empyema

Pia mater:
Viral meningitis
Bacterial meningitis
Chronic meningitis

Brain:
Encephalitis
Intracerebral abscess
Acute disseminated encephalomyelitis

Fig. 1 **Central nervous system infection.**

Table 1 **Cerebrospinal fluid findings**				
Parameter	Normal	Bacterial meningitis	Viral meningoencephalitis	TB meningitis
Appearance	Clear	Cloudy	Clear/cloudy	Clear/cloudy
Cell count (cells/mm)	<3 (mononuclear)	>500 predominantly neutrophils	<100 predominantly lymphocytes	<1500 predominantly lymphocytes
Protein (mg/dL)	30–45	>150	>100	>180
CSF/serum glucose ratio	0.6	<0.4	0.6	<0.6
Pressure (mmHg)	<18	>18	<18 (may be slightly increased)	>18
Grams stain	No organisms	Positive in 70–80%	No organisms	No organisms
Ziehl–Neelsen	–	–	–	Positive in 30–90%

Example of table: CSF findings in meningitis

with MRI, where available. Temporal lobe necrosis is often evident (Fig. 2). Electroencephalography is also abnormal. Polymerase chain reaction (PCR) amplification of viral nucleic acid in CSF has obviated the need for biopsy in recent times. PCR is thought to have a sensitivity of above 95% and a specificity of almost 100% in the diagnosis of HSE.

Treatment with intravenous aciclovir has greatly improved the outlook for HSE, but specific treatments are not available for many other viral encephalitides.

Tuberculous meningitis

Meningitis resulting from *Mycobacterium tuberculosis* (TBM) remains a common problem in Asia and sub-Saharan Africa. The high incidence of human immunodeficiency virus (HIV) infection in these areas of the world has greatly increased the problem of tuberculosis, so that it is now a public health disaster in large parts of the world.

TBM tends to present with symptoms of fever, weight loss and headache being present for several weeks prior to admission. Cranial nerve palsies are common. Clinical staging has been used to relate clinical presentation to expected prognosis with treatment. The patient is said to have stage 1 disease if rational with no focal neurological signs or hydrocephalus, stage 2 if there is confusion or focal neurology and stage 3 if the patient is stuporous or has hemiparesis.

Diagnosis is based upon clinical findings and CSF examination showing elevated protein, reduced glucose and elevated white cell counts, usually with lymphocytosis. Staining of spun CSF deposit for the presence of acid-fast bacilli can reveal the diagnosis in about a third of cases, and TB culture may be

positive in a few more, but many cases have no confirmatory diagnosis by detection of the bacilli. PCR for TB has also been disappointing in this respect. CT and MRI scans of the brain are frequently abnormal with basal meningitis and focal lesions.

Treatment usually consists of four-drug antituberculous therapy with rifampicin, isoniazid, ethambutol and pyrazinamide for the initial 2 months of treatment, then continuing with rifampicin and isoniazid for the remainder of treatment. There is no consensus on the total duration of treatment, and advice varies from 6 to 12 months. Adjunctive steroid treatment is normally given for stage 2 or 3 disease, such as prednisolone (1 mg/kg), reducing over 4–6 weeks.

Cerebral abscess and subdural empyema

Chronic infection of the paranasal sinuses or otitis media can result in intracranial infection. Infection spreads contiguously through bony structures, such as the petrous temporal bone, or through venous drainage emissaries. Intracranial infection is usually either abscess formation (Fig. 3) or subdural empyema.

Patients usually complain of the symptoms of sinusitis, congestion and nasal discharge, which have often been present for months or weeks. This is followed by progressive drowsiness, confusion, headaches and focal neurological signs, indicating intracranial involvement.

Abnormalities are usually evident on CT or MRI scans of the head, revealing opacification of sinuses, bony erosion and the presence of an empyema or abscess. Definitive microbiological

diagnosis can be made at surgical drainage of the abscess or empyema, which usually entails craniotomy. Typical organisms cultured include *Streptococcus milleri group, Strep. pneumoniae, Staphylococcus aureus, Haemophilus influenzae* and anaerobic bacteria.

Surgical drainage is advocated together with prolonged intravenous antibiotic therapy of 4–6 weeks' duration. Oral follow-on antibiotics can be given for a further 4–6 weeks.

Clinical case

A 36-year-old woman was admitted after having developed a left-sided weakness that had come on gradually over 2 days. Her family said that she had then become aphasic and they had been unable to get her out of bed. An MRI scan was carried out and revealed multiple demyelinating areas (Fig. 4). She had recently been diagnosed with her first episode of genital herpes. What is your diagnosis? Suggest a management plan.

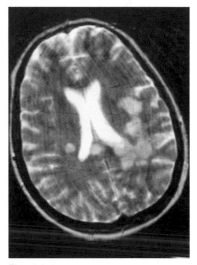

Fig. 4 **MRI scan showing multiple areas of demyelination.**

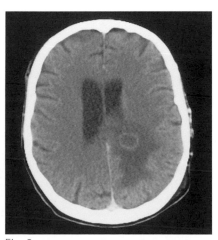

Fig. 3 **CT scan revealing cerebral abscess with surrounding oedema and mass effect.**

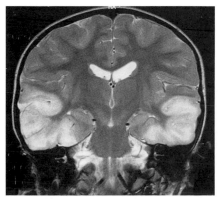

Fig. 2 **MRI scan of a patient with HSE.**

Summary points

- If you suspect meningitis, do not wait for scans or LP results: take a blood culture, then administer antibiotics.
- LP is contraindicated if intracranial abscess or empyema is suspected or shown on brain scanning.
- PCR of virus from the CSF is useful in identifying viral causes of encephalitis.
- Steroids may be useful adjuncts in the treatment of meningitis.
- Empyema, like other pus collections, should be drained.

Pneumonia

Community-acquired pneumonia

Community-acquired pneumonia (CAP) is a frequent cause of hospital admission, and the mortality of patients admitted to intensive care units (ICUs) with CAP is about 50%. *Streptococcus pneumoniae* is the most common pathogen and may be responsible for at least 40% of CAP, but aetiology is not identified in up to half the cases.

CAP typically presents abruptly with the triad of symptoms of fever, pleuritic chest pain and cough. Patients are usually pyrexial and dyspnoeic with chest signs such as crepitations and bronchial breathing located to one or more zones of the chest. Lobar consolidation is evident on chest radiographs (Fig. 1).

There is a spectrum of disease in CAP. Many patients may be treated at home with oral antibiotic therapy (Box 1). Those more severely affected require hospital admission for parenteral antibiotics and oxygen therapy (Box 1). Some of these require care in the ICU because of respiratory failure or severe sepsis. Assessment of severity is important and has prognostic implications. Using the CURB-65 score of severity, mortality rates from 2.4% to 83% are associated with the presence of one and four CURB markers respectively (Box 2).

Although CAP can affect healthy adults, a preponderance of people affected are old or have pre-existing medical conditions. Targeted history may suggest unusual pathogens. With caving and diving, the fungi *Histoplasma capsulatum* and *Scedosporium angiospermum* respectively have been implicated. Hunting in North America increases the risk for bacterial *Francisella tularensis* pneumonia. *Legionella pneumophila* pneumonia outbreaks have been described with exposure to hotel air conditioners and whirlpools. Overseas travel to Asia may be associated with viral pneumonia including severe acute respiratory syndrome (SARS) or H5N1 avian influenza. Farm visits and contact with newborn lambs or sheep placenta are associated with bacterial *Coxiella burnetti* (Q fever) pneumonia. Sick birds may transmit the bacterium *Chlamydia psittaci* (psittacosis). Alcoholic binges increase the risk for bacterial aspiration pneumonia with pathogens such as *Klebsiella pneumoniae*. Immunocompromised patients such as those with AIDS are at risk for fungal pneumonia such as *Pneumocystis carinii* and *Cryptococcus neoformans* pneumonia.

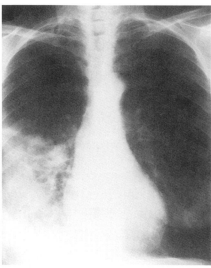

Fig. 1 **A chest radiograph with lobar consolidation of CAP.**

Box 1. *Initial management of the patient with CAP*

- Fluid resuscitation
- Oxygen therapy: aim to keep P_aO_2 >8 KPa (60 mmHg) and S_aO_2 >92%
- Antibiotics: intravenous for severe cases. Typically, a beta-lactam antibiotic, such as ampicillin, co-amoxiclav or cefuroxime, plus a macrolide such as erythromycin or clarithromycin. Alternatively, a fluoroquinolone, such as levofloxacin or moxifloxacin
- Investigations: arterial blood gases, C-reactive protein, chest radiograph, full blood count, blood glucose, renal and liver function, serum electrolytes, blood cultures, electrocardiograph
- Further investigations: bronchoscopy, pleural fluid aspiration, urine test for *Legionella* antigen detection

Notes of caution:
Point 1: Sputum culture is often recommended but difficult to interpret given the frequency of nasopharyngeal carriage of *Streptococcus pneumoniae*.
Point 2: *Mycobacterium tuberculosis* is a rare cause of respiratory failure. Have a high index of suspicion and request sputum or bronchial washing examinations for acid-fast bacilli.

Box 2. *Assessment of the severity of CAP*

Factors associated with a poor prognosis

Age over 50 years
Presence of coexisting disease
Hypoxaemia [p_aO_2 <8 kPa (60 mmHg), S_aO_2 <92%]
Multilobar/bilateral disease evident on chest radiograph

CURB-65 score (advocated by British Thoracic Society)

Confusion: abbreviated mental test score 8 or less
Urea: raised >7 mmol/L (blood urea nitrogen >20 mg/dL)
Respiratory rate: raised >30 breaths/min
Blood pressure: systolic <90 or diastolic <60 mmHg
65, age over
CURB-65 score of 3 or more defines severe CAP.

Hospital-acquired pneumonia

Pneumonia occurring after 48 h of hospital admission is known as hospital-acquired pneumonia (HAP). Approximately 1% of patients acquire HAP, but rates as high as 50% have been recorded in patients undergoing mechanical ventilation. The attributable mortality of HAP may be 30–50%.

HAP has a multifactorial aetiology, involving host factors such as immobility and lowered immunity due to intercurrent illness and premorbid conditions. Contributing factors are instrumentation of the respiratory tract during intubation or bronchoscopy and reduction of cough reflex owing to drugs and impaired consciousness. Foreign bodies, including tracheal tubes and tracheostomies, breach the usual physical barrier to the lungs and provide colonising bugs with a convenient portal of entry. Treatment with broad-spectrum antibiotics encourages colonisation of the respiratory tract with resistant flora found in hospitals, such as

Pseudomonas aeruginosa, methicillin-resistant *Staphylococcus aureus* (MRSA) and the Enterobacteriaceae. Aspiration of colonising bacteria is believed to be the usual mechanism of infection. Haematogenous seeding of the lungs is a less frequent aetiology.

Diagnosis of HAP is based upon clinical findings of fever, purulent sputum production and increasing oxygen requirements with laboratory evidence of leucocytosis and chest radiograph findings of new or worsening shadowing (Fig. 2). HAP should be distinguished from other conditions, which may present similarly in hospitalised patients, such as pulmonary embolism and congestive cardiac failure.

Obtaining sputum for microbiological review allows identification of possible pathogens. Non-directed bronchial lavage through a standard suction catheter passed down the endotracheal tube is straightforward and minimally invasive. Quantitative bacterial counts have been carried out on such specimens and have correlated with the likelihood of ventilator-associated pneumonia (VAP). Blood cultures may be positive in up to one-fifth of cases. More invasive techniques, including bronchoscopic lavage and protected brush specimens taken through a bronchoscope, are more sensitive and specific for the diagnosis of VAP, but require skilled operators and may not be available in all centres.

Empirical treatment of HAP should be guided by local policy. Typically, an antipseudomonal penicillin, such as ceftazidime or pipericillin–tazobactam, in combination with an aminoglycoside such as gentamicin would be suitable. Where MRSA prevalence is high, vancomycin should be added to this regimen (Box 3).

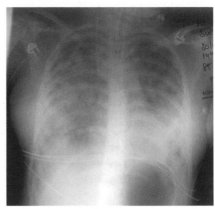

Fig. 2 **Chest radiograph of ventilator-associated pneumonia.**
Widespread air space shadowing is present in this case of severe ventilator-associated pneumonia.

Clinical case

A 52-year-old male smoker who works as an air-conditioning engineer presents with fever and cough. He is found to be in respiratory failure and is transferred to the ICU for intubation and mechanical ventilation. His chest radiograph is pictured (Fig. 3). What diagnoses are you suspecting and how would you investigate and manage this case?

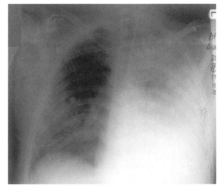

Fig. 3 **Chest radiograph of the patient described above.**

Box 3. *Virulent viral vectors of pneumonia*

Viral causes of pneumonia have hit the headlines in recent years.

SARS was first described in 2003 in Asia and is caused by the SARS coronavirus. Most cases have occurred in various countries in Asia and present with fever, cough and respiratory distress. Mortality rates were about 10%. No antiviral therapy has been shown to be effective. Strict adherence to contact and airborne precautions is required as health care workers treating affected patients have themselves become victims.

Strains of *avian influenza A* are causing chaos in poultry farms in south and east Asia. H5N1 is a particularly worrisome strain of influenza A. First seen in 1997 in Hong Kong, it is associated with severe disease with mortality in humans in excess of 60%. Currently, H5N1 does not seem to be readily transmissible from human to human, but should it reassort with one of the more common human influenzas, it may become a readily transmissible deadly virus, and the next influenza pandemic will be under way. Specific antiviral therapy is now available for influenza. Where the risk of severe infection is high, such as in patients with immunosuppression or chronic respiratory or cardiac disease, treatment early in the infection with neuraminidase inhibitors, such as zanamivir or oseltamivir, is indicated.

Local policy should be followed when viral pneumonia is suspected.

Summary points

- *Streptococcus pneumoniae* is the most common pathogen causing CAP.
- Pneumonia occurring after 48 h of hospital admission is known as hospital-acquired pneumonia.
- Assessing the severity of pneumonia helps the clinician to decide whether ICU admission is advisable.
- Detailed history may point to 'atypical' causes of pneumonia.
- SARS and influenza are two viral causes of severe pneumonia.

Infections associated with prosthetic material in the ICU

The range of prosthetic devices in use is ever increasing in sophistication and duration of use, from a few hours or days to lifelong placement. Septic complications can be common (ventriculostomy) or very unusual (arterial stents or coils).

General principles of infected prosthetic material include:

- Early infection is often associated with *Staphylococcus aureus* and other higher virulence organisms
- Later infection may be associated with lower virulence organisms of the skin flora
- Infections are often chronic and suppurative
- Infections are rarely cured without the removal of infected prosthetic material
- Infections often require prolonged intravenous therapy.

Intravascular cannulae and infection

There are multiple types of intravascular cannulae. The peripheral venous catheter is designed for short-term use. Such catheters are normally made of polyurethane or similar material and should be removed at 48–72 h or before if signs of inflammation are present (Box 1).

Central venous catheters, placed in femoral, jugular or subclavian veins, can be used for longer periods of time. Longer term central vein cannulae designed to remain in situ for months are tunnelled subcutaneously or located subcutaneously with a reservoir. Such catheters are used for

chemotherapy in cancer and for haemodialysis.

Pathogenesis of infection of intravascular cannulae

Infection typically occurs after 1–30/1000 days of use. Insertion of the device is associated with a breakdown of natural barriers to infection and is often mediated by the tracking of organisms along the external surface of the catheter. There may be contamination of the hub with distal spread of infection along the cannula lumen. In rare cases, there may be contamination of the infusate or haematogenous seeding of the device (Box 2 and Box 3).

Clinical signs of intravascular cannula infection

Infection can be localised, where there is erythema, pain and warmth of the cannula exit site. Local spread may

Box 2. Biofilm formation and intravascular cannula infection

Some organisms, particularly coagulase-negative staphylococci (CONS), are able to produce complex polysaccharides, which diffuse into the extracellular material and produce a slime or biofilm (Fig. 1). Slime helps organisms to colonise biomaterials and to resist the action of antibiotics, and is very difficult to remove other than by device removal.

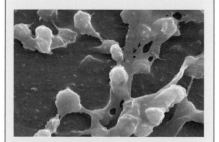

Fig. 1 **Staphylococci surrounded by a sticky biofilm** (CONS) (courtesy of Dr R.M. Donlan and Dr J. Carr).

Box 1. Factors associated with infection in intravascular cannulae

- Longer duration
- Break in asepsis during placement or use
- Manipulation of the device
- Composition (polytetrafluoroethylene worse than polyurethane)
- Central site, especially groin.

result in septic thrombophlebitis with induration of the vein, redness spreading away from the cannula, pus or abscess formation in tissues around and within the vein. Generalised infection and bacteraemia are associated with positive blood cultures and systemic upset.

Management of intravascular cannula infection

Microbiological sampling, blood cultures and pus collection (if possible) should be followed by commencement of antibiotic therapy if infection rather than inflammation is felt to be present. Broad-spectrum treatment with an agent that has good activity against common pathogens, such as cefuroxime, should be commenced. Local prevalence of methicillin-resistant *Staphylococcus aureus* (MRSA) or knowledge of previous infection may influence therapy in individual cases and result in broader therapy with vancomycin or other agents. In most cases, line removal will be necessary. Indications for line removal would include abscess formation at the line site, difficult to treat organisms [e.g. vancomycin-resistant Enterococci (VRE) or *Candida*] and failure of clinical or microbiological response within 48–72 h (Table 1).

Urinary catheter-associated infections

Urinary tract infection (UTI) is the most frequent hospital-acquired infection and is the most common diagnosis in elderly people hospitalised with bacteraemia. Following the placement of an indwelling urinary catheter (IUC), acquisition of infection occurs at a rate of approximately 5% per day, and 100% of people with long-term urinary catheters will have evidence of bacteriuria, the majority without symptoms (Box 4). The normal human urethra is free of bacteria, and sterility is maintained by the flushing action of voiding of urine and the resultant complete emptying of the bladder. IUCs are associated with UTI as they overcome these defences by acting as a foreign body entering the bladder on

Table 1 Causes of intravascular cannula infection

Coagulase-negative staphylococci
Staphylococcus aureus (including MRSA)
Enterococcus species
Candida species
Coliform species (including *Escherichia coli, Serratia marcescens, Enterobacter* species)
Acinetobacter baumanii
Pseudomonas aeruginosa

Box 3. Keep it clean! Aseptic technique for line insertion (Fig. 2)

Wear sterile gloves for line insertion, and gown and mask for central lines
Clean the skin with chlorhexidine or povidone–iodine
Use large sterile drapes
Cover the inserted line with clear polyurethane dressings so that it is visible
Always wear sterile gloves when manipulating the line
Catheters impregnated with antibiotics, such as doxycycline, and antibacterials, such as silver, are associated with lower infection rates.

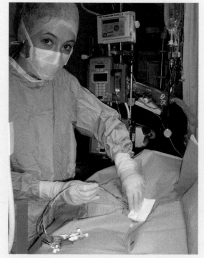

Fig. 2 **Keep it clean! Aseptic technique for line insertion.**

Box 4. Measures for the prevention of UTI in the patient with an IUC

- Aim for early removal of the IUC
- Always use a closed urinary system
- Aseptic technique should be maintained.

which a biofilm containing bacteria develops, which cannot then be eradicated. The organisms are then able to gain access to the bladder through ascension of the IUC.

The spectrum of organisms in IUC-associated infection is different from that in uncomplicated UTIs. Although *Escherichia coli* is still common, there is an increased prevalence of Gram-negative organisms with more resistant antibiotic profiles, such as *Enterobacter* species and *Pseudomonas aeruginosa*, as well as Gram-positive organisms, particularly MRSA and *Candida*.

The clinical presentation of UTI associated with IUCs can be varied, from asymptomatic bacteriuria to septic shock and death. The infection can be located within the bladder only (cystitis) or may spread to involve the kidneys (pyelonephritis) and prostate gland (prostatitis). Abscess formation can occur, usually perinephric or prostatic in location. Pyelonephritis and abscess formation tend to be associated with a more severe illness with systemic features of severe sepsis and positive blood cultures.

Definitive diagnosis of UTI in catheterised patients is difficult. Urine can be collected for microbiological examination by aseptic aspiration from the urinary catheter port. As biofilms are frequently present in such catheters, urine samples are frequently abnormal and often contain bacteria, thus the significance of positive cultures is difficult to determine. A clinical diagnosis is often required and is assisted by the exclusion of other sources of infection.

Suitable intravenous therapy includes a beta-lactam antibiotic with broad spectrum, such as cefuroxime, often in combination with an aminoglycoside antibiotic. Oral agents used for UTI include trimethoprim, nitrofurantoin and fluoroquinolones. If MRSA is suspected or isolated, vancomycin is the drug of choice.

Duration of therapy should be kept to a minimum of 5–7 days in less severe cases associated with an IUC, but should be continued for 14 days if pyelonephritis is suspected. Change of IUC is normally only required if it is blocked or malfunctioning. The need for further imaging of the urinary tract should be considered if structural abnormality is suspected.

Clinical case

Mrs MD is a 67-year-old lady with chronic renal failure in the ICU with severe community-acquired pneumonia. She has had a right jugular vein central line placed. Intravenous cefuroxime and erythromycin have been started. Her initial response to therapy was good. Four days later, she became septic and unwell. Her right jugular line was removed. A swelling was noted around the right side of the neck extending up to the face (Fig. 3). What is the likely diagnosis and what is the appropriate management?

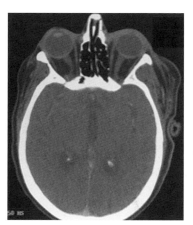

Fig. 3 **CT scan with extensive soft tissue swelling extending from neck to parotid area.**

Summary points

- Prosthetic material infection is a modern epidemic in medicine.
- Antibiotics alone are unlikely to cure implanted prosthetic material infections.
- Strict asepsis and hygiene is required when placing or manipulating an intravascular catheter.
- Urinary tract sepsis associated with long-term catheters can become complicated with abscess formation.

The immunocompromised patient in critical care

Reduction in host immunity, whether as a result of a disease process or a therapeutic procedure, is associated with an increased occurrence of infection in the affected host. This is particularly pertinent currently as major advances have taken place in the development of treatments for cancers and the transplantation of solid organs, resulting in growing numbers of people with impaired immunity. In addition, since its first descriptions in the early 1980s, a catastrophic pandemic of virally induced immunodeficiency (HIV, human immunodeficiency virus) is taking place, especially in areas of the world, such as Asia and sub-Saharan Africa, where resources for health care are often very poor.

The host–parasite relationship and the development of disease are dependent upon multiple factors. Two key aspects are the virulence of the pathogen, which is directly related to the development of infective disease, and the immunity of the host, which is indirectly related. High-virulence pathogens, such as severe acute respiratory syndrome (SARS), tend to cause disease whenever they meet a human host, whereas lower virulence organisms, such as *Streptococcus oralis* (part of the oral flora), only result in disease where there is impaired host immunity.

There are several important categories of impaired immunity; these include granulocytopenia and disorders of neutrophil function, cellular and humoral immune dysfunction and splenectomised patients, as illustrated by the cases opposite.

Granulocytopenia is a common complication of the treatment of haematological malignancy with chemotherapy or bone marrow transplantation. The risk of infection increases with falling granulocyte counts and is very high at counts below 500 cells/mm³ (0.5 cells×10⁹/L). Commonly, infection arises at sites such as the oropharynx, gastrointestinal tract and respiratory tract, and bloodstream invasion is common. The causative species are often those associated with normal flora, *Escherichia coli, viridans group streptococcus* and coagulase-negative staphylococcus.

Impaired cellular immunity occurs in HIV infection and lymphomas. It can also be a consequence of the use of cytotoxic drugs for the treatment of cancer and immunosuppressive drugs such as ciclosporin A for the prevention of rejection in organ transplantation. This type of immunodeficiency results in the predisposition to a range of opportunistic pathogens, many of which are reactivated latent pathogens. Common infections are toxoplasmosis, *Mycobacterium tuberculosis, Mycobacterium avium* complex, PCP and the herpes group viruses (cytomegalovirus, herpes simplex virus and varicella zoster virus).

Defects in humoral immunity due to antibody deficiency are commonly seen in haematological disorders such as chronic lymphocytic leukaemia, multiple myeloma and common variable hypogammaglobulinaemia. There is a high risk of bacterial infections, especially those that are encapsulated, such as *Haemophilus influenzae, S. pneumoniae* and *Neisseria meningitidis*. Recurrent respiratory tract infections and bacteraemia occur. Treatment with intravenous immunoglobulin may be given in severe cases.

Splenectomy, both primary due to excision of the spleen and secondary due to a number of other conditions, including sickle cell anaemia, is associated with a defect in the handling of encapsulated bacteria such as *S. pneumoniae, N. meningitidis* and *H. influenzae* type b (Hib). Splenectomised individuals are at risk of developing of overwhelming infection, which can result in multiorgan failure and death, within hours of the onset of symptoms. Prophylaxis against the development of severe sepsis involves the administration of penicillin or amoxicillin prophylaxis. Prophylaxis is normally given for a minimum of 2 years. Vaccination against *S. pneumoniae, N. meningitidis* and Hib should be offered. Patients should be educated about the risks and offered expectant early empiric therapy, such as amoxicillin tablets.

HIV and critical care

All patients should be regarded as potentially infected with blood-borne viruses, so there is no need for special precautions when dealing with patients with HIV infection. Universal precautions to implement include safe handling of

Clinical history 1

A 32-year-old man was diagnosed with acute myeloblastic leukaemia and commenced chemotherapy. After his second course, his neutrophil count dropped rapidly to 0.01 cells×10⁹/L (Fig. 1). Two days later, he felt very unwell and developed high swinging fevers and diarrhoea. On admission, he was found to have oral mucositis and was tachypnoeic. His blood pressure was 70/40 mmHg. He was transferred to the ICU. His blood pressure responded to fluid challenge and commencement of antibiotics (pipericillin–tazobactam with gentamicin). Blood cultures grew *Klebsiella pneumoniae*.

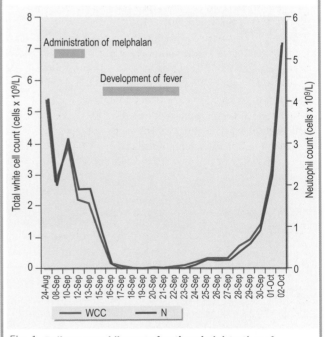

Fig. 1 **Daily neutrophil count after the administration of chemotherapy.**

Clinical history 2

A 51-year-old man was admitted to the ICU complaining of night sweats and increasing breathlessness. A chest radiograph (Fig. 2) was suggestive of PCP (*Pneumocystis carinii* pneumonia, now called *P. jiroveci*). HIV antibodies were detected, CD4 T-cell count was 6 cells/mm³ and HIV1 RNA was 750 000 copies/mL, indicating severe impairment of cellular immunity. Treatment with oxygen by face mask, steroids and sulphamethoxazole–trimethoprim (200 mg/kg) was commenced. After initial improvement, there was a sudden deterioration with respiratory distress and left shoulder tip pain. On examination, surgical emphysema was evident over the upper thorax. Chest radiograph confirmed bilateral pneumothoracies, a complication of severe PCP. Bilateral chest drains were placed, and endotracheal intubation was carried out urgently. Unfortunately, hypoxia was persistent and he died several hours after intubation.

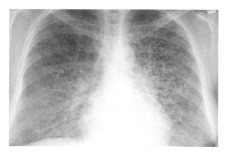

Fig. 2 **Chest radiograph** (courtesy of Dr M. Gotway).

Clinical history 3

A 78-year-old female was found unconscious at home. She had a history of chronic neck and back pain over the past 12 months. Examination revealed that she was unconscious (GCS of 5/15). She was pyrexial and had marked neck rigidity. There was increased tone and reflexes in the limbs but no other neurological findings. Bacterial meningitis or viral encephalitis was considered. Ceftriaxone 2 g intravenously twice daily was commenced, and she was transferred to the ICU. Resuscitation included elective endotracheal intubation and mechanical ventilation. A chest radiograph showed consolidation of the left lower lobe. A lumbar puncture was carried out revealing turbid cerebrospinal fluid (CSF). Laboratory analysis confirmed the presence of neutrophilia and Gram-positive organisms in the CSF, which proved to be *S. pneumoniae* (Fig. 3). CSF glucose was <1.0 mmol/L (serum 6.3 mmol/L) and protein 2132 mg/L. Treatment was changed to high-dose intravenous benzyl penicillin, according to susceptibility results. She made good progress and was discharged back to the haematology ward where bone marrow aspirate revealed >20% plasma cells, consistent with multiple myeloma.

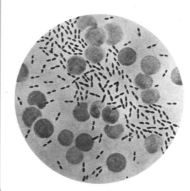

Fig. 3 **Gram stain showing neutrophils and Gram-positive cocci of *S. pneumoniae*** (courtesy of the CDC, Atlanta, GA).

Clinical history 4

A 26-year-old man was admitted to the ICU, having developed the blistering rash of chickenpox 48 h previously (Fig. 4). Tachypnoea and respiratory failure indicated chickenpox pneumonia. Endotracheal intubation and positive pressure ventilation were required. On the following day, a drop in blood pressure and haemoglobin was noted. Abdominal examination revealed marked splenomegaly, and ultrasound was consistent with splenic rupture. Urgent splenectomy was carried out. Following surgery, amoxicillin 250 mg was administered twice daily through a nasogastric tube. Plans were made for vaccination on recovery.

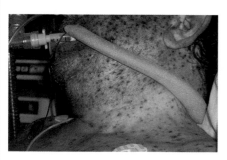

Fig. 4 **Rash of chickenpox.**

sharps, wearing of protective clothing (masks, goggles, gloves, gown) when handling body fluids, rigorous adherence to handwashing protocols and reporting any accidents with sharps or body fluids as soon as possible. It is good practice that all health care workers are vaccinated against hepatitis B virus.

Clinical case

What to do if you accidentally injure yourself with a sharp instrument?

Summary points

- Immunocompromise is an increasing problem in medicine.
- The chances of developing infection depend on the virulence of the pathogen and the nature of the immune response.
- Different infections occur according to which part of the immune system is compromised.
- Transmission of blood-borne viruses can be prevented by implementation of universal precautions.
- High-risk accidents with sharps may require the immediate administration of post-exposure prophylaxis (PEP).

Tropical medicine

Medicine in tropical areas deserves consideration for a number of reasons, not least because a large proportion of the world's population lives in tropical areas. Many tropical countries are resource poor, and spending on health may be only a few dollars per head of population per year, and even vaccine-preventable diseases, such as tetanus, diphtheria and measles, occur frequently. The returning traveller brings tropical infection to many other parts of the world. It is vital that clinicians working in non-tropical countries are aware of major tropical diseases, so that treatment opportunities are not lost. Patients with a history of travel to the tropics may present to the intensive care unit (ICU) with life-threatening illnesses whose cause and severity may not be appreciated.

There are a number of diseases, which, largely because of environmental limitation of vector species, are exclusive to tropical areas. Infections such as malaria and dengue fever result in high morbidity and mortality in local people. Global warming may have a significant effect on the epidemiology of these diseases with gradual expansion into new areas.

The pandemic of human immunodeficiency (HIV) infection cannot be underestimated, and the main burden of the epidemic is occurring in some of the poorest countries of the world. Sub-Saharan Africa is particularly affected. Common diseases, such as salmonellosis, pneumonia and tuberculosis, are burgeoning in such areas where immune competence is waning as a result of the high prevalence of HIV (Table 1).

Malaria

Malaria is a life-threatening parasitic disease, which is transmitted from person to person through the bite of a female *Anopheles* mosquito, which requires blood to nurture her eggs. Approximately 40% of the world's population, mostly in resource-poor countries, is at risk of malaria. Malaria is found throughout the tropical and subtropical regions of the world and causes more than 300 million acute illnesses and at least one million deaths annually. Ninety per cent of deaths due to malaria occur in sub-Saharan Africa, mostly among young children. Malaria kills an African child every 30 s.

There are four types of human malaria: *Plasmodium vivax*, *P. malariae*, *P. ovale* and *P. falciparum*. *P. vivax* and *P. falciparum* are the most common, and falciparum is the most deadly type of malaria infection.

The malaria parasite enters the human host when an infected *Anopheles* mosquito takes a blood meal. Inside the human host, the plasmodia evade the immune system, infect the liver and red blood cells and, finally, develop into a form that is able to infect a mosquito again when it bites an infected person.

Malaria symptoms appear about 9–14 days after the infectious mosquito bite. Typically, malaria produces fever, headache, vomiting and other flu-like symptoms. Malaria can kill by infecting and destroying red blood cells (anaemia) and by clogging the capillaries that carry blood to the brain (cerebral malaria) or other vital organs, causing renal failure, jaundice, coagulopathy and pulmonary oedema (Box 1).

ICU treatment of malaria includes:

- Eradicating the parasites
- Supporting the failing organs (e.g. ventilation, pressors, inotropes, fluid and blood, dialysis)
- Treating coexisting bacterial infection.

Dengue

Dengue is the most important mosquito-borne viral disease in the world. In the last 50 years, incidence has increased 30-fold. An estimated 2.5 billion people are at risk in over 100 endemic countries. Up to 50 million infections occur annually with 500 000 cases of dengue haemorrhagic fever (DHF) and 22 000 deaths, mainly among children.

Dengue fever and DHF are present in urban areas in the Americas, Southeast Asia, the eastern Mediterranean and the western Pacific, and dengue fever is present mainly in rural areas in Africa. Rapid population growth, rural–urban migration, inadequate basic urban infrastructure and increase in the volume of solid waste providing larval habitats in urban areas have resulted in burgeoning of the main mosquito vector, *Aedes aegypti* (Box 2). Increased air travel and breakdown of vector control measures contribute to the global burden of dengue and DHF.

Aedes aegypti and *Aedes albopictus* mosquitoes transmit four distinct, but closely related, viruses that cause dengue. Person–person spread of infection does not occur. Recovery from infection provides lifelong immunity against that serotype, but confers only partial and transient protection against subsequent infection by the other three types. There is good evidence that sequential infection increases the risk of more serious disease resulting in DHF.

Dengue fever causes a severe, flu-like illness that affects infants, young children and adults, but seldom causes death. There is a spectrum of disease from a mild febrile syndrome to the classical incapacitating disease with abrupt onset and high fever, severe headache, pain behind the eyes, muscle and joint pains, and rash.

DHF and dengue shock syndrome are potentially deadly complications of dengue that are characterised by high fever, bleeding diathesis and circulatory failure. Bleeding, associated with derangement of coagulation and thrombocytopenia, is evident in the skin where there may be bruising and a petechial purpuric skin rash. Potentially fatal gastrointestinal, cerebral and pulmonary haemorrhage

Table 1 **Economic indicators, population demographics and HIV rates in Uganda compared with the USA**		
	Uganda	**USA**
Life expectancy at birth (years)	49	77
Under-5 mortality rate (per 1000 live births)	147	9
Gross national income per capita (int.$)	1320	35 060
Per capita total expenditure on health (int.$)	57	4887
% of adults with HIV (low–high estimate)	4.1 (2.8–6-6)	0.6 (0.3–1.1)

Source: World Health Organization Statistical Information System (WHOSIS).

may occur. Fever usually continues for 2–7 days and can be as high as 40–41°C. In severe cases, there is development of hypotensive shock with circulatory failure associated with pleural effusions, oedema and increased haematocrit. Without treatment, death follows in 12–24 h in 20% of cases but, with intensive supportive therapy, mortality can be as low as 1%. The mainstay of treatment is maintenance of circulating blood volume with crystalloids.

Box 1. Multidrug-resistant malaria is here to stay!

WHO (World Health Organization) supports artemisinin-based combination therapies (ACTs)

There is now widespread global resistance of *P. falciparum* to conventional antimalarial drugs, such as chloroquine, sulphadoxine–pyrimethamine (SP) and amodiaquine.

There is hope for the future, however, thanks to the development of a new group of antimalarials, the artemisinin compounds (artesunate, artemether and dihydroartemisinin) from the Chinese herbal medicine 'qing hausu'. Artemesinins are active against multidrug-resistant *P. falciparum* malaria, produce a very rapid therapeutic response, are well tolerated by patients and reduce transmission of malaria through activity against gametocytes.

After a series of very encouraging studies of artemesinin, the WHO has recommended that all countries experiencing resistance to conventional monotherapies should use combination therapies containing artemisinin derivatives (ACTs) with lumefantrine, mefloquine, amodiaquine or sulphadoxine–pyrimethamine for falciparum malaria treatment.

Box 2. Aedes albopictus (Asian tiger mosquito) – the worldwide tyre traveller (Fig. 1)

Geographical expansion of the mosquito has been aided by international commercial trade, particularly in used tyres, which easily accumulate rain water. In recent years, *Aedes albopictus*, a dengue vector, has become established in the United States, Latin American and Caribbean countries, in parts of Europe and in one African country. The fear is that dengue fever may follow.

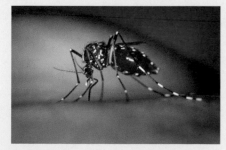

Fig. 1 **Aedes albopictus** (Asian tiger mosquito) (from the Centers for Disease Control).

Clinical case 1

A 29-year-old aid worker has been working in rural Sierra Leone, west Africa, for the past 3 months. He returns to the UK and is taken ill after a few days. He is admitted to the hospital, but deteriorates over several days and is admitted to the ICU, and barrier nursing is commenced. He is febrile and shocked and has a bleeding diathesis due to disseminated intravascular coagulation. He has leucopenia and raised C-reactive protein. Over the next few days, despite supportive therapy with fluid resuscitation, mechanical ventilation and broad-spectrum antibiotic therapy, he worsens with the development of jaundice, hepatitis and acute renal failure. Spontaneous bleeding is seen in the skin and from the endotracheal tube. A series of malaria films and blood cultures are negative. After an illness of 2 weeks, he dies of multiorgan failure. What is the likely aetiology of this fatal infection?

Clinical case 2

A 50-year-old woman has returned to the UK from the Indian subcontinent. She stayed with friends in their home in Karachi and attended a conference there. Four days after return, she developed a high fever; this was shortly followed by a purpuric skin rash, particularly over the extremities and affecting the palms and soles (Fig. 2). She becomes very unwell over the next 48 h in hospital with development of deranged liver function tests and renal failure. A chest radiograph is consistent with acute respiratory distress syndrome (ARDS). She has raised inflammatory markers and thrombocytopenia and leucopenia. She is admitted to the ICU when her blood pressure starts to drop. What is the likely diagnosis?

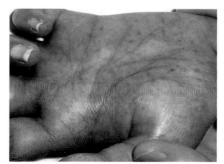

Fig. 2 **Purpuric rash on the palm.**

Summary points

- When a patient presents to the ICU with a history of travel, consider a tropical infection.
- Malaria is often a multidrug-resistant infection and treatment should include artemisinin.
- Dengue is the most important mosquito-borne viral disease in the world – and it's spreading!
- Viral haemorrhagic fevers occur in outbreaks. They have extremely high and rapid mortality.

Clever bugs and defunct drugs

The most resistant bacteria frequently arise in intensive care units (ICUs). Patients are vulnerable following surgery or trauma or having serious illness. Typically, they have multiple intravenous lines and endotracheal intubation overcoming natural barriers to infection. They are normally sedated or unconscious and require frequent attention from nursing and medical staff. Multiple episodes of infection may occur requiring recurrent use of broad-spectrum antibiotics. Such circumstances are ideal for the selection and transmission of resistant organisms.

It is estimated that there are 40 handwashing opportunities per hour for a nurse on an ICU. Compliance with hand hygiene is only about 50%. The use of alcohol hand rubs has the potential to improve hand hygiene as it is quick and effective. Placement of alcohol-based hand rubs at the end of beds and around wards can prompt medical and nursing staff to disinfect hands after patient contact. Portable alcohol dispensers can be given to staff.

Methods of resistance

Resistance develops in bacteria in response to antibiotics and is a quantitative phenomenon; the more the antibiotic is used, the more the resistance develops. Resistance (Fig. 1) generally spreads among bacteria on transferable elements, such as plasmids, transposons and insertion sequences (Fig. 2).

The post-antibiotic era

The combination of several factors hails the alarming prospect of a post-antibiotic era, when virtually untreatable organisms will be the norm in hospitals.
- Continuing unchecked use of broad-spectrum antibiotics
- Failure of control of infection
- Transmission of multiresistant organisms between patients
- Increasingly sophisticated medical management
- Patients living longer with chronic medical conditions.
Currently, in US hospitals, 50% of *Staphylococcus aureus* are methicillin resistant (MRSA), 30% of enterococci are vancomycin resistant (VRE), and 15–20% of *Pseudomonas aeruginosa* are resistant to fluoroquinolones and imipenem. There have been disturbing recent reports of a growing prevalence of community-acquired MRSA. Sadly, recent media reports have indicated that pharmaceutical industries are not prioritising the development of new antimicrobials. It is to be hoped that the tide will change and that research into the control of infection and the development of novel therapies receives the attention that is deserved before the situation becomes untenable.

MRSA

Staphylococcus aureus is part of the normal flora of the skin and anterior nares. It is a common cause of infection in humans, particularly of skin and soft tissue, bone and joint. Methicillin resistance develops in S. *aureus* due to the

acquisition of a large mobile genetic element, which carries the *mecA* gene. This gene encodes for PBP2´, which permits cell wall synthesis in the presence of beta-lactam antibiotics, including flucloxacillin and nafcillin. Strains of S. *aureus* with methicillin resistance are not necessarily more virulent than strains that are susceptible, but MRSA strains are more prevalent in hospitals because of epidemic spread and selection through the use of broad-spectrum antibiotics.

Acquisition of MRSA by a patient in hospital results in replacement of their normal staphylococcal flora with MRSA. MRSA colonisation can then be detected on skin (especially in moist places, such as armpits and groins), in the throat, on devices (such as intravenous or urinary catheters) and on any wounds or ulcers.

MRSA is generally treated with the glycopeptide antibiotics, vancomycin and teicoplanin. These antibiotics can only be given intravenously. Following identification of

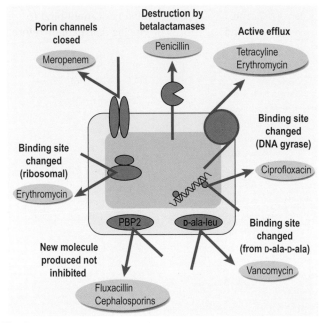

Fig. 1 **Mechanisms of resistance to antibiotics exhibited by bacteria.**

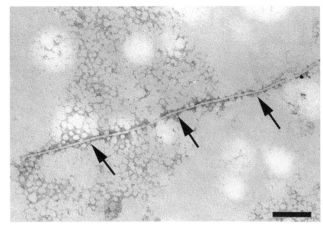

Fig. 2 **Pilus formation,** demonstrated by electron microscopy in *Haemophilus influenzae*, enables the spread of genetic material between bacteria (courtesy of Dr D.W. Crook).

MRSA bacteraemia, a course of 2–4 weeks of intravenous treatment is necessary as it is usually presumed that an endovascular source of infection has been established by *S. aureus*. Oral courses of therapy are not usually given for MRSA, but agents such as rifampicin, doxycycline, sulphamethoxazole–trimethoprim and fusidin may have a role depending on the susceptibility pattern of the strain.

VRE

Enterococci are part of the normal bowel flora. They are increasingly responsible for colonisation and infection in hospitals, as they are resistant to many groups of antibiotics. Enterococci usually show moderate innate resistance to penicillins, cephalosporins, clindamycin, aminoglycosides, sulphamethoxazole and fluoroquinolones. *Enterococcus faecalis* is normally susceptible to ampicillin, and *E. faecium* to vancomycin, but there has been epidemic spread, especially in US hospitals, of a strain of *E. faecium* with high-level resistance to vancomycin. Vancomycin resistance is due to the possession of the *vanA* gene, which mediates the replacement of D-alanyl-D-alanine linkages of the growing cell wall with D-alanyl-D-lactate. Glycopeptide antibiotics cannot bind to D-ala-D-lactate, and organisms producing *vanA* are therefore resistant.

Enterococci, including VRE, have low virulence, so tend to cause infections in hosts with compromised defences. Epidemics of infection occur in haematology, renal and intensive care units. High antibiotic use, especially with cephalosporins and vancomycin, is thought to be an important predisposing factor. Most affected cases have colonisation only, but about 10% will suffer a serious invasive infection, for which few therapeutic options are available. Some strains of VRE are susceptible to teicoplanin. Otherwise, treatment with chloramphenicol may be effective, and linezolid and quinupristin–dalfopristin are generally active. Occasional cases have been treated with very high doses of ampicillin (>300 mg/kg/day).

Simple measures can save lives. A study compared the use of 'gloves and gowns' with 'gloves only' donned when entering the rooms of patients colonised with VRE. It was estimated that 58 cases of VRE colonisation and six cases of VRE bacteraemia were averted by the use of 'gloves and gowns'.

Clinical pearl

New drugs for MRSA and VRE

In recent years, three agents with activity against resistant Gram-positive bacteria have been developed, Synercid® (dalfopristin–quinupristin, a streptogramin), linezolid (oxazolidinone) and daptomycin (cyclic lipopeptide). These agents are also active against many strains of VRE. Linezolid can be administered orally as well as intravenously, which represents a breakthrough in management. These agents are generally reserved for special cases, especially MRSA and VRE, following the recommendation of an infectious disease physician or clinical microbiologist, and sometimes represent the final therapeutic opportunity for some difficult to treat infections.

Clinical pearl

Feedback curtails inappropriate use of antibiotics

Giving physicians feedback on the appropriateness of their prescription of vancomycin resulted in an increase in adherence to guidelines from 17% to 71%, which was combined with a reduction in vancomycin use from 76 to 45 defined daily doses per 1000 admissions and no increase in mortality attributed to staphylococci.

Clinical case

A 50-year-old man was repatriated to his home hospital ICU after being involved in an accident overseas. He had suffered multiple injuries requiring surgery and had acquired ventilator-associated pneumonia. Samples taken on admission showed that he was colonised on intravenous line tips and in tracheal aspirates with *Acinetobacter baumanii* with resistance to cephalosporins, fluoroquinolones and imipenem. The isolate was susceptible only to amikacin and colistin. The index case was moved into a side room, and enhanced infection control precautions were commenced.

Over the next 4 weeks, 11 patients in the unit acquired the organism and an outbreak was declared. Over subsequent weeks, 34 patients were found to be colonised by the same strain of *A. baumanii*. How should this outbreak be managed?

Clinical pearl

VRSA (vancomycin-resistant *Staphylococcus aureus*)

■ For many years, the idea of spread of the *vanA* gene from VRE to *S. aureus* remained a theoretical nightmare. In 2002, just such an isolate was identified in a Michigan, USA, resident aged 40 years with diabetes, peripheral vascular disease and chronic renal failure on dialysis, who had been treated for chronic foot ulcerations with multiple courses of antimicrobial therapy, some of which included vancomycin. Since that time, another two cases have been described in the USA, all of which have the *vanA* gene. Treatment options are limited, but agents with some activity include linezolid, quinupristin–dalfopristin and trimethoprim–sulphamethoxazole. VRSA is fortunately still rare, but is clearly a reality, and it remains to be seen whether or not it will spread within hospitals in the way that MRSA has done. Chronic pyelonephritis may progress to chronic renal failure and endstage renal disease, but does not cause hypertension in later life.

Summary points

■ Resistance to antimicrobials is a major problem and may require the use of novel or toxic agents.

■ Infections acquired in ICUs are often caused by organisms, such as MRSA and VRE, with resistance to conventional antibiotics.

■ Knowledge of the local resistance patterns is important when choosing appropriate empirical therapy.

■ Early recognition of outbreaks and intervention to prevent transmission can limit the damage.

■ There is a pressing need for the development of new antimicrobial agents.

Special topics

Inflammation

Inflammation is the normal response to insults such as infection, trauma or foreign bodies. When controlled, inflammation can result in the clearance of infection or the repair of tissue. However, when unregulated, this process can cause damage to tissue that is otherwise normal. Several clinical syndromes concerning inflammation have been described. *Systemic inflammatory response syndrome* (SIRS) is widespread inflammation, clinically defined as the presence of two or more of the following criteria: (1) temperature (T) >38°C or T <36°C; (2) white blood count (WBC) >12 000 cells/cm³, WBC <4000 cells/cm³ or >10% immature; (3) heart rate (HR) >90 beats/min; (4) respiration rate (RR) >20 breaths/min or $P_a\text{CO}_2$ <32 mmHg. *Sepsis* is a clinical syndrome bearing the symptoms of SIRS secondary to an infectious aetiology. Sepsis is considered to be *severe sepsis* when complicated by hypotension, hypoperfusion or organ dysfunction. *Septic shock* is persistent severe sepsis despite adequate fluid resuscitation. *Multiple organ dysfunction syndrome* (MODS) may result from these inflammatory processes, and is largely responsible for their associated morbidity and mortality.

The rise and fall of the inflammatory response

Inflammatory actions are executed by a concerted action of immune cells and cytokines. When the inflammatory response is triggered, macrophages are activated to secrete cytokines such as tumour necrosis factor (TNF)α, interleukin (IL)-1 and IL-2 (Fig. 1). These mediators activate the immune system, recruiting activated leucocytes to the site of injury. Leucocytes release mediators that cause local inflammation including vasodilation and increased microvascular permeability. Chemical mediators including reactive oxygen species, nitric oxide and lysosomal proteases facilitate cellular death of microorganisms or affected cells. The process is amplified and fine tuned by cells of the adaptive immune system. Helper T cells (CD4 cells) develop inflammatory or anti-inflammatory profiles in response to their interactions with antigen-presenting cells (APCs). Macrophages that have ingested necrotic cells will induce a Th1 cell, whereas ingestion of apoptotic cells will induce a Th2 cell. Th1 cells secrete interferon-γ, activating macrophages, whereas Th2 cells secrete IL-10 and IL-4, which suppress macrophage activation.

The resolution of the inflammatory process is less well understood. Anti-inflammatory cytokines such as IL-10 and transforming growth factor (TGF)-β provide negative feedback, curbing the production of TNFα and IL-1. This suppresses macrophage activation, thereby encouraging anergy and apoptosis of activated immune cells. T cells become functionally inactivated secondary to a lack of co-stimulatory signalling. After removal of the initial insult, there is a decrease in inflammatory mediators, neutrophils and T cells die off, and macrophages leave the site of injury, allowing for tissue repair.

Insights into the activation of inflammation

The inflammatory response can be activated by a number of insults, with the classic example being bacteria. The discovery of *Toll-like receptors* (TLRs), membrane proteins with bacterial products as ligands, has furthered the understanding of

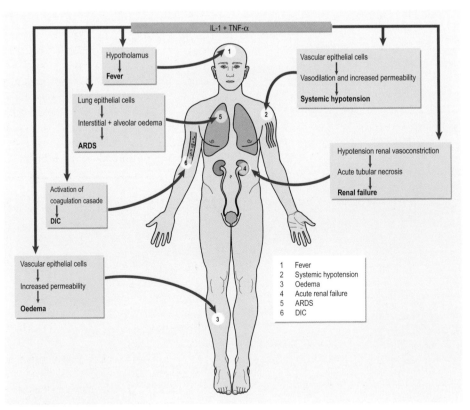

Fig. 1 **Clinical effects of inflammatory mediators** (SIRS).

mechanisms by which bacteria produce an inflammatory response. This discovery demonstrates that the innate immune system responds to specific signals and provides new therapeutic targets for clinical manipulation. TLR-4 is the co-receptor for CD14, which binds lipopolysaccharide (LPS), a molecule found in the outer membrane of Gram-negative bacteria. Activation of TLR-4 allows for signal transduction, leading to activation of APCs. LPS also activates the complement, coagulation and fibrinolytic cascades, and has been found to reproduce many of the manifestations of sepsis. TLR-2 binds to Gram-positive bacterial cell wall products such as peptidoglycan, lipoteichoic acid and lipoproteins, also leading to activation of the inflammatory response.

Injury, morbidity and mortality

While inflammatory syndromes are associated with increased morbidity and mortality, the mechanisms of cellular damage leading to organ dysfunction are not clear. It has been difficult to identify a common pathological process as the basis of MODS. One proposed mechanism of cell damage is hypoxia secondary to microvascular dysfunction. The release of mediators such as endothelin and platelet-activating factor causes vasoconstriction and impaired oxygen diffusion, leading to ischaemic cell injury. Another likely contributing factor is the direct effect of inflammatory cytokines, reactive oxygen species and endotoxin on cells. They cause cytopathic hypoxia, or decreased oxygen utilisation secondary to mitochondrial dysfunction. These mediators also lead to accelerated apoptosis in parenchymal cells. However, these cellular mechanisms do not fully explain the degree of organ dysfunction in MODS, and the cause of death in sepsis is often elusive.

This arena of research has produced exciting findings concerning the nature of inflammatory syndromes. Evidence has emerged that the compensatory anti-inflammatory response (CARS) and resultant immunosuppression may play a significant role in sepsis-induced mortality. There is a shift over time from a hyperinflammatory state to an immunosuppressive state (Fig. 2). This is supported by the fact that patients with sepsis exhibit features of an anti-inflammatory response, including a loss of delayed hypersensitivity, a decreased ability to clear infection and a predisposition to nosocomial infection. Autopsy studies have shown that patients who died of sepsis had decreased levels of B cells, CD4 cells and follicular dendritic cells, which suggests increased apoptosis of these cells secondary to a predominant anti-inflammatory response. Theoretically, this would result in decreased antibody production, macrophage

activation and antigen presentation. This has led to the concept that the inflammatory and anti-inflammatory response must be appropriately balanced in order to achieve homeostasis after an insult (Fig. 3). If the proinflammatory response predominates, the result will be SIRS and organ dysfunction. If the anti-inflammatory response predominates, the result may be immunosuppression, secondary infection and organ dysfunction. The concept has emerged of tailoring therapy to the time course of a patient's disease, where anti-inflammatory medications are given during the hyperinflammatory state, while immune-boosting therapies are given during the immunosuppressed state.

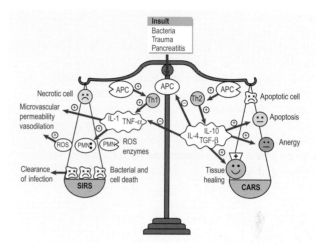

Fig. 3 **The balance of the inflammatory response.** After the initial insult, antigen-presenting cells (APCs) are activated. If they ingest necrotic cells, they induce Th1 cells. If they ingest apoptotic cells, they induce Th2 cells. Th1 cells induce inflammatory cytokines, which activate neutrophils (PMNs) to release reactive oxygen species (ROS) and enzymes. Th2 cells induce anti-inflammatory cytokines. The balance of these processes may determine a patient's clinical course.

Clinical case

A 58-year-old female presents with severe epigastric pain with associated fever, chills, nausea, vomiting and anorexia. Her vital signs are: T=38.5°C, HR=110 beats/min, BP=125/85 mmHg, RR=18 breaths/min, O₂ saturation=96% on room air. Acute pancreatitis is diagnosed. During the hospital stay, she is persistently febrile, with temperature ranging from 38°C to 39.5°C. Should her fever be treated?

Summary points

- Inflammation is a localised response to injury mediated by cytokines.
- An imbalance between proinflammatory and anti-inflammatory actions can result in SIRS.
- The discovery of Toll-like receptors has advanced the understanding of inflammatory response activation.
- Excessive effects of the CARS may be as harmful as those of the SIRS.
- Therapies aimed at blocking inflammation have been disappointing.
- Future therapies may be based on the pathogen, the time course of disease and a patient's genetic profile.

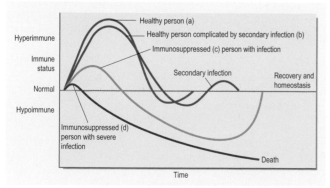

Fig. 2 **The temporal course of the inflammatory response.**

Burns

Unique considerations in burn care include airway compromise from inhalation injury, inadequate ventilation owing to burn eschar of the chest wall and profound fluid shifts secondary to insensible losses and tissue sequestration. Burnt patients often have other injuries, and a thorough history, physical examination and appropriate diagnostic studies are essential. Prevention of hypothermia and limitation of insensible fluid losses through the disrupted epithelial barrier are indicated. Burn units are warm and moist environments.

Burn size

Initial care and subsequent management of the burn wound is based upon its size. The size of the burn can be estimated by the 'rule of nines' (Fig. 1). In the adult, the surface area of the head, trunk and extremities is each approximated by a multiple of nine, with the perineum representing the final 1%. Paediatric burns require special assessment owing to different head and trunk proportions. Because of this, the patient's palm can be used to approximate 1% of body surface area. This fact is consistent regardless of patient age.

Burn depth

Burns are classified by size and depth of tissue injury. Wounds are separated into partial and full thickness. Partial thickness burns include first and second degree, while third-degree burns are referred to as full thickness (Fig. 2). Partial thickness implies some retained ability to re-epithelialise.

Fluid resuscitation

Extensive research since the 1960s has resulted in standardised formulae for the fluid management of burns victims. The most commonly used is called the Parkland formula. Fluid replacement is calculated as 4 mL per percentage body surface area burned per kilogram of body weight. The first half is given over 8 h, and the second half is given over the subsequent 16 h. Adequacy of resuscitation is monitored with clinical and laboratory data. Maintaining urine output of 0.5 mL/kg/h is a common goal for the adult patient. Clinical endpoints and acumen may be more sensible than slavish adherence to formulaic approaches.

Monitoring

Pulse oximetry is standard, but probe placement is often limited by the location of the burn. Probe placement on the tongue has been described. Arterial catheterisation can be helpful, particularly in the early post-burn period. Central venous catheters are more secure than peripheral lines in burn patients with limited access points, and facilitate multiple drug infusions and volume resuscitation. Ideally, catheters are placed through uninjured skin. Urine output is a helpful indicator of adequacy of resuscitation.

Inhalation injury

Inhalation injury results from thermal and chemical injury to the airway. Hot gases and toxic products of combustion lead to airway epithelial disruption and an inflammatory response. Life-threatening airway oedema might be present and must be considered. History of a closed space fire or clues such as singed facial hair or black sputum should prompt early tracheal intubation. Pulmonary infection is common owing to the impaired epithelial defences.

Carbon monoxide toxicity

Inhaled CO is toxic because it has 250 times more avid binding to haemoglobin than oxygen. Not only does CO prevent haemoglobin from carrying oxygen, it also shifts the oxyhaemoglobin dissociation curve to the left, decreasing oxygen unloading in the periphery. Oxygen delivery is thus

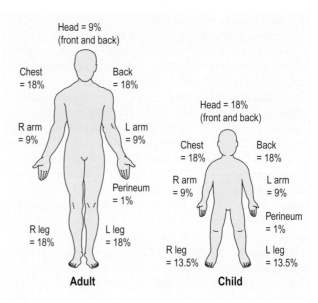

Fig. 1 **The rule of nines can help estimate the size of the burn wound.**

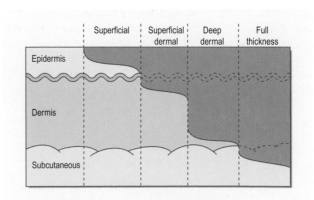

Fig. 2 **A diagram of burn wound depth.** Clinical determination between deep dermal (second degree) and full-thickness (third degree) burns can be difficult and may not be immediately apparent. Reassessment is often necessary.

impaired by two mechanisms. An elevated carboxyhaemoglobin level confirms the diagnosis. Therapy consists of high inspired oxygen concentration. Hyperbaric oxygen therapy may be helpful.

Wound care

Burns disrupt the vital protective functions of the skin. Burnt, non-viable skin is a potential medium for infecting microorganisms. This combination renders burn patients at high risk of infectious complications. Burns are initially treated with topical antimicrobial agents, such as silver sulphadiazine or mupiricin. Each has advantages and disadvantages. The key to modern burn care is early burn excision and skin grafting. This decreases infectious complications. New biological dressings have made possible early excision even in situations where there is limited autologous skin for grafting.

Escharotomy

Circumferential burns are particularly problematic. Most commonly, the extremities are involved. The burnt tissue acts as a tourniquet around progressively swelling tissues. Tissue perfusion can be limited. When the chest wall is involved, it becomes non-compliant and can contribute to respiratory failure in the spontaneously breathing patient, or cause marked airway pressure elevations and hypercapnia in mechanically ventilated patients. Escharotomy is the required therapy.

Patients are also at risk of abdominal compartment syndrome. The abdominal wall fascia is relatively non-compliant. With intra-abdominal fluid sequestration, intra-abdominal pressure rises. This can limit ventilation in the same way as chest wall burns. In addition, intra-abdominal hypertension leads to hypoperfusion of the kidneys and gut and limits venous return to the heart. Subsequent decreased cardiac output further limits splanchnic perfusion. Renal failure and mesenteric ischaemia occur if the intra-abdominal hypertension is not relieved. This is accomplished with decompressive laparotomy.

Electrical burns

With electrical burns, the majority of damaged tissue is not readily apparent. Entrance and exit sites of the current path can usually be assessed. Muscle and nervous tissue are most susceptible to injury owing to low resistance compared with bone and internal organs. Muscle damage can be extensive. Rhabdomyolysis and renal failure are possible. Serum creatinine kinase, urine myoglobin and urine output are helpful in monitoring progress. Extremity compartment syndromes can occur and may require fasciotomy. Patients should be evaluated for cardiac arrhythmias.

Chemical burns

Management of chemical burns begins with removal of clothing and the offending agent. Personal protective equipment for health care personnel is important. Acid and alkali burns are initially irrigated with water after removal of dry chemical debris. Hydrofluoric acid burns may require local infiltration with calcium gluconate or application of calcium gluconate gel. After aggressive lavage, the patient is covered with clean linens and hypothermia is avoided.

Petrol and phenol burns are also initially managed with copious water irrigation. Both agents can produce significant systemic derangements in addition to the cutaneous effects. Petrol causes lipid degeneration in the renal tubules and hepatocytes, and also denatures surfactant. Systemic effects of phenol include red cell haemolysis, renal tubular damage and hepatic centrilobular necrosis. Both agents can cause seizure.

Injury from hot tar is limited to the cutaneous injury, but removing the offending agent is difficult. Hydrocarbon solvents are avoided.

Pain control

Burn victims can experience exquisite pain and may require high doses of opiates. Judicious use of short-acting narcotics and ketamine may be useful for dressing changes.

Clinical case

A 40-year-old man is involved in an explosion and subsequent fire at a large industrial warehouse. He is calm and interactive upon arrival and reports no significant past medical history. He is intubated owing to concern for inhalation injury. What management is indicated?

Summary points

- If there is any possibility of airway or inhalation injury, consider early intubation!
- Assess for occult injury.
- Prevent hypothermia and desiccation.
- Clean, dress and cover the burn wounds.
- Infectious complications are common.

Obstetric critical care

Critical illness during pregnancy is relatively uncommon, and generally ranges from one to nine occurrences in 1000 gestations. Obstetric disorders account for the majority of intensive care unit (ICU) admissions among obstetric patients, particularly in the postpartum period. The antepartum ICU admissions result from a wide variety of medical conditions that show wide geographical variation. Respiratory illness, trauma and drug abuse are more common in developed countries, while malaria, human immunodeficiency virus (HIV)-related illness, viral hepatitis, valvular heart disease and burns are more common in underdeveloped regions of the world. Advanced maternal age (> 40 years), multiparity and multiple gestations are associated with higher ICU admission rates. Among ICU patients, obstetric patients generally have better outcomes than non-pregnant patients, although global variations in health care systems, medical illnesses and obstetric diseases contribute to disparate rates of maternal mortality.

Physiological changes in pregnancy
(Fig. 1)

A number of adaptive processes occur during pregnancy to support placental blood flow and oxygen delivery. A major component of this is expansion of maternal blood volume to levels about 40–45% above baseline. Cardiac output begins to rise in early pregnancy and remains elevated throughout. Systemic vascular resistance is lower, primarily due to the low-resistance placental vascular bed, and stroke volume is increased owing to greater left ventricular compliance and end-diastolic volume. Extracellular fluid accumulation occurs as well, contributing to peripheral oedema near term. Red cell mass increases only 20–30% above baseline, leading to progressive haemodilution and decreased blood viscosity as blood volume expands. Fetal oxygen extraction is facilitated by the presence of fetal haemoglobin (Hgb F), which is 80–90% saturated at an oxygen tension of 30–35 mmHg.

Oxygen consumption is increased, although minute ventilation, stimulated by progesterone, increases to a greater degree, producing a mild respiratory alkalosis. Decreased functional residual capacity occurs owing to elevation of the diaphragm, especially in the supine position. This, combined with increased oxygen consumption, significantly limits oxygen reserve and leads to rapid desaturation during periods of hypoventilation.

Glomerular filtration rate (GFR), creatinine clearance and urinary volume are all increased in pregnancy to handle the excretory demands of increased maternal metabolism. The increased GFR may lead to glycosuria, although response to a glucose load should be assessed to rule out gestational diabetes.

Increasing size of the gravid uterus displaces the intra-abdominal contents and increases intra-abdominal pressure. Progesterone-related smooth muscle relaxation in the gastrointestinal tract leads to decreased motility and lower oesophageal sphincter laxity.

Critical illness considerations specific to pregnancy

Peripartum haemorrhage
The two primary causes of antepartum haemorrhage are placenta praevia, in which the placenta is abnormally implanted in the lower uterus, and abruptio placentae, in which the placenta separates from its bed. Placenta praevia generally produces recurrent painless bleeding during the third trimester of pregnancy, but may lead to significant bleeding at the time of delivery. Placental abruption is a threat to both the fetus and the mother, leading to shock, fetal demise and possible disseminated intravascular coagulation (DIC). Management is restoring adequate circulating blood volume and delivery of the fetus. Postpartum haemorrhage may occur related to retained placental tissue or uterine inversion, both of which should be recognised and corrected at the time of delivery. The third and most common cause of postpartum haemorrhage is uterine atony, which requires mechanical compression and pharmacological treatment with oxytocin or potent smooth muscle and vascular constrictors.

Tocolytic-induced pulmonary oedema
A well-recognised complication of tocolytic therapy for preterm labour is pulmonary oedema. Cardiac dysfunction, volume overload, capillary leak syndrome and decreased colloid oncotic pressure have all been postulated as potential aetiological factors, although the exact mechanism remains unknown. Treatment consists of supplemental oxygen, discontinuation of tocolytic therapy and aggressive diuresis.

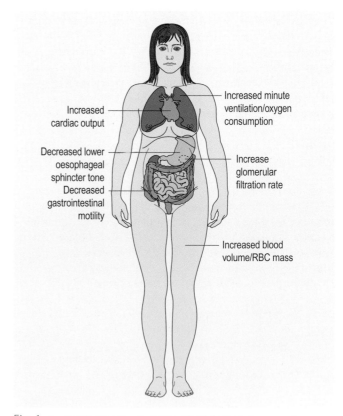

Fig. 1 **Anatomic drawing depicting physiological changes of pregnancy.**

Amniotic fluid embolism

Although uncommon, amniotic fluid embolism is associated with significant maternal mortality. It is associated with increased maternal age, multiparity, protracted labour, fetal distress and placental disruption, and may occur with either vaginal or caesarean delivery. The usual presentation is rapid clinical deterioration with acute dyspnoea, hypoxaemia and hypotension, potentially progressing to cardiopulmonary arrest. The pathophysiology is thought to be related to products of arachidonic acid metabolism, and the clinical manifestations include pulmonary hypertension, cardiac dysfunction and pulmonary oedema. Treatment is supportive.

Pre-eclampsia

Pre-eclampsia affects up to 5–10% of pregnancies and generally occurs in the late second or third trimester. It is a multisystem disease characterised by the triad of hypertension (≥ 140/90), proteinuria (> 300 mg/24 h) and non-dependent oedema. Approximately 2–10% of pre-eclamptic patients develop a more severe form of the condition known as eclampsia with progressive hypertension, multiorgan system dysfunction and neurological changes including seizures and coma. Pathophysiology is characterised by microangiopathic changes in the vascular endothelium related to excessive levels of thromboxane relative to prostacyclin, leading to vasoconstriction, hypoperfusion, tissue hypoxia and activation of inflammatory and coagulation pathways. Intravascular volume is generally decreased, while salt and water retention lead to increased oedema.

Two syndromes, haemolysis, elevated liver enzymes, low platelet count (HELLP) and acute fatty liver of pregnancy (AFLP), are considered to be variants of the pre-eclamptic state. Both entities have been linked to specific defects in fetal fatty acid oxidation. Distinction between these syndromes is difficult owing to similarities in presentation and overlap in laboratory findings (Table 1). AFLP is less common than HELLP and tends to be more acute in onset with profound hepatic failure, hypoglycaemia, encephalopathy, gastrointestinal bleeding and eventual maternal death. HELLP is associated with liver enzyme abnormalities, but hepatic synthetic function is generally preserved and thrombocytopenia predominates. Further complicating matters are the clinical similarities between these two entities and haemolytic uraemic syndrome (HUS) and thrombotic thrombocytopenic purpura (TTP).

Treatment of pre-eclampsia is largely supportive, with termination of the pregnancy the only definitive therapy. Control of hypertension in pre-eclampsia is necessary to prevent maternal hypertensive injury, particularly to prevent cerebral haemorrhage. Caution should be exercised to avoid lowering the blood pressure excessively (diastolic < 90) to avoid inadequate perfusion to the fetus. Magnesium sulphate is recommended for both hypertension management and eclamptic seizure prophylaxis with therapeutic levels of approximately 4–8 mEq/L (see Clinical pearl). Deep tendon reflexes and respiratory rate should be monitored frequently during therapy to detect increasing plasma magnesium concentrations and avoid overdose. Seizures may require emergency measures including airway management, supplemental oxygen therapy and respiratory support, phenytoin or benzodiazepine therapy and immediate delivery. Hypovolaemia and oliguric acute renal failure often complicate pre-eclampsia, and occasionally necessitate invasive monitoring when there is poor response to fluid challenges. Once the diagnosis of HELLP or AFLP is made, delivery should be considered to improve maternal outcome.

Table 1 **Distinguishing features of HELLP and AFLP**		HELLP	AFLP
Early			
	Platelet count	50K–150K	> 100K
	LDH level	600–1400 IU/L	Normal
	Bilirubin/PT levels	Normal	Abnormal
			Uric acid elevated
Late			
	Platelet count	< 50K	< 100K
	LDH level	> 1400 IU/L	< 600 IU/L
	Bilirubin/PT levels	Abnormal	Abnormal
			Hypoglycaemia

LDH, lactate dehydrogenase; PT, prothrombin time.

Clinical pearl

Magnesium sulphate (plasma level 4–8 mEq/L) is effective initial therapy for prevention of convulsions
Magnesium decreases muscle membrane excitability and reduces uterine hyperactivity
Magnesium has a mild antihypertensive effect
Plasma levels of magnesium > 10–25 mEq/L may lead to muscle weakness, respiratory paralysis and cardiac arrest.

Clinical case

A 37-year-old primigravida, at 34 weeks' gestation, presents with right upper quadrant tenderness and a 3-week history of rapid weight gain. Blood pressure is 180/110 mmHg. How would you proceed?

Summary points

- The principles for emergency management of the pregnant patient are the same as for any patient…Airway, Breathing, Circulation.
- Maintaining adequate oxygenation and circulation in the mother is necessary for the well-being of the fetus.
- Airway management in the pregnant patient may be more difficult, and oxygen desaturation may occur more quickly than in the general adult population.
- Patients at gestational age 20 weeks or greater should be positioned in the left lateral tilt position to displace the gravid uterus, minimise inferior vena cava compression and preserve cardiac output.

Toxicity: poisonings and overdoses

Poisoning results from exposure to a toxin. Overdose occurs when a drug exceeds its therapeutic concentration, becoming a toxin. Toxicity is the harm that results from poisoning and overdoses. A cluster of symptoms and signs characteristic of toxicity – a toxidrome – may be evident (Table 1). The toxidrome produced by anticholinergic agents, tricyclic antidepressants and antihistamines is characterised as 'Hot as a hare, mad as a hatter, blind as a bat, red as a beet and dry as a bone.'

The initial priority is to provide life support and resuscitation. Many toxins depress mental status, and tracheal intubation is indicated. Hydration and vasoactive agents may be required. Thiamine, dextrose and naloxone are often given empirically. Some toxins have antidotes. Management of toxicity includes attempts to decrease absorption, increase clearance and treat complications.

Diagnosis

The time of exposure is helpful. Important aspects of examination include pupil size and reactivity, temperature and skin features. Tachycardia and hypertension occur with sympathomimetic and anticholinergic agents. Tricyclic antidepressant toxicity includes sympathomimetic and anticholinergic effects. Neurological signs include depressed mental status (e.g. ethanol), agitation (e.g. anticholinergics) or seizures (e.g. insulin). Muscle rigidity is part of the neuroleptic malignant syndrome, while dyskinesias are seen with cocaine.

Laboratory

Important tests include serum electrolytes, arterial blood gases, serum anion gap and serum osmolar gap. There is increased anion gap metabolic acidosis with ethanol, ethylene glycol, formaldehyde, metformin and salicylate poisonings.

Serum concentrations are important for paracetamol (acetaminophen), methanol, ethylene glycol, salicylate, theophylline and digoxin poisonings.

Reducing exposure

Exposure can sometimes be limited with activated charcoal and gut irrigation. Activated charcoal binds toxins in the gut including carbamazepine, dapsone, phenobarbital, quinine and theophylline. Gut irrigation can be used for substances not well absorbed by activated charcoal, such as iron, lithium, sustained-released medicines or illicit drug packets. The elimination of toxins cans be enhanced by urinary alkalinisation with salicylates and phenobarbital, by haemodialysis and by haemoperfusion.

Paracetamol (acetaminophen)

Paracetamol is the most common pharmaceutical overdose and can result in life-threatening hepatic injury. Toxicity is

Table 1 **Typical toxidromes**	
Anticholineric agents	**Cholinergic agents (e.g. organophosphates)**
Hyperthermia	Salivation, slow heart, sweating, small pupils
Psychosis	Lacrimation
Blurred vision	Urination
Flushing	Diarrhoea
Dry skin	Gastrointestinal cramps
	Emesis

secondary to accumulation of the toxic metabolite N-acetyl-p-benzoquinonimine (NAPQI). The toxic threshold of paracetamol is 150 mg/kg in adults and can be less in susceptible patients. At-risk groups include patients with chronic alcoholism, poor nutrition and those with induced cytochrome P450 enzymes (e.g. patients taking phenytoin or phenobarbital) (Fig. 1) Manifestations of toxicity occur in stages. Symptoms of hepatotoxicity occur 48–96 h after ingestion and include coagulopathy and encephalopathy.

N-acetylcysteine (NAC) mitigates paracetamol toxicity through multiple routes. The serum paracetamol concentration should be obtained at or after 4 h following ingestion and compared with the levels expected to cause hepatotoxicity on the Rumack–Matthew nomogram. It is prudent to administer NAC until liver injury has been excluded. The nomogram is of limited utility with multiple ingestions, chronic use or extended release preparations.

Benzodiazepines

Benzodiazepines cause respiratory and mental status depression, which may proceed to coma. Treatment includes flumazenil, a benzodiazepine antagonist. Flumazenil is contraindicated in patients at risk of seizures or who chronically take benzodiazepines. Repeat flumazenil doses may be necessary because of its short half-life.

Amphetamines

Methamphetamine and 3,4-methylenedeoxyamphetamine, also known as ecstasy, are commonly abused. They increase catecholamines, resulting in hypertension, tachyarrhythmias, hyperthermia, agitation and mydriasis. Toxic effects include rhabdomyolysis, myocardial ischaemia, stroke, intracranial haemorrhage, seizures and hepatotoxicity. Treatment is supportive.

Cocaine

Cocaine intoxication results in sympathomimetic effects. Central nervous system (CNS) effects include agitation, psychosis and seizures. Other adverse effects include hypertension, arrhythmias, myocardial ischaemia, heart failure, intracranial haemorrhage, cerebral infarct, aortic dissection and respiratory complications. Hyperthermia and

Table 2 **Common toxins and antidotes**

Agent (common source)	Signs and symptoms of intoxication	Treatments
Beta-blockers	Bradycardia, conduction defects, hypotension	Atropine, glucagon, pacing
Calcium channel blockers	Bradycardia, hypotension, atrioventricular block, nausea	Calcium gluconate
Carbon monoxide (smoke inhalation)	Hypoxaemia, headache, dizziness, mental status changes	Oxygen, intubation and mechanical ventilation
Cyanide (sodium nitroprusside, plastics, plants, smoke inhalation)	Coma, seizures, hypotension, bradycardia, lactic acidosis	Oxygen, amyl and sodium nitrites, sodium thiosulphate
Digoxin/cardiac glycosides	Arrythmias, gastrointestinal symptoms, visual symptoms	Digoxin Fab (Digibind)
Insulin	Coma and seizures	Glucose, glucagon
Organophosphates (insecticides)	Bronchospasm, respiratory failure, weakness, paralysis	Atropine, pralidoxime

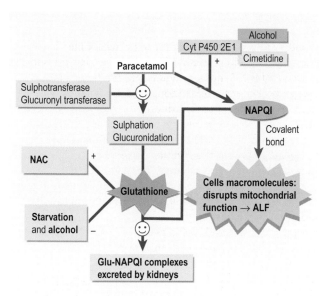

Fig. 1 **Paracetamol-induced hepatotoxicity.** *N*-acetyl-*p*-benzoquinonimine (NAPQI) is a toxic metabolite of paracetamol. NAPQI causes acute liver failure (ALF). NAPQI is mopped up by glutathione. Cytochrome P450 2E1 catalyses NAPQI production from paracetamol; this is upregulated by alcohol and other P450 inducers and downregulated by cimetidine and other P450 inhibitors. *N*-acetylcysteine (NAC) increases glutathione, which binds to NAPQI facilitating its excretion.

rhabdomyolysis may occur. Hypertension and angina are treated with nitrates, calcium channel blockers or labetalol. Beta-blockers alone should be avoided because of unopposed alpha-mediated vasoconstriction. Cocaine may promote platelet aggregation; aspirin is indicated. Seizures should be treated with benzodiazepines.

Salicylates

The most common salicylate is aspirin. At toxic concentrations, salicylates uncouple oxidative phosphorylation and inhibit the Krebs cycle, leading to multiorgan dysfunction. Symptoms and signs include tinnitus, nausea, vomiting, seizures, respiratory alkalosis (via direct central stimulation) and increased anion gap metabolic acidosis. Gastrointestinal bleeding, hypoglycaemia, renal failure and liver failure may occur. Clinical features usually present with salicylate levels of > 40 mg/dL, but occur at lower concentrations with chronic poisoning. In symptomatic patients, or patients with serum concentrations > 35 mg/dL, sodium bicarbonate is used to alkalinise the urine, increasing renal clearance. Haemodialysis may be needed.

Opioids

Opioid intoxication causes respiratory depression, miosis and sedation. Respiratory compromise may also occur via aspiration or non-cardiogenic pulmonary oedema. Pethidine (meperidine) and propoxyphene can cause seizures. Naloxone antagonises opioids and can be administered intravenously, intramuscularly, sublingually or via a tracheal tube. Naloxone may precipitate acute opioid withdrawal with a risk of seizures and pulmonary oedema. Repeat doses or a continuous infusion are often necessary owing to naloxone's short half-life.

Other poisons

Other poisonings are shown in Table 2. The assistance of a poison centre is helpful.

Clinical case
A farm worker presents with slurred speech and mental status changes. He has pinpoint pupils, muscle fasciculations, decreased tone, wheezing, a heart rate of 35/min, shallow breathing and pronounced sweating. What should be done?

Summary points
- Initial management is emergency resuscitation.
- Treatments include antidotes, attempts to decrease absorption and enhance elimination, and treatment of complications.
- A poison centre may advise on specific management.

Deliberate attacks: chemicals, radiation and bioterrorism

Outbreaks of illness occasionally occur as a result of malign intent. This has been of media interest in recent times because of an upsurge in international terrorism and also as a result of several well-documented episodes, such as the release of Sarin into the Tokyo subway by the terrorist group Aum Shinrikyo and anthrax spores being sent in the US mail.

Health personnel have a key role in the process of recognition, investigation, management and response to such incidents, and it is essential that they are well informed and confident of their actions and role. A number of sources of information are useful in this respect, including the Centers for Disease Control and Prevention, USA, and the Health Protection Agency of the UK.

An *outbreak* is said to occur when the number of cases observed exceeds that expected over a given time period and when those cases are linked by epidemiological, microbiological, toxicological or radiological features. A single case of a serious unusual illness e.g. inhalational anthrax, is of concern for public health and is referred to as an *incident*.

An outbreak of illness may be the result of natural or accidental processes, but deliberate release should be considered. Deliberate release may be overt, with immediate acute recognition, or covert, with delayed recognition.

Chemical agents

Chemical agents from several groups can be released deliberately and result in injury to health. The major groups are fluoroacetic acid derivatives, carbamates, organochlorines, organophosphates, nerve gases, cyanides, arsenicals, mercurials, selenium salts, lung-damaging gases (chlorine, phosgene) and mustard gases. The main effects of these agents are recorded in Fig. 1.

Biological agents

A variety of serious infectious diseases have the potential to be used for biological warfare or terrorism. The major ones are listed below, but other possible agents are haemorrhagic fever viruses (Ebola, Marburg, Congo-Crimean haemorrhagic virus), tularaemia,

Q fever, Brucella and alphaviruses (Venezuelan equine encephalitis).

Anthrax (*Bacillus anthracis*)
Fig. 2a is a chest radiograph showing pneumonia and mediastinal widening due to inhalational anthrax (although not an example of a confirmed case of inhalation anthrax). Fig. 2b shows cutaneous anthrax, a painless vesicle progressing to a black eschar with extensive surrounding oedema. Fig. 2c shows a Gram stain of *Bacillus anthracis*.

Plague (*Yersinia pestis*)
This can be either pneumonic, with rapidly progressive severe pneumonia, or bubonic, with swollen, painful, tender lymphadenopathy associated with erythema and oedema.

Smallpox (*Variola major*)
Fig. 3 shows the distribution of the rash of smallpox showing vesicular rash (Fig. 3a) preferentially affecting the extremities (Fig. 3b).

Botulinum toxin
Acute-onset descending flaccid paralysis with cranial nerve involvement.

Consciousness is maintained, and there is no fever or sensory impairment.

Radiation exposure

Exposure to radiation may result from external irradiation of the body due to a nuclear or 'dirty' bomb or can occur after ingestion of radioactive material due to contamination of watercourses or food. The traumatic effects of blast injury may also be evident in affected individuals.

Whole-body irradiation
Prodrome: nausea, vomiting, fever and diarrhoea.
Illness: infection, bleeding and mucositis. Diarrhoea, sore throat.

Early biological warfare

The Black Death (probably *Yersinia pestis* pandemic) of 1346, which killed about a third of the population of Europe, reputedly started as a result of the Tartars catapulting the corpses of plague victims over the walls of besieged Genoa.

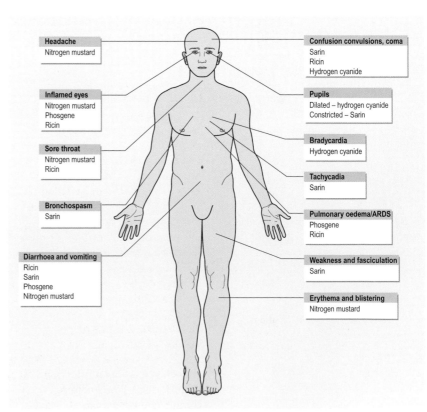

Fig. 1 **Effects of the major groups of chemical agents on the human body.**

Labels on figure:

Headache — Nitrogen mustard

Inflamed eyes — Nitrogen mustard, Phosgene, Ricin

Sore throat — Nitrogen mustard, Ricin

Bronchospasm — Sarin

Diarrhoea and vomiting — Ricin, Sarin, Phosgene, Nitrogen mustard

Confusion convulsions, coma — Sarin, Ricin, Hydrogen cyanide

Pupils — Dilated – hydrogen cyanide, Constricted – Sarin

Bradycardia — Hydrogen cyanide

Tachycadia — Sarin

Pulmonary oedema/ARDS — Phosgene, Ricin

Weakness and fasciculation — Sarin

Erythema and blistering — Nitrogen mustard

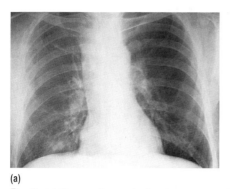

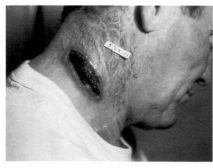

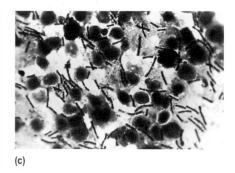

(a)   (b)   (c)

Fig. 2 **(a) Chest radiograph showing pneumonia and mediastinal widening** (courtesy of American College of Physicians). **(b) Cutaneous anthrax:** (from Centers for Disease Control). **(c) Gram stain of *Bacillus anthracis*** (from Centers for Disease Control).

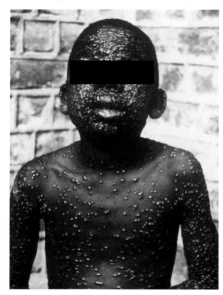

(a)

Table 1 **Specific measures in the management of cases**		
Agent	Treatment	Post-exposure prophylaxis
Anthrax	Ciprofloxacin* for 60 days	Ciprofloxacin for 60 days†
Plague	Gentamicin or streptomycin†	Ciprofloxacin for 7 days†
Botulism	Trivalent antiserum (A, B and E) single injection intravenously	
Smallpox	Supportive	Vaccination

*Rifampicin and clindamycin have been added for severe cases. May be susceptible to penicillin.
†Alternative is doxycycline.

Local exposure

Erythema, oedema, blistering, desquamation of skin. Necrosis or gangrene of extremities.

Admission of cases

Persons affected by possible intentional release of chemicals, infective agents or radiation are likely to need hospital assessment and treatment. Many health care facilities will have a 'major incident protocol', which staff should be familiar with and will be able to implement when necessary.

Health and safety

Containment of the problem, with prevention of spread of toxic or infectious material to other persons, is paramount. Decontamination (in the 'hot zone') of persons is essential following exposure to hazardous material. The clothes of the affected person are removed, and they are encouraged to shower using soap and water prior to entry to the hospital environment. Personal protective equipment (PPE) must be used when working in the decontamination area.

Diagnostic sampling

Samples of blood or other material should be taken for diagnostic purposes. 'High-risk' labelling of specimens should be carried out. Blood cultures, urine samples and clotted blood samples should be taken for microbiological

analysis. Further sampling, such as sputum, throat swab, bronchial washings, swabs of lesions and cerebrospinal fluid analysis, may be carried out when appropriate to the case. Blood and urine are collected for toxicological analysis.

Containment

Where the diagnosis is uncertain, it would seem appropriate to nurse patients in side rooms or in cohorts where possible. The universal, or standard, precautions should be followed. Similarly, cleaning of clinical areas, disinfection and sterilisation of equipment is carried out according to standard precautions.

Additional precautions may be required for certain cases, such as smallpox where strict isolation and respiratory mask precautions by staff for up to 30 days is necessary.

Management of cases

Some specific measures are listed in Table 1.

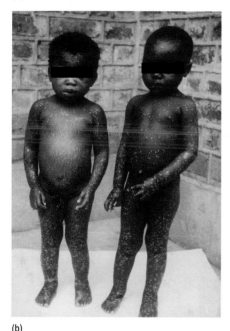

(b)

Fig. 3 **Distribution of rash of smallpox** showing vesicular rash **(a)** preferentially affecting the extremities **(b)**. (From Centers for Disease Control.)

Summary points

■ Health care workers may be the first to recognise a deliberate incident or outbreak of illness, and a high index of suspicion is required.

■ Advance planning is key, so that a rapid response to decontaminate victims and contain the agent can be swiftly implemented.

Advanced cardiac life support

Many advances in emergency cardiac care (ECC) have been made in the 40 years since the introduction of modern cardiopulmonary resuscitation (CPR), leading to improved outcomes for cardiac arrest victims. The desire for a standardised international approach lead to the Guidelines 2000 Conference, the first such conference at which participating international experts and leaders concentrated on critical review and debate of all published evidence to create the new science- and evidence-based international guidelines.

What's new?

Highlights of significant revisions in resuscitation concepts and principles in the new guidelines for adult basic life support include:

1 *Phone first*. Rescuers should 'phone first' for unresponsive adults. Most adults with sudden (witnessed) non-traumatic cardiac arrest are found to be in ventricular fibrillation (VF). For these victims, the time from collapse to defibrillation is the single greatest determinant of survival. Whenever two or more rescuers are present, one rescuer remains with the victim to provide CPR, while the second rescuer activates the emergency medical response system. Early CPR is the best treatment for cardiac arrest until the arrival of advanced cardiovascular life support (ACLS) care and defibrillation capability. Early CPR prevents VF from deteriorating to asystole, may increase the chance of defibrillation, contributes to the preservation of heart and brain function and significantly improves survival.

2 *Decreased emphasis on the pulse check*. Many responders, including health care providers, may fail to provide chest compressions or defibrillation if they incorrectly determine the presence of a pulse. Additionally, rescuers require far too much time to perform the pulse check. Lay rescuers are no longer taught to check for a pulse; instead, they should evaluate for signs of circulation including spontaneous breathing, coughing or moving.

Health care providers should continue to check for a pulse, limiting the pulse check to no longer than 10 s.

3 *Minimise disruptions in chest compressions*. Every time chest compressions are stopped (e.g. for ventilation or pulse checks), multiple compressions are required to re-establish adequate blood flow to the brain, heart and other vital organs.

4 *Proficiency in bag-mask ventilation is mandatory*. The ability to provide competent bag-mask ventilation is of greater importance than skill in tracheal intubation.

5 *Verify and secure endotracheal tubes*. When tracheal intubation is performed, the guidelines require that validated secondary techniques, in addition to primary evaluation with physical examination, be used to confirm proper endotracheal position immediately following tube placement and whenever the patient is moved or transported. Likewise, validated techniques or devices should be used to prevent tracheal tube dislodgement.

A is for airway

Establishing a patent airway is fundamental to emergency cardiovascular care and resuscitation. Rescue breathing (ventilation using exhaled air) will deliver approximately 16–17% inspired oxygen concentration to the patient, ideally producing alveolar oxygen tension of 80 mmHg. During cardiac arrest, tissue hypoxia occurs due to inadequate pulmonary blood flow and high peripheral oxygen extraction secondary to low cardiac output.

The number of breaths delivered to initiate rescue breathing/ventilation varies throughout the world, and there are no data to suggest the superiority of one number over the other. In the USA, two breaths are recommended while, in Europe, Australia and New Zealand, two to five breaths are provided to initiate resuscitation. Delivery of fewer breaths will shorten the time to assessment of circulation/pulse and attachment of an automated external defibrillator (AED), but delivery of a greater number of breaths

may help to correct hypoxia and hypercarbia. In the absence of data to support one approach over another, it is acceptable to deliver from two to five initial breaths according to local custom and teaching.

During rescue breathing, gastric distension is likely to occur. Delivering smaller tidal volumes may minimise this risk, and current recommendations are to deliver slow breaths that will make the chest visibly rise. Supplemental oxygen should be provided as soon as possible and will allow for smaller tidal volumes.

The recommended compression–ventilation ratio is 30:2. If the patient is intubated with a cuffed endotracheal tube, chest compressions should be performed at a rate of 100/min and ventilations without interruption of chest compressions at a rate of 8–10/min.

Rapid defibrillation

Defibrillation in less than 5 min is a high-priority goal. For a person in VF, the probability of successful defibrillation and subsequent survival to hospital discharge is directly and negatively related to the time interval between onset of VF and delivery of the first shock. If restoration of spontaneous circulation occurs after 8–10 min following cardiac arrest, the frequency of significant, permanent neurological damage becomes unacceptably high. Responding and shocking as fast as possible is a central objective of all emergency medical response systems. Chest compressions should be used while preparing for defibrillation and never used in place of defibrillation when indicated. Current recommendations call for one shock (not three) with 360 joules or the biphasic equivalent. Chest compressions should resume immediately after defibrillation with *no* pulse check.

Chest compressions

During cardiac arrest, coronary perfusion pressure gradually rises with the performance of sequential compressions and is greater after 15 uninterrupted chest compressions than it is after five chest compressions. The current recommended ratio of 30 compressions to two ventilations during CPR provides more chest compressions per minute than the previous ratio of 15:2. Evidence suggests that adult cardiac arrest resuscitation is more likely to be successful with a higher number of chest compressions during CPR, even when victims receive fewer ventilations. Once a protected airway is established, compressions should be continuous at a rate of 100 compressions/min. To optimise cardiac output, the patient's chest is compressed to a depth of about 50 mm at the lower half of the sternum (Fig. 1). There is a dual mechanism to explain efficacy: direct cardiac compression between the thoracic spine and intermittent increases in intrathoracic pressure. It is important to release pressure completely between compressions to allow for filling. These manoeuvres may generate systolic pressures of 60–80 mmHg and a cardiac output approximately one-third of normal.

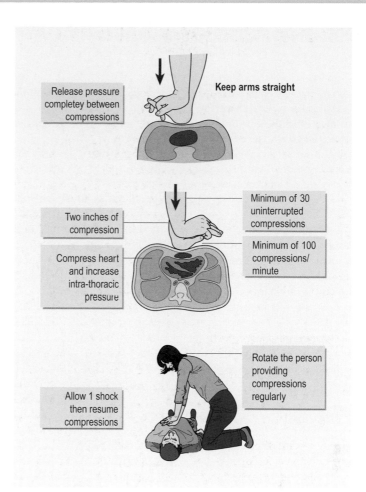

Fig. 1 **Chest compressions.**

The team

Emergency cardiovascular care responders will need to organise quickly into a functional team. The team leader is generally identified as possessing broad clinical and organisational skills. The team leader should be decisive and composed and keep the team focused on the ABCs (airway, breathing and circulation). The roles of other team members should be specifically assigned (start intravenous access, ventilate, intubate, defibrillate) to maintain organisation and ensure that necessary steps are completed. A controlled 'code' requires that the resuscitation room remain quiet so that all personnel can hear without shouting or repetitious commands. Team members should:

- State the vital signs every 5 min or with any change in the monitored parameters
- State when procedures and medications are completed
- Request clarification of any orders
- Provide primary and secondary assessment information.

A member of the team should be identified to keep record of interventions and times.

The team leader should communicate his or her observations and should actively seek suggestions from team members. Frequent evaluation and modification of

treatment will be necessary, particularly in unstable situations.

The pre-arrest period

Often, emergency responders may be called upon to care for those patients 'on their way to a cardiac arrest' or those recovering in the immediate post-resuscitation period. Examples of clinical conditions requiring such immediate care include acute coronary syndromes, hypotension and shock, acute pulmonary oedema, brady- or tachyarrhythmias and acute ischaemic stroke. Rapid and effective management of these patients may prevent full cardiopulmonary arrest from occurring. Many hospitals now employ emergency response teams to intervene in unstable patients before cardiac arrest occurs.

 Clinical tip
End-tidal CO_2 detection is extremely useful:
- It confirms that the endotracheal tube is not in the oesophagus
- It confirms the adequacy of chest compressions; the better the cardiac output, the higher the end-tidal CO_2.

Summary points
- There is an attempt to create international consensus in resuscitation guidelines.
- Chest compressions should be rapid, vigorous and sustained, with brief breaks for defibrillation.
- Defibrillate early.
- A leader should oversee and assign tasks to team members.
- In hospital, emergency response teams may be able to avert cardiac arrests.

Ethics: limiting and withdrawing treatment

Intensivists treat patients who have a high risk of dying *without* intensive therapies and a good chance of recovery *with* them. Identifying those patients who will benefit most from intensive therapies is a necessarily inexact science, particularly for any individual patient in the early stages. Usual clinical practice includes accepting this uncertainty and beginning heroic therapies on some very high-risk patients. Many intensive care units (ICUs) experience ~ 10–20% ICU mortality.

Increasingly, death in the ICU is preceded by a process of limiting and withdrawing treatment after recognition by the health care professionals and family [and sometimes the patient (Hall and Rocker 2000)] that continuing or escalating treatment is not in the patient's best interest. Withdrawal of treatment is usually, but not inevitably, followed by the death of the patient. Intensivists and intensive care nurses have had to become proficient in caring for patients who are very likely to die and for their families. The intensivist's responsibilities include those listed in Box 1.

Care of the patient and family

It is not uncommon for intensive care staff to focus on a curative or restorative objective and to overlook equally important objectives such as avoidance of suffering, maintaining patient dignity and 'sharing the chaotic journey' with the patient and family. Initially, the level of treatment may be very high, and meticulous attention to the details of treatment is essential to ensure that the patient is given the best opportunity to recover. However, focusing exclusively on the cure can delay the appreciation by staff, the patient and the family that a cure is not possible. The psychological and spiritual needs of the patient and the family may then be overlooked until shortly before death, when it is very difficult to meet these needs (Box 2). If 'curative' and 'palliative' objectives are simultaneously and conscientiously attended to from the moment of ICU admission (acknowledging that the relative priority of these objectives may shift during the course of the patient's illness), there will be far fewer difficulties for all concerned in the processes of withholding or withdrawing certain treatments should that become appropriate. Early involvement of others who may assist the patient and their family (e.g. social workers, palliative care specialists, chaplains and others) is facilitated by not having to define a time before which 'cure' is the only objective and after which 'comfort' is the only objective (Streat 2005a).

Assessment of prognosis

Most intensive care patients have a relatively straightforward course and a low risk of death. Certain patients, however [typically those with severe central nervous system (CNS) disorders, sepsis or multiple organ failure], have an initially unpredictable course and a high risk of complications, long-term severe disability or death.

Even moderate CNS-mediated disability often results in loss of cognitive, emotional, social and psychological well-being, as well as leading to unemployability and social isolation (Streat 2005b). Severe CNS-mediated disability also involves dependence upon others for activities of daily living. Positive predictive values for poor outcome of 70–100%, typically ~ 95%, occur with various findings associated with severe CNS damage. In severe traumatic brain injury, these include Glasgow coma score (GCS) 3 or bilaterally absent pupillary responses or bilaterally absent somatosensory evoked potentials (SEPs) or GCS ≤ 8 associated with either age > 60 years or hypotension (systolic blood pressure < 90 mmHg) and hypoxia or some computerised tomography (CT) features (Brain Trauma Foundation 2000). In hypoxic–ischaemic encephalopathy (Streat 2005b), they include persistent abnormal flexion (or worse) or status myoclonus or burst suppression on electroencephalography or fixed pupils or absent short-latency SEPs. In other catastrophic cerebral situations (e.g. stroke, encephalitis and acute demyelination), the adverse prognostic features are less well characterised statistically, but persistent coma, especially when associated with signs of progressive or structural brainstem dysfunction, is an ominous sign (Wijdicks and Rabinstein 2004) (see pp. 64 and 66). Similarly, in sepsis and multiple organ failure, equivalently predictive characteristics are less well quantified, but adverse features include high illness severity, advanced age, limiting co-morbidity, progressive multiple organ failure, inability to control the source of sepsis, patient preferences and the intensivist's opinion as to prognosis (see p. 140).

Establishing a good relationship

A relationship of mutual trust and respect enables the health care team and the family together to address difficult and painful issues, including limiting or withdrawing intensive therapies, the death of the patient and the option of organ or tissue donation. This should begin very early in the critical illness by way of a family meeting, which may be the first of several 'bad news' meetings in the days that follow. Family

---

Box 1. Intensivist's responsibilities

- Care of the patient and the family
- Assessment of prognosis
- Establishing a relationship of mutual trust and respect
- Formulating a medical recommendation to limit or withdraw treatment when appropriate
- Facilitating consensus between the team and the family
- Withdrawing treatment.

Box 2. Spiritual needs

Many modern physicians seem to have lost the understanding that death is a fact of life and will always occur. Some act as if life were eternal or at least, can always be meaningfully prolonged. In doing so indiscriminately, much unnecessary suffering is created among close family members.

Ake Grenvik

meetings should be attended by whoever the family defines themselves to include, by the intensivist and an intensive care nurse, and perhaps by a chaplain or social worker if the family wish. These meetings should occur away from the bedside, in a separate private room large enough to accommodate all the participants and should be protected from interruption. During these meetings, many aspects of the behaviour of the intensivist and nurse are crucial to establishing the necessary relationship. They include evident compassion (Cuthbertson et al 2000) of all staff for the patient and the family, use of plain speech, provision of consistent information, ensuring unhurried discussion, allowing silence, listening attentively to what the family say (Curtis et al 2005) and answering all questions truthfully and fully. By not being the 'bearer of bad news', the intensive care nurse remains available to support the family during and after the receipt of information from the intensivist.

Formulating a medical recommendation

In patients with severe CNS disorders, the extent of damage is assessed both clinically and with relevant investigations. Reliable clinical assessment of CNS function is possible only when the patient is free from sedation and other potentially confounding factors. Several days of intensive treatment may be required until it is appropriate to perform a sedative-free clinical assessment and subsequently formulate an opinion on prognosis.

In patients with sepsis or multiple organ failure, it is necessary to assess the extent of underlying co-morbidity and prior functional impairment, the severity of illness and its evolution with treatment (Streat 2005a), the adequacy of surgical source control and antibiotic treatment and any potentially treatable factors. This usually requires a period of intensive treatment and observation over several days. It is often appropriate to discuss limiting or withdrawing treatment from patients who are progressively deteriorating despite apparently appropriate treatment.

It is reasonable for the intensivist to recommend that treatment be limited or withdrawn when the death of the patient is imminent, or when the extent of CNS damage is such that survival is likely not to be in the patient's best interests or in accord with their preferences, or when the burden of ongoing treatment is probably not in the patient's best interests or in accord with their preferences.

Facilitating consensus

It is essential that all members of the treating team share a common view on prognosis and on what treatment is reasonable before the options of limiting treatment or withdrawing treatment are discussed with the patient and/or the patient's family. As none of the patients with severe brain damage (and perhaps only 5% of those with multiple organ failure) are capable of being involved in decision-making at this time, decisions about the appropriateness, intensity and duration of treatment are almost always made by others.

After consensus is established among the treating team, the intensivist or other appropriate senior clinician should meet with the family, convey information and introduce the consensus opinion of the team about limitation or withdrawal of treatment. The intensivist should first describe

the sequence of events from the onset of the illness until the present. When severe brain damage has occurred, the intensivist should explain the nature, extent and likely functional consequences of that damage. This should be in plain speech and in readily understood everyday terms, e.g. the nature of personality change, the domains of cognitive impairment, the likelihood of unemployability, specific focal neurological deficits if any and the likely level of interaction, speech, responsiveness and dependency. In multiple organ failure, the explanation should include the unfavourable clinical course, the lack of treatable factors, high likelihood of death and the ongoing burden of intensive treatments. After ensuring that the family have understood this information and have had any resultant questions answered, the intensivist should introduce the consensus recommendation that intensive therapies be limited or withdrawn and then invite discussion. Framing the discussion as 'seeking consensus with a recommendation' in the context of shared decision-making rather than 'asking for permission to stop treatment' is recommended. The values and previously expressed preferences of the patient are discussed, along with the clinical information and views of the treating team and family members. Despite the inherent prognostic uncertainties, intensivists and patients' families often decide together to limit or withdraw treatment. Intensivists must document such discussions and decisions in the patient's clinical record.

Withdrawing treatment

Desirable components of good end-of-life care in the ICU include good communication and continuity of care, control of distressing symptoms, attention to the emotional and spiritual needs of all involved and ensuring that the family have unrestricted access to the patient.

Treatments and investigations that are commonly withdrawn (Hall and Rocker 2000) include mechanical or inotropic circulatory support, renal replacement therapy, blood products, antibiotics, mechanical ventilatory support, the endotracheal tube, investigations and physiological monitoring.

Care for the patient and their family is however never withdrawn – the ambience usually becomes less technological and more *caring*. Attention becomes focused on ensuring that the needs of the patient and the family are met. Symptom control commonly involves the use of opioids or sedatives (Hall and Rocker 2000).

> ### *Summary points*
>
> - Predicting benefit from intensive therapy is uncertain.
> - An obsessive focus on 'cure' can impair patient dignity, leaving unmet psychological and spiritual needs.
> - Attempts at cure and palliation should overlap.
> - Talk to the family *early*, establishing trust and mutual respect.
> - Let the family define who attends family meetings.
> - *Listen*, show compassion and use plain speech.
> - Establish team consensus, then explain the prognosis and the team's recommendations, and *then* seek family consensus.
> - Certain treatments are withdrawn, but *care* is never withdrawn.

Trauma

Trauma is disturbingly common in the modern world and disproportionately affects the young. Common goals in the management of trauma patients include effective resuscitation from shock, prevention of secondary injuries to compromised organs, early surgical therapy for amenable injuries and prevention of complications.

Initial evaluation

Groups such as the American College of Surgeons have standardised the evaluation of trauma patients. A range of injuries may present requiring various investigations and interventions (Fig. 1). The priorities are airway patency and maintenance, adequacy of oxygenation and ventilation, and evaluation of circulatory function. These are frequently referred to as the 'ABCs'.

Airway can be compromised by injury (e.g., facial fractures, laryngeal trauma, expanding haematoma from carotid artery laceration) or by obtundation owing to brain injury or intoxication.

Breathing can be affected by chest wall trauma, lung parenchymal injury, pneumothorax or haemothorax, spinal cord injury, diaphragm injury and drugs and alcohol.

Circulatory failure or shock occurs most commonly with haemorrhage. Control of the bleeding source is often required. Initial volume resuscitation is with isotonic solutions, although there is research interest in hypertonic solutions. Blood products are reserved for specific indications. There is debate regarding colloid versus crystalloid resuscitation and optimal endpoints of resuscitation. Other forms of shock are less obvious. Cardiogenic shock can occur from direct injury to the coronary arteries, cardiac valves or papillary muscles. The possibility of pre-existing ischaemic or valvular heart disease should be considered. Obstructive shock – limitation of venous return or prevention of arterial outflow – can occur with pericardial tamponade, tension pneumothorax, abdominal compartment syndrome or massive pulmonary embolism. Neurogenic shock is an infrequent cause of hypotension with spinal cord injury and severe brain injury. Distributive shock can be caused by sepsis later in a trauma

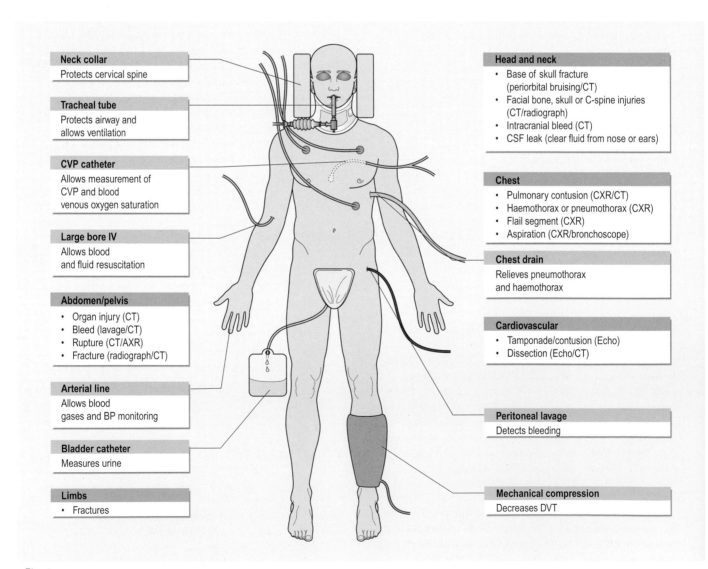

Neck collar
Protects cervical spine

Tracheal tube
Protects airway and allows ventilation

CVP catheter
Allows measurement of CVP and blood venous oxygen saturation

Large bore IV
Allows blood and fluid resuscitation

Abdomen/pelvis
- Organ injury (CT)
- Bleed (lavage/CT)
- Rupture (CT/AXR)
- Fracture (radiograph/CT)

Arterial line
Allows blood gases and BP monitoring

Bladder catheter
Measures urine

Limbs
- Fractures

Head and neck
- Base of skull fracture (periorbital bruising/CT)
- Facial bone, skull or C-spine injuries (CT/radiograph)
- Intracranial bleed (CT)
- CSF leak (clear fluid from nose or ears)

Chest
- Pulmonary contusion (CXR/CT)
- Haemothorax or pneumothorax (CXR)
- Flail segment (CXR)
- Aspiration (CXR/bronchoscope)

Chest drain
Relieves pneumothorax and haemothorax

Cardiovascular
- Tamponade/contusion (Echo)
- Dissection (Echo/CT)

Peritoneal lavage
Detects bleeding

Mechanical compression
Decreases DVT

Fig. 1 **Trauma patients:** injuries, investigations and interventions.

patient's hospital course. Acute adrenal insufficiency from trauma is rare.

Disability is next. This essentially refers to evaluation of central nervous system (CNS) injury. Finally, *Exposure* and *Events* help to remind health workers to perform a thorough physical examination and record important historical points regarding the mechanism of injury.

Team approach to trauma care

A multidisciplinary approach to trauma management is essential. It is important to identify all injuries and to formulate care plans. The intensivist's role is to coordinate sometimes conflicting priorities among the other providers and to maintain a global perspective on the patient's progress. For example, delaying definitive long bone fracture fixation under general anaesthesia until intracranial hypertension is controlled may be prudent.

Common problems in the trauma ICU

Respiratory failure, ventilator-associated pneumonia, decubitus ulcers, delirium, malnutrition and deep venous thrombosis (DVT) occur commonly. Patients with cervical spinal cord injury frequently have respiratory insufficiency or failure owing to impaired mechanics and are at high risk of pneumonia and DVT. Brain injury and penetrating pancreatic injury both predispose to malnutrition. Dysphagia and gastric dysmotility are associated with the former, while ileus, intra-abdominal abscess and malabsorption syndromes can result from the latter.

Thromboembolic disease in trauma

Trauma patients almost universally have all three factors of Virchow's triad: stasis, endothelial injury and hypercoagulability. Spine, extremity and severe abdominal solid organ injuries are frequently managed with transient periods of immobilisation before definitive therapy. Endothelial injury may result from direct vascular injury such as a stab wound to a femoral artery. In addition, there is accumulating evidence that the inflammatory response to severe injury even without direct vascular injury may incite or exacerbate endothelial damage. This may also play a role in the development of the hypercoagulable state of trauma patients.

Fatal PE is an important preventable cause of death in trauma patients. Pharmacological prophylaxis with low-molecular-weight heparins is superior to unfractionated heparin. However, contraindications to anticoagulant medications abound in the early phases of injury. These include intracranial haemorrhage, major solid organ injury, spine injury with the potential for epidural haematoma and severe pelvic and long bone fractures. Lower extremity sequential compression devices, graduated stockings, pneumatic foot pumps and other devices have been employed with varying success in DVT prophylaxis. Trauma patients with known DVT and PE should ideally receive therapeutic anticoagulation. Because of the long list of absolute and relative contraindications to anticoagulation, trauma patients with DVT are sometimes candidates for prophylactic inferior vena cava filter placement.

Nutritional support

One of the key factors in wound healing is nutrition. The ideal amount and composition of nutritional support in trauma patients is elusive. Recent research suggests that feeding patients additional calories according to the severity of injury may be deleterious. Similarly, early institution of total parenteral nutrition (TPN) when the gastrointestinal (GI) tract is dysfunctional has its detractors. Supplying 20–25 kcal/kg/day is probably a reasonable goal for most patients. Gastric feeds are tolerated by most patients. Severe brain injury and direct injury to the upper GI tract may require small bowel feeds. If it appears unlikely that a patient will not tolerate enteral nutritional support for more than 1 week, then TPN should be considered. Patients with multiple injuries have frequent interruption of tube feeds for investigations. Trauma patients rarely receive their prescribed nutritional support.

Other key factors in trauma management

In the trauma ICU, several general principles are applicable. Optimal sedation and analgesia are essential. This can be difficult with extraordinary pain or previous narcotic use. Peptic ulcer prophylaxis is especially important in severe brain injury and burns. Periodic interruption of sedation is useful for early liberation from mechanical ventilation and for assessment of neurological function in brain-injured patients. DVT prophylaxis may be more critical than in general ICU patients. There is a high risk of bedsores. This is compounded by immobility, musculoskeletal injury, poor wound care, malnutrition, hyperglycaemia, obesity and smoking history. Regular turning to relieve pressure points and the use of protective beds may decrease the risk of bedsores. A daily review of key management issues can expedite recovery and facilitate communication among team members.

> ### Clinical case
> A 44-year-old male involved in a high-speed motor vehicle collision has a spinal cord injury at the C5 level, pulmonary contusions and pelvic fracture. He is admitted, sedated and mechanically ventilated with 'logroll only' activity restrictions. Operative stabilisation of his spine and pelvis will be delayed until his pulmonary contusion improves. What are the management goals and what may complicate his stay?

> ### Summary points
> - Initial thorough review of injuries and periodic assessment are essential to prevent missed injuries and delayed diagnoses.
> - Sepsis and venous thromboembolism are major causes of morbidity and late mortality in patients who survive the immediate post-injury period.

Reference material

References and further reading

The history of intensive care

Hanson CW, Durbin CG, Maccioli GA, Deutschman CS, Sladen RN, Pronovost PJ, Gattinoni L. (2001) The anesthesiologist in critical care medicine: past, present, and future. *Anesthesiology* 95(3): 781–788.

Jude JR, Kouwenhoven WB, Knickerbocker GG. (1961) Cardiac arrest. Report of application of external cardiac massage on 118 patients. *JAMA* 178: 1063–1070.

Lax E (2004) *The Mould in Dr Florey's Coat*. New York: Henry Holt & Co.

Safar P, Escarraga LA, Elam JO. (1958) A comparison of the mouth-to-mouth and mouth-to-airway methods of artificial respiration, with the chest pressure arm lift methods. *N Engl J Med* 258: 671–677.

Severinghaus JW, Astrup P, Murray JF. (1998) Blood gas analysis and critical care medicine. *Am J Respir Crit Care Med* 157(4): S114–S122.

Swan HJ, Ganz W, Forrester J. (1970) Catheterization of the heart in man with use of a flow-directed balloon-tipped catheter. *N Engl J Med* 283(9): 447–451.

Trubuhovich RV. (2004) Further commentary on Denmark's 1952–53 poliomyelitis epidemic, especially regarding mortality; with a correction. *Acta Anaesthesiol Scand* 48(10): 1310–1315.

Zoll PM, Linenthal AJ, Gibson W, Pall MH, Normal LR. (1956) Termination of ventricular fibrillation in man by externally applied electric countershock. *N Engl J Med* 254: 727–732.

What is intensive care?

Baldock G, Foley P, Brett S. (2001) The impact of organisational change on outcome in an intensive care unit in the United Kingdom. *Intens Care Med* 27(5): 865–872.

Ferdinande P. Members of the Task Force of the European Society of Intensive Care Medicine (1997) Recommendations on minimal requirements for Intensive Care Departments. *Intens Care Med* 23: 226–232.

Haupt MT, Bekes CE, Brilli RJ, Carl LC, Gray AW, Jastremski MS, Naylor DF, Rudis M, Spevetz A, Wedel SK, Horst M. (2003) Guidelines on critical care services and personnel: recommendations based on a system of categorization of three levels of care. *Crit Care Med* 31(11): 2677–2683.

Landrigan CP, Rothschild JM, Cronin JW, Kaushal R, Burdick E, Katz JT, Lilly CM, Stone PH, Lockley SW, Bates DW, Czeisler CA. (2004) Effect of reducing interns' work hours on serious medical errors in intensive care units. *N Engl J Med* 351(18): 1838–1848.

Evidenced-based intensive care

Cook DJ, Sibbald WJ, Vincent JL, Cerra FB. (1996) Evidence based critical care medicine; what is it and what can it do for us? Evidence Based Medicine in Critical Care Group. *Crit Care Med* 24: 334–337.

Dellinger RP, Carlet JM, Masur H, Gerlach H, Calandra T, Cohen J, Gea-Banacloche J, Keh D, Marshall JC, Parker MM, Ramsay G, Zimmerman JL, Vincent JL, Levy MM. (2004) Surviving Sepsis Campaign guidelines for management of severe sepsis and septic shock. *Crit Care Med* 32: 858–873.

Guyatt GH, Haynes RB, Jaeschke RZ, Cook DJ, Green L, Naylor CD, Wilson MC, Richardson WS. (2000) Users' Guides to the Medical Literature: XXV. Evidence-based medicine: principles for applying the Users' Guides to patient care. Evidence-Based Medicine Working Group. *JAMA* 284: 1290–1296.

McAlister FA, Straus SE, Guyatt GH, Haynes RB. (2000) Users' Guides to the Medical Literature: XX. Integrating research evidence with the care of the individual patient. Evidence-Based Medicine Working Group. *JAMA* 283: 2829–2836.

Vincent JL. (2004) Evidence-based medicine in the ICU: important advances and limitations. *Chest* 126: 592–600.

Critical care transport

Beckmann U. (2004) Incidents relating to the intra-hospital transfer of critically ill patients. *Intens Care Med* 30: 1579–1585.

Duke GJ. (2001) Outcome of critically ill patients undergoing interhospital transfer. *Med J Aust* 174: 122–125.

Fromm RE Jr. (2000) Critical care transport. *Crit Care Clin* 16(4): 55–57.

Gebremichael M. (2000) Interhospital transport of the extremely ill patient: The mobile intensive care unit. *Crit Care Med* 28(1): 79–85.

Gooden C. (2003) Anesthesia for magnetic resonance imaging. *Int Anesthesiol Clin* 41(2): 29–37.

Warren J. (2004) Guidelines for the inter- and intrahospital transport of critically ill patients. *Crit Care Med* 32(1): 256–262.

Drug interactions

Cupp MJ, Tracy TS. (1998) Cytochrome P450: new nomenclature and clinical implications. *Am Fam Phys* 57(1): 107–116.

Drug Interactions. Cytochrome P450 System. Division of Clinical Pharmacology, Indiana University Department of Medicine. URL: http://medicine.iupui.edu/flockhart/clinlist.htm (up-to-date overview of clinically relevant interactions).

To Err Is Human: Building a Safer Health System (2000) Institute of Medicine (Ch. 2, p. 26).

Clinical excellence

Bossuyt PM, Reitsma JB, Bruns DE *et al.* (2003) The STARD statement for reporting studies of diagnostic accuracy: explanation and elaboration. *Clin Chem* 49: 17–18.

Klein JG. (2005) Five pitfalls in decisions about diagnosis and prescribing. *Br Med J* 330(7494): 781–783.

Perow C. (1999) *Normal Accidents. Living with High-risk Technologies*. Princeton, NJ: Princeton University Press.

Sackett D. (2004) *Clinical Epidemiology*. Philadelphia, PA: Lippincott Williams & Wilkins.

The airway in ICU

Hauswald M, Sklar DP, Tandberg D *et al.* (1991) Cervical spine movement during airway management: cinefluoroscopic appraisal in human cadavers. *Am J Emerg Med* 9: 535–538.

http://www.das.uk.com/guidelines/cvci.html

http://www.das.uk.com/guidelines/ddl.html

Vascular access in the ICU

MacLennan N, Nixon C, Lai J.

Better Anaesthesia Through Sonography – A Guide to Practical Perioperative Ultrasound. www.bats.ac.nz.

Hind D, Calvert N, McWilliams R, Davidson A, Paisley S, Beverley C, Thomas S. (2003) Ultrasonic locating devices for central venous cannulation: meta-analysis. *Br Med J* 327(7411): 361.

Ruesch S, Walder B, Tramer MR. (2002) Complications of central venous catheters: internal jugular versus subclavian access – a systematic review. *Crit Care Med* 30: 454–460.

Randolph AG, Cook DJ, Gonzales CA, Pribble CG. (1996) Ultrasound guidance for placement of central venous catheters: a meta-analysis of the literature. *Crit Care Med* 24: 2053–2058.

Fibreoptic bronchoscopy in the ICU

Honeybourne D, Babb J, Bowie P *et al.* (2001) British Thoracic Society guidelines on diagnostic flexible bronchoscopy. *Thorax* 56: I1–I21.

Mehta AC, Prakash UB, Garland R, Haponik E, Moses L, Schaffner W, Silvestri G. (2005) American College of Chest Physicians and American Association for Bronchoscopy consensus statement: prevention of flexible bronchoscopy-associated infection. *Chest* 128(3): 1742–1755.

Prakash UBS. (1993) Does the bronchoscope propagate infection? *Chest* 104: 552–559.

Cerebrospinal fluid, lumbar puncture and lumbar drain

Donald PR, Schoeman JF. (2004) Tuberculous meningitis. *N Engl J Med* 351(17): 1719–1720.

Johnston M, Zakharov A, Papaiconomou C, Salmasi G, Armstrong D. (2004) Evidence of connections between cerebrospinal fluid and nasal lymphatic vessels in humans, non-human primates and other mammalian species. *Cerebrospinal Fluid Res* 1(1): 2.

Mechanical ventilation

Caramez MP, Borges JB, Tucci MR, Okamoto VN, Carvalho CR, Kacmarek RM, Malhotra A, Velasco IT, Amato MB. (2005) Paradoxical responses to positive end-expiratory pressure in patients with airway obstruction during controlled ventilation. *Crit Care Med* 33(7): 1519–1528.

Girault C, Daudenthun I, Chevron V, Tamion F, Leroy J, Bonmarchand G. (1999) Noninvasive ventilation as a systematic extubation and weaning technique in acute-on-chronic respiratory failure: a prospective, randomized controlled study. *Am J Respir Crit Care Med* 160: 86 92.

Hedenstierna G, Edmark L, Aherdan KK. (2000) Time to reconsider the pre-oxygenation during induction of anaesthesia. *Minerva Anesthesiol* 66(5): 293–296.

Herriger A, Frascarolo P, Spahn DR, Magnusson L. (2004) The effect of positive airway pressure during pre-oxygenation and induction of anaesthesia upon duration of non-hypoxic apnoea. *Anaesthesia* 59(3): 243–247.

O'Croinin D, Ni Chonghaile M, Higgins B, Laffey JG. (2005) Bench-to-bedside review: permissive hypercapnia. *Crit Care* 9(1): 51–59.

Richards G, White H, van Schalkwyk J. (1999) Lung recruitment (your 'ARDS' patient need not die hypoxaemic). www.anaesthetist.com/icu/organs/lung/recruit/index.htm

van Schalkwyk J. (2001) New approaches to ventilation. www.anaesthetist.com/anaes/vent/newvent.htm

The Acute Respiratory Distress Syndrome Network. ARDSnet study group. (2000) Ventilation with lower tidal volumes as compared with traditional tidal volumes for acute lung injury and the acute respiratory distress syndrome. *N Engl J Med* 342(18): 1301–1308.

Renal replacement therapy

Burn DJ, Bates D. (1998) Neurology and the kidney. *J Neurol Neurosurg Psychiat* 65: 810–821.

Kapadia FN. (2003) Special issues in the patient with renal failure. *Crit Care Clin* 19(2): 233–251.

Maxvold N, Bunchman T. (2003) Renal failure and renal replacement therapy. *Crit Care Clin* 19(3): 563–575.

Vanholder R, Van Biesen W, Lameire N. (2001) What is the renal replacement method of first choice for intensive care patients? *J Am Soc Nephrol* 12(2): S40–S43.

Mechanical circulatory support

DeBakey ME. (1971) Left ventricular bypass pump for cardiac assistance. Clinical experience. *Am J Cardiol* 27: 3–11.

Gemmato CJ, Forrester MD, Myers TJ, Frazier OH, Cooley DA. (2005) Thirty-five years of mechanical circulatory support at the Texas Heart Institute. *Tex Heart Inst J* 32: 168–177.

Mert M, Akcevin A, Yildiz CE, Suzer K. (2005) Postoperative mechanical circulatory support with Biomedicus centrifugal pump. *Asian Cardiovasc Thorac Ann* 13(1): 38–41.

Circulation

Landry DW, Oliver JA. (2001) The pathogenesis of vasodilatory shock. *N Engl J Med* 345(8): 588–595.

Landry DW, Oliver JA.(2004) Insights into shock. *Sci Am* 290(2): 36–41.

Oxygen delivery

Anonymous. (1996) Practice guidelines for blood component therapy: A report by the American Society of Anesthesiologists Task Force on Blood Component Therapy. *Anesthesiology* 84: 732–747.

Hsia C. (1998) Mechanisms of disease: respiratory function of hemoglobin. *N Engl J Med* 338: 239–247.

Leach RM, Treacher DF. (2002) The pulmonary physician in critical care 2: oxygen delivery and consumption in the critically ill. *Thorax* 57: 170–177.

Marino P. (1998) *The ICU Book*, 2nd edn. Philadelphia, PA: Lippincott Williams & Wilkins.

Meier J, Kemming G, Kisch-Wedel H, Wölkhammer S, Habler O. (2004) Hyperoxic ventilation reduces 6-hour mortality at the critical hemoglobin concentration. *Anesthesiology* 100: 70–76.

Rivers E, Nguyen B, Havstad S, Ressler J, Muzzin A, Knoblich B, Peterson E, Tomlanovich M, the Early Goal-Directed Therapy Collaborative Group. (2001) Early goal-directed therapy in the treatment of severe sepsis and septic shock. *N Engl J Med* 345: 1368–1377.

West J. (2001) *Pulmonary Physiology and Pathophysiology: An Integrated, Case-Based Approach.* Philadelphia, PA: Lippincott Williams & Wilkins.

ICU acid–basics

Buck RP *et al.* (2002) Measurement of pH. Definition, standards, and procedures. *Pure Appl Chem* 74(11): 2169–2200. www.iupac.org/publications/pac/2002/pdf/7411x2169.pdf

van Schalkwyk J. (1999) *A basic approach to body pH.* www.anaesthetist.com/icu/elec/ionz/Stewart.htm

Stewart PA. (1981) *How to Understand Acid–base.* Elsevier North Holland. Now available online at www.acidbase.org/

Carbon dioxide

Laffey JG, Kavanagh BP. (1999) Carbon dioxide and the critically ill – too little of a good thing? *Lancet* 354(9186): 1283–1286.

Laffey JG, Kavanagh BP. (2002) Hypocapnia. *N Engl J Med* 347(1): 43–53.

Laffey JG, Engelberts D, Duggan M, Veldhuizen R, Lewis JF, Kavanagh BP. (2003) Carbon dioxide attenuates pulmonary impairment resulting from hyperventilation. *Crit Care Med* 31(11): 2634–2640.

Laffey JG, Jankov RP, Engelberts D, Tanswell AK, Post M, Lindsay T, Mullen JB, Romaschin A, Stephens D, McKerlie C, Kavanagh BP. (2003) Effects of therapeutic hypercapnia on mesenteric ischemia–reperfusion injury. *Am J Respir Crit Care Med* 168(11): 1383–1390.

Laffey JG, O'Croinin D, McLoughlin P, Kavanagh BP. (2004) Permissive hypercapnia – role in protective lung ventilatory strategies. *Intens Care Med* 30(3): 347–356.

Thermal disorders

Bouchama A, Knochel JP. (2002) Heat stroke. *N Engl J Med* 346(25): 1978–1988.

Ginsberg MD, Busto R. (1998) Combating hyperthermia in acute stroke: a significant clinical concern. *Stroke* 29(2): 529–534.

http://www.athleteproject.com

Feeding and starving in the ICU

Detsky A, McLaughlin J, Baker J *et al.* (1987) What is subjective global assessment of nutritional status? *J Parenteral Enteral Nutr* 11(1): 8–13.

Harris J, Benedict F. (1919) *A Biometric Study of Basal Metabolism in Man.* Washington, DC: Carnegie Institute of Washington.

Kleiber M. (1947) Body size and metabolic rate. *Physiol Rev* 27: 511–541.

Electrolyte abnormalities

Adrogue HJ, Madias NE. (2000) Hypernatremia. *N Engl J Med* 342(20): 1493–1499.

Adrogue HJ, Madias NE. (2000) Hyponatremia. *N Engl J Med* 342(21): 1581–1589.

Gennari FJ, Segal AS. (2002) Hyperkalemia: an adaptive response in chronic renal insufficiency. *Kidney Int* 62(1): 1–9.

Gennari FJ. (2002) Disorders of potassium homeostasis. Hypokalemia and hyperkalemia. *Crit Care Clin* 18(2): 273–288.

Scheinman SJ, Guay-Woodford LM, Thakker RV, Warnock DG. (1999) Genetic disorders of renal electrolyte transport. *N Engl J Med* 340(15): 1177–1187.

Fluid therapy in the ICU

Arieff AI. (1999) Fatal postoperative pulmonary edema: pathogenesis and literature review. *Chest* 115(5): 1371–1377.

Finfer S, Bellomo R, Boyce N, French J, Myburgh J, Norton R, SAFE Study Investigators. (2004) A comparison of albumin and saline for fluid resuscitation in the intensive care unit. *N Engl J Med* 350(22): 2247–2256.

Holte K, Klarskov B, Christensen DS, Lund C, Nielsen KG, Bie P, Kehlet H. (2004) Liberal versus restrictive fluid administration to improve recovery after laparoscopic cholecystectomy: a randomized, double-blind study. *Ann Surg* 240(5): 892–899.

Needham DM, Detsky AS, Stewart TE. (2001) Recent evidence for intravenous fluid choice in patients with severe infection. *Intens Care Med* 27(3): 609–612.

Nisanevich V, Felsenstein I, Almogy G, Weissman C, Einav S, Matot I. (2005) Effect of intraoperative fluid management on outcome after intraabdominal surgery. *Anesthesiology* 103(1): 25–32.

Blood and blood components

Cable R, Carlson B, Chambers L, Kolins J, Murphy S, Tilzer L, Vassallo R, Weiss K, Wissel M. (2002) *Practice Guidelines for Blood Transfusion: A Compilation from Recent Peer-Reviewed Literature.* American Red Cross. www.aabb.org

Kuriyan M, Carson JL. (2004) Blood transfusion risks in the intensive care unit. *Crit Care Clin* 20(2): 237–253.

Raghavan M, Marik PE. (2005) Anemia, allogenic blood transfusion, and immunomodulation in the critically ill. *Chest* 127(1): 295–307.

Roa SR, Jollis JG, Harrington RA, Granger CB, Newby LK, Armstrong PW, Moliterno DJ, Lindblad L, Pieper K, Topol EJ, Stamler JS, Califf RM. (2004) Relationship of blood transfusion and clinical outcomes in patients with acute coronary syndromes. *JAMA* 292(13): 1555–1562.

Spahn DR, Dettori N, Kocian R, Chassot P. (2004) Transfusion in the cardiac patient. *Crit Care Clin* 20(3): 269–279.

Neurological assessment

Claassen J, Mayer SA. (2002) Continuous electroencephalographic monitoring in neurocritical care. *Curr Neurol Neurosci Rep* 2: 534–40.

Mednick AS, Mayer SA. (2002) Critical care management of neurologic catastrophes. *Adv Neurol* 90: 87–101.

Rafanan AL *et al.* (2000) Head computed tomography in medical intensive care unit patients: clinical indications. *Crit Care Med* 28: 1306–1309.

Smith MC. (2001) Quantification of neurologic function. *Crit Care Med* 29(10): 2036–2037.

The Brain Trauma Foundation. The American Association of Neurological Surgeons. (2000) The joint section on neurotrauma and critical care. Initial management. *J Neurotrauma* 17: 463–469.

Central nervous system injury

Ball PA. (2001) Critical care of spinal cord injury. *Spine* 26(24 Suppl): S27–S30.

Bayir H, Clark RS, Kochanek PM. (2003) Promising strategies to minimize secondary brain injury after head trauma. *Crit Care Med* 31(1 Suppl): S112–S117.

Bracken MB, Holford TR. (1993) Effects of timing of methylprednisolone or naloxone administration on recovery of segmental and long-tract neurological function in NASCISJ *Neurosurg* 79: 500–507.

Hurlbert RJ. (2001) The role of steroids in acute spinal cord injury: an evidence-based analysis. *Spine* 26(24 Suppl.): S39–S46.

Winslow C, Rozovsky J. (2003) Effect of spinal cord injury on the respiratory system. *Am J Phys Med Rehabil* 82(10): 803–814.

www.asia-spinal injury. org/(Follow links to Publications then Dermatome Chart.)

Weakness in the ICU

Adnet F, Dhissi G, Borron SW (2001) Complication profiles of adult asthmatics requiring paralysis during mechanical ventilation. *Intens Care Med* 27(11): 1729–1736.

Coakley JH, Nagendran K, Yarwood GD, Honovar M, Hinds CJ (1998) Patterns of neurophysiological abnormality in prolonged critical illness. *Intens Care Med* 24(8): 801–807.

De Jonghe B, Sharshar T, Lefaucheur JP, Authier F-J (2002) Paresis acquired in the intensive care unit: a prospective multicenter study. *JAMA* 288(22): 2859–2867.

Ford EV. (1995) Monitoring neuromuscular blockade in the adult ICU. *Am J Crit Care* 4(2): 122–130.

Hund E. (1999) Myopathy in critically ill patients. *Crit Care Med* 27(11): 2544–2547.

Wagenmakers AJ. (2001) Muscle function in critically ill patients. *Clin Nutr* 20(5): 451–454.

Seizures

Bleck TP, Smith MC, Pierre-Louis SJC *et al.* (1993) Neurologic complications of critical medical illness. *Crit Care Med* 21: 98–103.

Marik PE, Varon J.(2004) The management of status epilepticus. *Chest* 126(2): 582–591.

Tomson T, Beghi E, Sundqvist A, Johannessen SI. (2004) Medical risks in epilepsy: a review with focus on physical injuries, mortality, traffic accidents and their prevention. *Epilepsy Res* 60(1): 1–16.

Varelas PN, Mirski MA. (2001) Seizures in the adult intensive care unit. *J Neurosurg Anesthesiol* 13(2): 163–175.

Altered mental states

Jenkins DH. (2000) Substance abuse and withdrawal in the intensive care unit. *Surg Clin North Am* 80(3): 1033–1053.

(2002) Cohen I, Gallagher T, Polman A, Dasta J, Abraham E, Papadokos, P. Management of the agitated intensive care unit patient. *Crit Care Med* 30(1): S97–123.

Misra S, Ganzini L. (2003) Delirium, depression and anxiety. *Crit Care Clin* 19(4): 771–787.

Pisani MA, McNicoll L, Inouye SK. (2003) Cognitive impairment in the intensive care unit. *Clin Chest Med* 24(4): 727–737.

Analgesia in the ICU

Bruce J, Drury N, Poobalan AS, Jeffrey RR, Smith WC, Chambers WA. (2003) The prevalence of chronic chest and leg pain following cardiac surgery: a historical cohort study. *Pain* 104(1–2): 265–273.

Peng PW, Tumber PS, Gourlay D. (2005) Review article: perioperative pain management of patients on methadone therapy. *Can J Anaesth* 52(5): 513–523.

Vickers AP, Jolly A. (2006) Naltrexone and problems in pain management. *Br Med J* 332(7534): 132–133.

ICU sedation

Capuzzo M, Pinamonti A, Cingolani E, Grassi L, Bianconi M, Contu P, Gritti G, Alvisi R. (2001) Analgesia, sedation, and memory of intensive care. *J Crit Care* 16(3): 83–89.

Mullins ME, Barnes BJ. (2002) Hyperosmolar metabolic acidosis and intravenous lorazepam. *N Engl J Med* 347(11): 857–858.

Ramsay MAE, Savage TM, Simpson BR *et al.* (1974) Controlled sedation with alphaxalone/alphadolone. *Br Med J* 2: 656.

Rudis MI, Sikora CA, Angus E *et al.* (1997) A prospective, randomized, controlled evaluation of peripheral nerve stimulation versus standard clinical dosing of neuromuscular blocking agents in critically ill patients. *Crit Care Med* 25(4): 575–583.

Organ donation

Cuthbertson SJ, Margetts MA, Streat SJ. (2000) Bereavement follow-up after critical illness. *Crit Care Med* 28(4): 1196–1201.

Frigerio M, Gronda EG, Mangiavacchi M, Andreuzzi B, Colombo T, De Vita C, Oliva F, Quaini E, Pellegrini A. (1997) Restrictive criteria for heart transplantation candidacy maximize survival of patients with advanced heart failure. *J Heart Lung Transplant* 16(2): 160–168.

Streat S. (2004) Moral assumptions and the process of organ donation in the intensive care unit. *Crit Care* 8: 382–388.

Wijdicks EFM. (2001) The diagnosis of brain death. *N Engl J Med* 344(16): 1215–1221.

Wood KE, Becker BN, McCartney JG, D'Alessandro AM, Coursin DB. (2004) Care of the potential organ donor. *N Engl J Med* 351(26): 2730–2739.

Monitoring the cardiovascular system

Fick A. (1870) *Über die Messung des Blutquantums in den Herzventrikeln.* Wurzburg: Sitx. der Physik-Med. ges, p. 16.

Gnaegi A, Feihl F, Perret C. (1997) Intensive care physicians' insufficient knowledge of right-heart catheterization at the bedside: time to act? *Crit Care Med* 25: 213–220.

Kramer A, Zygun D, Hawes H, Easton P, Ferland A. (2004) Pulse pressure variation predicts fluid responsiveness following coronary artery bypass surgery. *Chest* 126(5): 1563–1568.

Rizvi K, Deboisblanc BP, Truwit JD, Dhillon G, Arroliga A, Fuchs BD, Guntupalli KK, Hite D, Hayden D, NIH/NHLBI ARDS Clinical Trials Network. (2005) Effect of airway pressure display on interobserver agreement in the assessment of vascular pressures in patients with acute lung injury and acute respiratory distress syndrome. *Crit Care Med* 33(1): 98–103; discussion pp. 243–244.

Stephan F, Flahault A, Dieudonne N, Hollande J, Paillard F, Bonnet F. (2001) Clinical evaluation of circulating blood volume in critically ill patients – contribution of a clinical scoring system. *Br J Anaesth* 86(6): 754–762.

Ischaemic heart disease

Antman E. (2004) ACC/AHA Guidelines for the management of patients With ST-elevation myocardial infarction. *J Am Coll Cardiol* 44(3): E1–E211.

Atwater B. (2005) Platelet glycoprotein IIb/IIIa receptor antagonists in non-ST segment elevation acute coronary syndromes: a review and guide to patient selection. *Drugs* 65(3): 313–324.

Braunwald E. (2002) ACC/AHA 2002 Guideline update for the management of patients with unstable angina and non–ST-segment elevation myocardial infarction. *J Am Coll Cardiol* 40(7): 1366–1374.

Giugliano R. (2005) 2004 ACC/AHA guideline for the management of patients with STEMI: the implications for clinicians. *Nature Clin Pract Cardiovasc Med* 2(3): 114–115.

Kamineni R. (2004) Acute coronary syndromes: initial evaluation and risk stratification. *Prog Cardiovasc Dis* 46(5): 379–392.

www.acc.org/qualityandscience/clinical/guidelines/stemi/Guideline1/index.pdf

www.acc.org/qualityandscience/clinical/guidelines/unstable/incorporated/UA_incorporated.pdf

Heart failure in the ICU

Casey C, Knight BP. (2004) Cardiac resynchronization pacing therapy. *Cardiology* 101(1–3): 72–78.

Massie B, Shah N. (1997) Evolving trends in the epidemiologic factors of heart failure: rationale for preventive strategies and comprehensive disease management. *Am Heart J* 133(6): 703–712.

Mebazaa A, Karpati P, Renaud E, Algotsson L. (2004) Acute right ventricular failure – from pathophysiology to new treatments. *Intens Care Med* 30(2): 185–196.

Perrone S, Kaplinsky E. (2005) Calcium sensitizer agents: a new class of inotropic agents in the treatment of decompensated heart failure. *Int J Cardiol* 103(3): 248–255.

Zile M, Brutsaert D. (2002) New concepts in diastolic dysfunction and diastolic heart failure: Part I. *Circulation* 105: 1387–1393.

Zile M, Brutsaert D. (2002) New concepts in diastolic dysfunction and diastolic heart failure: Part II. *Circulation* 105: 1503–1508.

Arrhythmias

Delacretaz E. (2006) Clinical practice. Supraventricular tachycardia. *N Engl J Med* 354(10): 1039–1051.

Hall MC, Todd DM. (2006) Modern management of arrhythmias. *Postgrad Med J* 82(964): 117–125.

Mangrum JM, DiMarco JP. (2000) The evaluation and management of bradycardia. *N Engl J Med* 342(10): 703–709.

Pacing

American Society of Anesthesiologists Task Force on Perioperative Management of Patients with Cardiac Rhythm Management Devices. (2005) *Anesthesiology* 103(1): 186–198.

Kusumoto FM, Goldschlager N. (1996) Cardiac pacing. *N Engl J Med* 334(2): 89–97.

Kusumoto FM, Goldschlager N. (2002) Device therapy for cardiac arrhythmias. *JAMA* 287(14): 1848–1852.

McPherson CA, Manthous C. (2004) Permanent pacemakers and implantable defibrillators: considerations for intensivists. *Am J Respir Crit Care Med* 170(9): 933–340.

Rosanio S *et al.* (2005) Benefits, unresolved questions, and technical issues of cardiac resynchronization therapy for heart failure. *Am J Cardiol* 96(5): 710–717.

Cardiac surgery

Adam DH, Antman EM. (2001) Medical management of the patient undergoing cardiac surgery. In: Braunwald E, Zipes DP, Libby P (eds) *Heart Disease: A Textbook of Cardiovascular Medicine*, 6th edn. Philadelphia, PA: W.B. Saunders.

Patel H, Pagani FD. (2003) Extracorporeal mechanical circulatory assist. *Cardiol Clin* 21: 29–41.

Skiles JA, Griffin BP. (2000) Transesophageal echocardiographic (TEE) evaluation of ventricular function. *Cardiol Clin* 18(4): 681–697.

www.anaesthetist.com (for an introduction to echocardiography)

Pulmonary hypertension

Chatterjee K, De Marco T, Alpert JS. (2002) Pulmonary hypertension: hemodynamic diagnosis and management. *Arch Intern Med* 162(17): 1925–1933.

Gilbert B, Langleben D, Bernarrd H. (2003) Pulmonary artery hypertension: pathophysiology and anesthetic approach. *Anesthesiology* 99(6): 1415–1432.

McNeil K, Dunning J, Morrell NW. (2003) The pulmonary physician in critical care. 13: The pulmonary circulation and right ventricular failure in the ITU. *Thorax* 58(2): 157–162.

Nazzareno G, Werner S, Naeije R, Simonneau G, Rubin LJ. (2004) Comparative analysis of clinical trials and evidence-based treatment algorithm in pulmonary artery hypertension. *J Am Coll Cardiol* 43(12S1): S81–88.

Valvular and congenital heart disease

Russell IA, Rouine-Rapp K, Stratman G, Miller-Hance WC. (2006) Congenital heart disease in the adult: a review with internet-accessible transesophageal echocardiographic images. *Anesth Analg* 102: 694–723.

Stayer SA, Andropoulos DB, Russell IA. (2003) Anesthetic management of the adult patient with congenital heart disease. *Anesthesiol Clin N Ann* 21: 53–673.

The Task Force on the Management of Valvular Heart Disease of the European Society of Cardiology. (2007) Guidelines on the management of valvular heart disease. *European Heart J* 28(2): 230–268.

Respiratory failure

Antonelli M *et al.* (1998) A comparison of noninvasive positive-pressure ventilation and conventional mechanical ventilation in patients with acute respiratory failure. *N Engl J Med* 339: 429–435.

Bersten AD *et al.* (1991) Treatment of severe cardiogenic pulmonary edema with continuous positive airway pressure delivered by face mask. *N Engl J Med* 325: 1825–1830.

Brochard L *et al.* (1995) Noninvasive ventilation for acute exacerbations of COPD. *N Engl J Med* 333: 817–822.

Estaban E *et al.* (2004) Noninvasive positive-pressure ventilation for respiratory failure after extubation. *N Engl J Med* 350: 2452–2460.

Polkey M, Moxham J. (2001) Clinical aspects of respiratory muscle dysfunction in the critically ill. *Chest* 119: 926–939.

Truwit J, Bernard G. (2004) Noninvasive ventilation – don't push too hard. *N Engl J Med* 350: 2512–2515.

Ware L, Matthay M. (2000) The acute respiratory distress syndrome. *N Engl J Med* 342: 1334–1349.

Asthma

Levy B, Kitch B, Fanta C. (1998) Medical and ventilatory management of status asthmaticus. *Intens Care Med* 24: 105–117.

Miller T, Barbers R. (1999) Management of the severe asthmatic. *Curr Opin Pulmon Med* 5(1): 58–62.

Papiris S, Kotanidou A, Malagari K, Roussos C. (2002) Clinical review: severe asthma. *Crit Care* 6(1): 30–44.

Tamul P, Peruzzi W. (2004) Assessment and management of patients with pulmonary disease. *Crit Care Med* 32(4 Suppl.): S137–S45.

Chronic obstructive pulmonary disease

Barnes PJ. (2000) Chronic obstructive pulmonary disease. *N Engl J Med* 343(4): 269–280.

Barnes PJ. (2004) Corticosteroid resistance in airway disease. *Proc Am Thorac Soc* 1(3): 264–268.

Niewoehner E *et al.* (1999) Effect of systemic glucocorticoids on exacerbations of chronic obstructive pulmonary disease. *N Engl J Med* 340(25): 1941–1947.

The ICU chest radiograph

Grainger RG, Allison D, Dixon AK (eds). (2001) Grainger & Allison's Diagnostic Radiology: A Textbook of Medical Imaging, 4th edn. New York: Churchill Livingstone.

Mettler RG. (2005) Essentials of Radiology, 2nd edn. Philadelphia, PA: Elsevier.

Trotman-Dickenson B. (2003) Radiology in the intensive care unit. *J Intens Care Med* 18(4): 198–210.

Renal failure

Abernethy VE, Lieberthal W. (2002) Acute renal failure in the critically ill patient. *Crit Care Clin* 18(2): 203–222.

Hladunewich M, Rosenthal MH. (2000) Pathophysiology and management of renal insufficiency in the perioperative and critically ill patient. *Anesthesiol Clin North Am* 18(4): 773–789.

Schrier RW, Wang W, Poole B, Mitra A. (2004) Acute renal failure: definitions, diagnosis, pathogenesis, and therapy. *J Clin Invest* 114(1): 5–14.

Thadhani R, Pascual M, Bonventre JV. (1996) Acute renal failure. *N Engl J Med* 334(22): 1448–1460.

Gastrointestinal bleeding

Beejay U, Wolfe MM. (2000) Acute gastrointestinal bleeding in the intensive care unit. The gastroenterologist's perspective. *Gastroenterol Clin North Am* 29(2): 309–336.

Conrad SA. (2002) Acute upper gastrointestinal bleeding in critically ill patients: causes and treatment modalities. *Crit Care Med* 30(6 Suppl.): S3655–S3658.

Kupfer Y, Cappell MS, Tessler S. (2000) Acute gastrointestinal bleeding in the intensive care unit. The intensivist's perspective. *Gastroenterol Clin North Am* 29(2): 275–307.

nobelprize.org/nobel_prizes/medicine/laureates/2005/press.html

Gastrointestinal motility disorders

Cleary RK. (1998) *Clostridium difficile*-associated diarrhoea and colitis: clinical manifestations, diagnosis and treatment. *Dis Colon Rectum* 41: 1435–1449.

Dietz DW. Small bowel obstruction. In: Fazio VW, Church JM, Delaney CP (eds) 2005 *Current Therapy in Colon and Rectal Surgery*, 2nd edn. Philadelphia, PA: Elsevier Mosby.

Toursarkissian B, Thompson RW. (1997) Ischemic colitis. *Surg Clin North Am* 77: 461–470.

Young-Fadok. Constipation. In: Fazio VW, Church JM, Delaney CP (eds) *Current Therapy in Colon and Rectal Surgery*, 2nd edn. Philadelphia, PA: Elsevier Mosby.

Cholecystitis and pancreatitis

Nathens AB *et al.* (2004) Management of the critically ill patient with severe acute pancreatitis. *Crit Care Med* 32: 2524–2536. *This is a review of recommendations of an international consensus conference.*

UK Working Party on Acute Pancreatitis. (2005) UK guidelines for the management of acute pancreatitis. *Gut* 54: 1–9.

Werner J *et al.* (2005) Management of acute pancreatitis: from surgery to interventional intensive care. *Gut* 54: 426–436. *This is a good update of recent changes in management strategies.*

Liver failure

Dargan PI, Jones AL. (2002) Acetaminophen poisoning: an update for the intensivist. *Crit Care* 6(2): 108–110.

Krasko A, Deshpande K, Bonvino S. (2003) Liver failure, transplantation, and critical care. *Crit Care Clin* 19(2): 155–183.

Marrero J, Martinez FJ, Hyzy R. (2003) Advances in critical care hepatology. *Am J Respir Crit Care Med* 168(12): 1421–1426.

Rahman T, Hodgson H. (2001) Clinical management of acute hepatic failure. *Intens Care Med* 27(3): 467–476.

Williams R, Wendon J. (1994) Indications for orthotopic liver transplantation in fulminant liver failure. *Hepatology* 20: S5–S10.

Endocrine function in the ICU

Marik PE, Varon J, Fromm RM. (2002) The management of severe asthma. *Chest* 122: 1784–1796.

Mechanick JI. (2002) Endocrine and metabolic issues in the management of the chronically critically ill patient. *Crit Care Clin* 18(3): 619–641.

Nylen ES. (2004) *J Intens Care Med* 19(2): 67–82.

Van den Berghe G. (2000) *Eur J Endocrinol* 143: 1–13.

Diabetes mellitus in the ICU

Hogan P, Dall T, Nikolov P, American Diabetes Association. (2003) Economic costs of diabetes in the US in 2000. *Diabetes Care* 26(3): 917–932.

Ljungqvist O, Nygren J, Soop M, Thorell A. (2005) Metabolic perioperative management: novel concepts. *Curr Opin Crit Care* 11(4): 295–299.

Umpierrez GE, Cuervo R, Karabell A, Latif K, Freire AX, Kitabchi AE. (2004) Treatment of diabetic ketoacidosis with subcutaneous insulin aspart. *Diabetes Care* 27(8): 1873–1878.

Endocrine emergencies

Arlt W, Allolio B. (2003) Seminar: adrenal insufficiency. *Lancet* 361: 1881–1893.

Chiasson J, Aris-Jilwan N, Bélanger R, Bertrand S, Beauregard H, Ékoé J, Fournier H, Havrankova J. (2003) Diagnosis and treatment of diabetic ketoacidosis and the hyperglycemic hyperosmolar state. *Can Med Assoc J* 168: 859–866.

Cooper M, Stewart P. (2003) Current concepts: corticosteroid insufficiency in acutely ill patients. *N Engl J Med* 348: 727–734.

Marino P. (1998) *The ICU Book*, 2nd edn. Philadelphia, PA: Lippincott Williams & Wilkins.

Stoelting R, Dierdorf S. (2002) *Anesthesia and Co-Existing Disease*, 4th edn. New York: Churchill Livingstone.

Tietgens S, Leinung M. (1995) Thyroid storm. *Med Clin North Am* 79: 169–184.

Wall C. (2000) Myxedema coma: diagnosis and treatment. *Am Fam Phys* 62: 2485–2490.

Clotting and bleeding: a delicate balance

Bernard GR *et al*. (2001) Efficacy and safety of recombinant human activated protein C for severe sepsis. *N Engl J Med* 344(10): 699–709.

Bernard GR *et al*. (2003) Safety assessment of drotrecogin alfa (activated) in the treatment of adult patients with severe sepsis. *Crit Care* 7(2): 155–163.

Mammen E.F. (1998) Antithrombin: its physiological importance and role in DIC. *Semin Thromb Hemost* 24(1): 19–25.

Rintala E *et al*. (1998) Protein C in the treatment of coagulopathy in meningococcal disease. *Crit Care Med* 26(5): 965–968.

Roberts HR, Monroe DM, Escobar MA. (2004) Current concepts of hemostasis: implications for therapy. *Anesthesiology* 100(3): 722–730.

Bleeding in the ICU

Karkouti K *et al*. (2006) A propensity score case–control comparison of aprotinin and tranexamic acid in high-transfusion-risk cardiac surgery. *Transfusion* 46(3): 327–338.

Mannucci PM. (2005) Management of von Willebrand disease in developing countries. *Semin Thromb Hemost* 31(5): 602–609.

Mayer SA *et al*. (2005) Recombinant activated factor VII for acute intracerebral hemorrhage. *N Engl J Med* 352: 777–785.

Roberts HR, Monroe DM 3rd, Hoffman M. (2004) Safety profile of recombinant factor VIIa. *Semin Hematol* 41(1 Suppl. 1): 101–108.

Thrombosis in the ICU

Caprini JA, Glase CJ, Anderson CB, Hathaway K. (2004) Laboratory markers in the diagnosis of venous thromboembolism. *Circulation* 109(12 Suppl. 1): I4–I8.

Geerts W, Selby R. (2003) Prevention of venous thromboembolism in the ICU. *Chest* 124(6 Suppl.): S357–S363.

Hirsh J, Heddle N, Kelton JG. (2004) Treatment of heparin-induced thrombocytopenia: a critical review. *Arch Intern Med* 164(4): 361–369.

Marik PE, Andrews L, Maini B. (1997) The incidence of deep venous thrombosis in ICU patients. *Chest* 111(3): 661–664.

Streiff MB. (2003) Vena caval filters: a review for intensive care specialists. *J Intens Care Med* 18(2): 59–79.

Warkentin TE, Kelton JG. (2001) Temporal aspects of heparin-induced thrombocytopenia. *N Engl J Med* 344(17): 1286–1292.

Prevention and treatment of infections

Alliance for Prudent Use of Antibiotics: www.tufts.edu/med/apua/Practitioners/healthcare.html

British National Formulary (UK): www.bnf.org

Guidelines for antibiotic use: Infectious disease societies of America (www.idsociety.org)

Pittet D, Allegranzi B, Sax H, Dharan S, Pessoa-Silva CL, Donaldson L, Boyce AM. (2006) WHO Global Patient Safety Challenge, World Alliance for Patient Safety. Evidence-based model for hand transmission during patient care and the role of improved practices. *Lancet Infect Dis* 6(10): 641–652.

Plowman R, Graves N, Griffin N, Roberts JA, Swan A, Cookson BD, Taylor L. (2000) Socio-economic burden of hospital-acquired infection. London: Public Health Laboratory Service (www.hpa.org.uk).

Scottish Intercollegiate Guidelines Network: www.sign.ac.uk/guidelines/published/index.html

Silvestri L, Van Saere HK, Milanese M, Gregori D, Gullo A. (2007) Selective decontamination of the digestive tract reduces bacterial bloodstream infection and mortality in critically ill patients. Systematic review of randomized controlled trials. *J Hosp Infect* 65(3): 187–203.

The Sanford guide (USA): www.sanfordguide.com/

Therapeutic Guidelines (Australia): www.tg.com.au/home/index.html

Treatment of CAP: British Thoracic Society (www.brit-thoracic.org.uk)

Sepsis and septic shock

Annane D, Sébille V, Charpentier C, Bollaert PE, François B, Korach JM, Capellier G, Cohen Y, Azoulay E, Troché G, Chaumet-Riffaut P, Bellissant E. (2002) Effect of treatment with low doses of hydrocortisone and fludrocortisone on mortality in patients with septic shock. *JAMA* 288(7): 862–871.

Beale RJ et al. (2004) Vasopressor and inotropic support in septic shock: an evidence-based review. *Crit Care Med* 32: S455–465.

Bernard GR et al. (2001) Efficacy and safety of recombinant human activated protein C for severe sepsis. *N Engl J Med* 344(10): 699–709.

Dellinger RP *et al*. (2004) Surviving Sepsis Campaign: Guidelines for management of severe sepsis and septic shock. *Crit Care Med* 32(3): 858–873.

Jacobi J. (2006) Corticosteroid replacement in critically ill patients. *Crit Care Clin* 22(2): 245–253.

Reid IA. (1997) Role of vasopressin deficiency in the vasodilation of septic shock. *Circulation* 95(5): 1108–1110.

Riedemann NC et al. (2003) Novel strategies for treatment of spesis. *Nature Med* 9: 517–524.

Rivers E *et al*. (2001) Early goal-directed therapy in the treatment of severe sepsis and septic shock. *N Engl J Med* 345(19): 1368–1377.

Van den Berghe G *et al*. (2001) Intensive insulin therapy in critically ill patients. *N Engl J Med* 345(19): 1359–1367.

Central nervous system infection

van de Beek D. (2004) Clinical features and prognostic factors in adults with bacterial meningitis. *N Engl J Med* 351(18): 1849–1859.

Bernardini GL. (2004) Diagnosis and management of brain abscess and subdural empyema. *Curr Neurol Neurosci Rep* 4(6): 448–456.

Fan E. (2004) West Nile virus infection in the intensive care unit: a case series and literature review. *Can Respir J* 11(5): 354–358.

Flores-Cordero JM. (2003) Acute community-acquired bacterial meningitis in adults admitted to the intensive care unit: clinical manifestations, management and prognostic factors. *Intens Care Med* 29(11): 1967–1973.

Hayes EB. (2005) Epidemiology and transmission dynamics of West Nile virus disease. *Emerg Infect Dis* 11(8): 1167–1173.

Sejvar JJ. (2006) Manifestations of West Nile neuroinvasive disease. *Rev Med Virol* 16(4): 209–224.

Thwaites GE. (2005) Tuberculous meningitis: many questions, too few answers. *Lancet Neurol* 4(3): 160–170.

Tyler KL. (2004) Update on herpes simplex encephalitis. *Rev Neurol Dis* 1(4): 169–178.

Pneumonia

Anonymous. (2001) Guidelines for the management of community acquired pneumonia in adults. British Thoracic Society. Thorax 56: Suppl. IV. www.brit-thoracic.org.uk

Fine MJ, Auble TE, Yealy DM *et al.* (1997) A prediction rule to identify low risk patients with community-acquired pneumonia. *N Engl J Med* 336: 243–250.

Fujitani S, Yu VL. (2006) Quantitative cultures for diagnosing ventilator-associated pneumonia: a critique. *Clin Infect Dis* 43(Suppl 2): S106–113.

Lim WS, MacFarlane JT, Boswell TC et al. (2001) SCAPA: Study of Community Acquired Pneumonia Aetiology in adults admitted to hospital: implications for management guidelines. *Thorax* 56: 296–301.

Mandell LA, Bartlett JG, Dowell SF et al. (2000) Update of practice guidelines for the management of community acquired pneumonia in immunocompetent adults. IDSA guidelines. *Clin Infect Dis* 37: 1405–1433.

Infections associated with prosthetic material in the ICU

Lindsay D, von Holy A. (2006) Bacterial biofilms within the clinical setting: what healthcare professionals should know. *J Hosp Infect* 64(4): 313–325.

McGee DC, Gould MK. (2003) Preventing Complications of Central Venous Catheterization. *N Engl J Med* 348(12): 1123–1133.

Nicolle LE. (2000) Urinary tract infection in long-term-care facility residents. *Clin Infect Dis* 31(3): 757–761. Epub 2000 Oct 4.

Safdar N, Fine JP, Maki DG. (2005) Meta-analysis: methods for diagnosing intravascular device-related bloodstream infection. *Ann Intern Med* (2005) 142(6): 451–466.

The immunocompromised patient in critical care

Corbett EL, Steketee RW, ter Kuile FO, Latif AS, Kamali A, Hayes RJ. (2002) HIV-1/AIDS and the control of other infectious diseases in Africa. *The Lancet* 359(9324), 2177–2187.

Corey L, Boeckh M. (2002) Persistent fever in patients with neutropaenia. *N Engl J Med* 346(4): 222–224.

Fishman, JA, Rubin, RH. (1998) Infection in organ transplant recipients. *N Engl J Med* 338: 1741.

Kovacs JA, Masur H. (2000) Prophylaxis against opportunistic infections in patients with human immunodeficiency virus infection. *N Engl J Med* 342(19): 1416–1429.

Mandell GL, Bennett JE, Dolin R (eds) (2004) Mandell, Douglas, and Bennett's Principles and Practice of Infectious Diseases (Principles & Practice of Infectious Diseases), 6th edn. New York: Churchill Livingstone.

Pizzo PA. (1999) Fever in immunocompromised patients. *N Engl J Med* 341: 893.

Sepkowitz K. (2005) Treatment of Febrile Neutropenic Infection. *Clin Infect Dis* 40: S253–S256.

Simon V, Ho DD, Abdool Karim Q. (2006) HIV/AIDS epidemiology, pathogenesis, prevention, and treatment. *The Lancet* 368(9534), 489–504.

Viscoli C, Vernier O, Machetti M. (2005) Infections in patients febrile neutropenia: epidemiology, microbiology, and risk stratification. *Clin Infect Dis* 40: S240–S245.

Tropical medicine

Anderson KB, Chunsuttiwat S, Nisalak A, Mammen Mp, Libraty DH, Rothman AL, Green S, Vaughn DW, Ennis FA, Endy TP. (2007) Burden of symptomatic dengue infection in children at primary school in Thailand: a prospective study. *The Lancet* 369 (9571), 1452–1459.

Ashley EA, white NJ. Artemisinin-based combinations. *Curr Opin Infect Dis* 18(6): 531–536.

Cook GC, Zumla AI (eds) (2002) Manson's Tropical Diseases. Philadelphia, PA: Saunders WB.

Guzmán MG, Kouri G. (2002) Dengue: an update. *The Lancet Infectious Diseases* 2(1), 33–42.

Jensenius M, Fournier PE, Raoult D. (2004) Rickettsioses and the international traveler. *Clin Infect Dis* 2004 39(10): 1493–1499. Epub 2004 Oct 22.

Quinn TC. (1996) Global burden of the HIV pandemic. *The Lancet* 348 (9020), 99–106.

Rigau-Pérez JG. (2006) Severe dengue: the need for new case definitions. *The Lancet Infectious Diseases* 6(5), 297–302.

Smithuis F, Kyaw MK, Phe O, Aye KZ, Htet L, Barends M, Lindegardh N, Singtoroj T, Ashley E, Lwin S, Stepniewska K, White NJ. (2006) Efficacy and effectiveness of dihydroartemisinin-piperaquine versus artesunate-mefloquine in falciparum malaria: an open-label randomised comparison. *The Lancet* 367 (9528) 2075–2085).

White N. (2004) Sharing malarias. *The Lancet* 363 (9414), 1006.

White N, Nosten F, Björkman A, Marsh K, Snow RW. (2004) WHO, the Global fund, and medical malpractice in malaria treatment. *The Lancet* 363 (9415) 1160.

http://www.cdc.gov/ncidod/dhqp/bp_vhf_interimGuidance.html

Website of Health Protection Association (HPA) of UK: http://www.hpa.org.uk/infections/topics_az/VHF/ACDP_VHF_guidance.pdf

Website of Centers for Disease Control and Prevention (CDC) of USA: http://www.cdc.gov/ncidod/dhqp/bp_vhf_interimGuidance.html

http://www.who.int/GlobalAtlas/home.asp

Clever bugs and defunct drugs

CDC. (2002) *Staphylococcus aureus* resistant to vancomycin, United States. *MMWR* 51: 565–567.

Fridkin SK et al. (2005) Methicillin-resistant Staphylococcus aureus disease in three communities. *N Engl J Med* 352(14): 1436–1444.

Kumana CR, Ching TY, Kong Y, Ma EC, Kou M, Lee RA, Cheng VC, Chiu SS, Seto WH. (2001) Curtailing unnecessary vancomycin usage in a hospital with high rates of methicillin-resistant *Staphylococcus aureus* infections. *Br J Clin Pharmacol* 52(47): 427–432.

Puzniak LA, Gillespie KN, Leet T, Kollef M, Mundy LM. (2004) A cost–benefit analysis of gown use in controlling vancomycin-resistant Enterococcus transmission: is it worth the price? *Infect Control Hosp Epidemiol* 25(57): 418–424.

Wenzel RP. (2004) The antibiotic pipeline – challenges, costs and values. *N Engl J Med* 351(6): 523–526.

Inflammation

Annane D, Bellissant E, Cavaillon JM. (2005) Septic shock. *Lancet* 365(9453): 63–78.

Ayala A, Chung C-S, Grutkoski PS, Sony GY (2003) Mechanisms of immune resolution. *Crit Care Med* 31(8 Suppl.): S558–571.

Bone RC. (1991) The pathogenesis of sepsis. *Ann Intern Med* 115: 457.

Bone RC. (1996) Immunologic dissonance: a continuing evolution in our understanding of the systemic inflammatory response syndrome (SIRS) and the multiple organ dysfunction syndrome (MODS). *Ann Intern Med* 125: 680.

Dellinger RP, Carlet JM, Masur H, Gerlach H, Calandra T, Cohen J, Gea-Banacloche J, Keh D, Marshall JC, Parker MM et al. (2004) Surviving Sepsis Campaign guidelines for management of severe sepsis and septic shock. *Crit Care Med* 32: 858–873.

Henson PM. (2005) Dampening inflammation. *Nature Immunol* 6(12): 1179–1181.

Hotchkiss RS, Karl IE. (2003) The pathophysiology and treatment of sepsis. *N Engl J Med* 348(2): 138–150.

Riedemann NC, Guo RF, Ward PA. (2003) Novel strategies for the treatment of sepsis. *Nature Med* 9: 517.

Rivers E, Nguyen B, Havstad S et al. (2001) Early goal-directed therapy in the treatment of severe sepsis and septic shock. *N Engl J Med* 345: 1368.

Serhan CN, Savill J. (2005) Resolution of inflammation: the beginning programs the end. *Nature Immunol* 6(12): 1191–1197.

Burns

(1992) *Can J Anaesth* 39(5 Pt 1): 454–457.

Sheridan RL. (2002) Burns. *Crit Care Med* 30: S500–14.

www.burnsurgery.org/Modules/pulmonary/sec3.htm

www.nda.ox.ac.uk/wfsa/html/u10/u1010_02.htm

www.worldwidewounds.com/2002/november/Latarjet/Burn-Pain-At-Dressing-Changes.html

Obstetric critical care

Chamberlain G. ABC of labour care: obstetric emergencies. (1999) *Br Med J* 318: 1342–1345.

Karnad DR. Critical illness and pregnancy: review of a global problem. (2004) *Crit Care Clin* 20: 555–576.

Naylor DF. Critical care obstetrics and gynecology. (2003) *Crit Care Clin* 19: 127–149.

Rizk NW. Obstetric complications in pulmonary and critical care medicine. (1996) *Chest* 110(3): 791–809.

Steingrub JS. Pregnancy-associated severe liver dysfunction. (2004) *Crit Care Clin* 20: 763–776.

Toxicity: poisonings and overdoses

Mokhlesi B et al. (2003) Adult toxicology in critical care. Part I: general approach to the intoxicated patient. *Chest* 123: 577–592.

Mokhlesi B et al. (2003) Adult toxicology in critical care. Part II: specific poisonings. *Chest* 123: 897–922.

Trujillo MH et al. (1998) Pharmacologic antidotes in critical care medicine: a practical guide for drug administration. *Crit Care Med* 26(2): 377–391.

Zimmerman JL. (2003) Poisonings and overdoses in the intensive care unit: general and specific management issues. *Crit Care Med* 31: 2794–2801.

Deliberate attacks: chemicals, radiation and bioterrorism

Ala'Aldeen D. (2001) Risk of deliberately induced anthrax outbreak. *Lancet* 358: 1386–1388.

Baker DJ. (2002) Management of casualties from terrorist chemical and biological attack: a key role for the anaesthetist (editorial). *Br J Anaesth* 89(2): 211–214.

Beeching NJ, Dance DAB, Miller ARO, Spencer RC. (2002) Biological warfare and bioterrorism (review). *Br Med J* 324: 336–339.

Gosden C, Gardener D. (2005) Weapons of mass destruction – threats and responses. *Br Med J* 13: 397–400.

Kerrod E, Geddes AM, Regan M, Leach S. (2005) Surveillance and control measures during smallpox outbreaks. *Emerg Infect Dis* 11(2): 291–297.

White SM. (2002) Chemical and biological weapons: Implications for anaesthesia and intensive care. *Br J Anaesth* 89(2): 306–324.

Advanced cardiac life support

Guidelines 2005 for Cardiopulmonary Resuscitation and Emergency Cardiovascular Care. *Circulation* 112(22 Suppl 1): 1–23.

circ.ahajournals.org/cgi/content/full/102/suppl_1/I-136#top

circ.ahajournals.org/content/vol112/22_suppl/

Ethics: limiting and withdrawing treatment

Brain Trauma Foundation. Management and prognosis of severe traumatic brain injury. February 2000, updated May 2003. Available at www.braintrauma.org/

Curtis JR, Engelberg RA, Wenrich MD, Shannon SE, Treece PD, Rubenfeld GD. (2005) Missed opportunities during family conferences about end-of-life care in the intensive care unit. *Am J Respir Crit Care Med* 171(8): 844–849.

Cuthbertson SJ, Margetts MA, Streat SJ. (2000) Bereavement follow-up after critical illness. *Crit Care Med* 28(4): 1196–1201.

Hall RI, Rocker GM. (2000) End-of-life care in the ICU: treatments provided when life support was or was not withdrawn. *Chest* 118(5): 1424–1430.

Streat SJ. (2005a) Illness trajectories are also valuable in critical care. *Br Med J* 330(7502): 1272.

Streat SJ. (2005b) When do we stop? *Crit Care Resusc* 7: 227–232.

Wijdicks EF, Rabinstein AA. (2004) Absolutely no hope? Some ambiguity of futility of care in devastating acute stroke. *Crit Care Med* 32(11): 2332–2342.

Trauma

Eastern Association for the Surgery of Trauma. Practice guidelines for the management of venous thromboembolism in trauma patients. www.east.org/tpg/dvt.pdf

Eastern Association for the Surgery of Trauma. Practice guidelines for nutritional support of the trauma patient. www.east.org/tpg/nutrition.pdf

Conversion factors

Abbreviated conversion table: US medical units to SI units

Chemistry	US Units	SI Units	Multiplication factor to convert US to SI units
Ammonia	µg/dL	µmol/L	0.554
Bilirubin total	mg/dL	µmol/L	17.1
Bilirubin direct	mg/dL	µmol/L	17.1
BUN	mg/dL	mmol/L	0.357
Calcium	mg/dL	mmol/L	0.25
CO_2 partial pressure (Pco_2)	mmHg	kPa	0.133
Cholesterol	mg/dL	mmol/L	0.026
Cortisol	µg/dL	nmol/L	27.6
Creatinine	mg/dL	µmol/L	88.4
Fibrinogen	mg/dL	mmol/L	0.01
Glucose	mg/dL	mmol/L	0.055
Glutathione	mg/dL	mmol/L	0.032
Iron total	µg/dL	µmol/L	0.179
Iron binding capacity	µg/dL	µmol/L	0.179
Lactic acids (as lactate)	mg/dL	mmol/L	0.111
Magnesium	mEq/L	mmol/L	0.5
Oxygen partial pressure (Po_2)	mmHg	kPa	0.133
Phosphorus	mg/dL	mmol/L	0.323
Progesterone	ng/L	nmol/L	0.0318
Salicylates	mg/dL	mmol/L	0.072
Testosterone	ng/dL	nmol/L	0.035
Thyroxine (T4)	µg/dL	nmol/L	13
Triglycerides	mg/dL	mmol/L	0.011
Uric acid	mg/dL	mmol/L	0.059

Clinical case answers

Evidenced-based intensive care

There are several problems, the most obvious being:

1. Confounding variable: the intervention group also received fluid, which is known to decrease renal injury in this setting.
2. Surrogate marker: the difference between the groups was in creatinine, which is a surrogate marker of renal function. This may have been a transient blip, and renal function may have been no different between the groups.
3. Power: this study was inadequately powered to detect safety differences between the groups. Many studies examining drugs may shed light on efficacy, but seldom on safety. Typically, many thousands of patients are required before any comment can be made on safety.

Critical care transport

Adequate preparation for transport to the MRI scanner will include ensuring that you will have adequate non-ferromagnetic monitoring capabilities for the duration of transport and MRI scan, as well as an ability to safely continue the administration of vasoactive infusions via MRI-compatible infusion pumps or microdrip infusion devices. You will need to confirm an adequate oxygen supply in an aluminium cylinder and, if mechanical ventilation is necessary, you will need to establish that a suitable ventilator is available in the MRI suite. In this patient with a history of rheumatic heart disease, atrial fibrillation and prior valve replacement, you will need to verify she has no contraindication to MRI such as a non-MRI-compatible prosthetic heart valve or pacemaker.

Drug interactions

The patient responded well to naloxone infusion, which had to be managed extremely carefully to minimise the risk of precipitating opiate withdrawal.

Amiodarone is a moderately powerful inhibitor of several CYP isoforms. It is likely that, in this case, the amiodarone inhibited the metabolism of the methadone, precipitating opiate toxicity. The metabolism of methadone is complex, involving both CYP 2B6 and CYP 3A4. Interactions have also been described between methadone and drugs such as azole antifungals.

The literature is replete with well-characterised drug interactions, for example patients who develop polymorphic ventricular tachycardia when given the combination of cisapride and erythromycin. We chose the above scenario because many real-life cases are less well characterised. If you are not familiar with the metabolism of a particular drug, check! For many drugs, we don't even know which enzyme is predominantly responsible for their metabolism; for others, metabolism varies from individual to individual! You should therefore be continually on the alert for potential new interactions.

Clinical excellence

Clinical inputs corroborate the diagnosis of diabetic ketoacidosis: history of diabetes, recent illness and failure to take insulin; and multimodal sensory inputs (touch, smell,

sight). The corresponding model is the one outlined on p. 124, and dictates further management and investigation – including fluid and insulin replacement, management of associated infection and performing relevant investigations, the results of which are likely to alter therapy. In managing the patient, you enter an ongoing process of assessment for responses to therapy, treatment alterations depending on the response, and vigilance for error.

Monitoring in the ICU

The fit cyclist probably has a resting heart rate of about 40/min, and may well normally have a blood pressure of 90/60 mmHg. In scenario A, inappropriate 'resuscitation' might harm the patient. In scenario B, the patient is likely to be seriously unwell. Have you missed the ruptured spleen?

The airway in ICU

The patient has bitten and permanently deformed the tube. Replace the tube with one that is not armoured and, in future, prevail upon the anaesthetist to get rid of the armoured tube *before* the patient comes to the ICU!

Vascular access in the ICU

The patient needs a cardiothoracic surgeon and major surgery to remove the guidewire. A clear case where prevention is far better. Rather than exhorting everyone to be more diligent, you could design a better system that would help prevent it being possible that the guidewire is able to be left in the patient! Until then always double check it has been removed.

Fibreoptic bronchoscopy in the ICU

It is likely that the view through the FOB will be of the vocal cords. The situation described is consistent with a tracheal tube that has migrated out of the larynx. With the resultant leak, the pilot balloon has been overinflated. This has resulted in further migration outward of the tracheal tube. The reason that the tube is at 25 cm at the lips may be that a staff member tried to advance the tracheal tube but, with the overinflated balloon, the tube curled in the back of the pharynx instead of advancing into the larynx. The safest method of advancing this tracheal tube to an appropriate position is to advance the FOB into the larynx such that its tip is about 4 cm above the carina. Then the pilot balloon of the tracheal tube can be deflated, and the tracheal tube may be advanced over the FOB until its tip reaches just beyond the tip of the FOB.

Cerebrospinal fluid, lumbar puncture and lumbar drain

Features are entirely compatible with early tuberculous meningitis, particularly the high protein. The high neutrophil count does *not* exclude tuberculous meningitis.

Mechanical ventilation

Disconnect the patient from the ventilator and listen to the satisfying 'woosh'. The problem is 'auto-PEEP' due to air trapping, which is causing high pressures and cardiovascular collapse. The solution is to dramatically lower the respiratory rate, even to less than five breaths per minute, allowing a very long expiration time.

Renal replacement therapy

This patient may be experiencing dialysis disequilibrium syndrome, which may occur with rapid (or overzealous) correction of uraemia. Symptoms include cramps, headache and nausea. Signs include delirium, blunted mental status, seizures and muscle irritability (myoclonus). This syndrome arises because of an osmotic gradient that develops between the plasma and brain during rapid dialysis. Intracellular acidosis occurs in the brain in association with an increase in unmeasured organic acids. This generates an osmotic gradient and leads to a shift of water into the brain parenchyma, producing encephalopathy, raised intracranial pressure and cerebral oedema. Prevention of dialysis disequilibrium syndrome is achieved by 'slow' dialysis. A further preventative measure includes the addition of an osmotically active solute (e.g. urea, glycerol, mannitol or sodium) to the dialysate. It is important to exclude other possible acute causes of altered mental function such as intracranial bleed, hypotension, hypoxia, arrhythmia, hypoglycaemia or myocardial infarction. Dialysis can rapidly correct acid–base abnormalities but may concomitantly cause electrolyte abnormalities. Rapid correction of metabolic acidosis may cause potassium to shift cells. If there is insufficient potassium in the dialysis fluid, hypokalaemia may result.

Mechanical circulatory support

The options were to give her more time (unlikely to have a good outcome), give her a heart transplant (not currently in the best condition to recover from this type of surgery) or to trial an adult left ventricular assist device (to allow her to recover enough to cope with transplant surgery). She had the LVAD implanted and, after a 5-week intensive care stay, including 2 weeks of inotropic support and 1 week of renal replacement therapy, she has gone home and is on the transplant waiting list.

Circulation

There are numerous indicators of (intravascular) hypovolaemia, including the pulsus paradoxus, the pulse pressure variation, the echocardiography findings and the relatively low central venous pressure. The wide pulse pressure, the bounding peripheral pulses, the warmth and the suspicion of infection are all strongly suggestive that there is a component of vasodilatory plus distributive shock. The relatively low cardiac index in this setting coupled with the echocardiography findings point to a component of cardiogenic shock. This patient's circulatory problems are complex. Immediate treatment priorities entail a combination of fluids (at least a few litres) and vasoconstrictor drugs [e.g. noradrenaline (norepinephrine) or adrenaline (epinephrine) with the possible addition of vasopressin or terlipressin].

Oxygen delivery

1. $DO_2 = 279$ mL/min. His metabolic acidosis and low SVO_2 imply that tissue perfusion is inadequate.
2. Transfuse to increase haemoglobin, improve cardiac output (CO), increase F_IO_2 and/or improve oxygenation (e.g. diuresis for pulmonary oedema, intubation to decrease work of breathing, etc.)
3. Increased SVO_2, decreased lactate, normalized pH.

Scenario	F_IO_2	P_aO_2 [mmHg (kPa)]	S_aO_2 (%)	Hb (g/L)	C_aO_2 (mL/L)	Q (L/min)	DO_2 (mL/min)	% change in DO_2
Normal values	0.21	100 (13.3)	98	140	187	5.5	1027	
Patient	0.5	65 (8.7)	92	65	82	3.4	279	−73
Increased F_IO_2	1.0	400 (53.3)	98	65	97	3.4	330	+18
Increased haemoglobin	0.5	65 (8.7)	92	100	125	3.4	426	+53
Increased CO	0.5	65 (8.7)	92	65	82	5.0	410	+47

The following table illustrates differences between this patient and a normal person. Interventions to increase oxygen delivery and their impacts are shown.

ICU acid–basics

Do nothing but wait.

Carbon dioxide

Case 1: The patient has a dangerous alkalaemia secondary to inappropriate hyperventilation. With this degree of alkalaemia, perfusion to vital organs, such as the heart and the brain, may be compromised. Prolonged administration of 100% oxygen is harmful and was not indicated for this patient.

Case 2: Dr Blowslow set the mechanical ventilator in such a way that lung distension and pressure transmitted to the alveoli was limited. This approach may be associated with improved outcome when patients have an acute lung injury or ARDS. There is an acidaemia associated with hypoventilation. But the oxygenation is adequate. In view of the fact that the patient is stable haemodynamically, it is probably appropriate to tolerate mild hypercapnia and acidaemia in an attempt to protect the lungs from further injury.

Thermal disorders

Warm the patient with a forced air warmer or equivalent. He will feel more comfortable, and you can supply the energy externally, rather than stressing his metabolic and cardiovascular system by making him produce the energy to warm himself up. He is awake and so external cooling will mean that he has to make even more energy to warm himself up. Remember that shivering will increase his metabolic rate by 100% and so stress his cardiovascular system to the point of causing a myocardial infarction.

Feeding and starving in the ICU

The respiratory quotient (RQ) of over 1.0 is due to de novo lipogenesis in the liver, which is causing hypercarbia. The high RQ and hyperglycaemia clearly show that the patient is being overfed. Feed the patient less!

Electrolyte abnormalities

It is likely that the patient has hypoparathyroidism and resulting hypocalcaemia following thyroidectomy. Hyperventilation may have worsened things; with alkalaemia, there is increased binding of calcium to albumin and the free, ionised calcium decreases. A rapid blood transfusion may also have contributed; the citrate in stored blood binds calcium. A blood gas should be sent, ventilation should be decreased, intravenous calcium should be given, and blood should be sent for determination of electrolytes (calcium, phosphate, magnesium, sodium and potassium) and parathyroid hormone concentration.

Fluid therapy in the ICU

This is not an easy problem and opinions would differ. This patient is clearly dehydrated. But fluid administration with leaky pulmonary capillaries may further damage the transplanted lungs, which have already sustained an injury. A reasonable approach may be to treat the hypotension with a pressor agent such as phenylephrine and even consider promoting diuresis. It is imperative to monitor renal function carefully and to reassess this bold approach at frequent intervals. If this patient develops progressive pulmonary failure, it is likely that he will die. Renal replacement therapy is available to treat acute tubular necrosis.

Blood and blood components

The most likely diagnosis is transfusion-related acute lung injury (TRALI). TRALI is a form of non-cardiogenic pulmonary oedema. It is a transfusion reaction caused by antibodies against recipient leucocyte HLA antigens or priming lipids. It occurs more commonly with products that have leucocytes, such as platelets and fresh frozen plasma. As a result, there is acute leakage of fluid and protein from an increase in permeability of the pulmonary circulation. It usually occurs within hours after a transfusion. The mainstay of treatment is continuous positive airway pressure, which usually buys sufficient time while the oedema resolves. Intubation coupled with respiratory and circulatory support may be required, as in this case, if oxygenation deteriorates. Other possible diagnoses include pulmonary oedema from fluid overload, anaphylactoid reactions to the transfusions, and other cardiac and pulmonary diseases such as acute myocardial infarction and pulmonary embolism.

Neurological assessment

The initial priorities include resuscitation, airway security, oxygenation and ventilation. A focused neurological examination as part of a systematic evaluation must be performed. A best Glasgow Coma Score should be recorded. Pulse oximetry, capnography and ECG telemetry are employed. Additional monitors such as arterial and central venous catheters or intracranial pressure monitors should be considered. After initial stabilisation, analgesia and sedation should be achieved with short-acting agents to avoid confounding repeat neurological examinations. Diagnostic studies, such as CT scans, should be reviewed. Consultation with a neurosurgeon is warranted.

Central nervous system injury

GCS = 5/10 .This is scored out of 10 because verbal assessment is deferred. Eye opening = 1/4, motor = 4/6. Verbal assessment is deferred because the tracheal tube makes this assessment impossible. CPP = 80–28 = 52 mmHg.

Manoeuvres to raise MAP, to lower ICP and to decrease cerebral oxygen requirements include:

1. Drain ventriculostomy intermittently.
2. Volume resuscitation to optimise cardiac output.
3. Induce osmotic diuresis with mannitol.
4. Sedation with thiopentone or propofol (and consider neuromuscular blockade).
5. Ventilation to normocapnia.
6. Elevate head of bed 30°.
7. Consider vasopressors [phenylephrine or noradrenaline (norepinephrine)].
8. Consider mild hypothermia.
9. Maintain normoglycaemia.

Weakness in the ICU

Steroids plus neuromuscular blocking agents (NMBAs) constitute a particularly pernicious drug combination in the development of prolonged weakness. Features of this myopathy include prolonged weakness, elevated creatine kinase (CPK) concentrations, myopathic features on electromyography, normal nerve conduction and sensation, and reduced deep tendon reflexes. Muscle biopsy tends to show type 1 and/or 2 fibre atrophy without inflammation. Some recently reported cases revealed thick myosin myofilament loss. Concomitant use of NMBAs and corticosteroids should be avoided if possible. This syndrome ('necrotising myopathy of intensive care') provides one of the differential diagnoses for ICU-acquired weakness. The myopathy appears to have several interdependent causes, and it is proposed that these should be classified as myonecrosis 'priming' factors (glucocorticoids, myotropic infections, sepsis) and 'triggering' factors (non-depolarising muscle blocking agents).

Seizures

The patient has status epilepticus, as he has experienced more than 10 min of continuous seizure activity. The immediate priority includes ensuring adequate ventilation and oxygenation. Check vital signs (ABCs). After assessing the ABCs, obtain intravenous (IV) access. Obtain a targeted history, especially in the case of a trauma, diabetes or possible toxicity. Send blood samples for testing, including blood gas, glucose, electrolytes, renal function, liver function and toxic screen. Administer IV lorazepam in 0.1 mg/kg. Follow up with thiamine 100 mg and 50% glucose 25 mg IV. Consider loading with phenytoin 25 mg/kg IV. If the seizures do not subside, propofol or thiopentone infusions may be required. With depressed consciousness, tracheal intubation and assisted ventilation may be required. Phenytoin is a dangerous drug with a narrow therapeutic window. There is no evidence to support its use for longer than a week following trauma. Daily phenytoin levels should be obtained to ensure that it is in the therapeutic range.

Altered mental states

There are multiple causes for delirium. In any patient, a careful history and physical examination are necessary, noting any focal neurological signs. Consulting with family members may be helpful, because alcohol withdrawal is a possible diagnosis that needs to be ruled out. The medication list should be reviewed, noting any possible psychoactive medications. Blood tests to evaluate glucose control, electrolytes, haemoglobin, renal and liver function and calcium should be obtained. Evidence of infection in the lungs, blood and urine should be sought. The blood results may reveal a metabolic abnormality, such as hyponatraemia, or organ dysfunction, such as renal failure. Empirical treatment for alcohol withdrawal (glucose, thiamine, vitamins and benzodiazepines) may be life saving. Sedation and replacing the tracheal tube may be indicated if the agitation is severe and the patient may be unable to protect his lungs from soiling. This may also be prudent if the patient has to travel for a special investigation, such as a CT scan. A brain scan may be indicated, especially if there are localising neurological signs.

Analgesia in the ICU

Call in an expert to help you manage this difficult problem. Non-opiate-based analgesia should be used. See Vickers and Jolly (2006).

Monitoring the cardiovascular system

Do a transoesophageal echocardiogram. In the case in question, TOE was repeatedly declined by the cardiologists consulted but, at autopsy, extensive endocarditis was found on the mitral valve.

Ischaemic heart disease

In this gentleman with a history of atherosclerotic vascular disease, chest 'heaviness', new-onset AF and a new LBBB, the immediate concern must be acute myocardial ischaemia. A brief and focused history and physical examination would help to identify risk factors and other potential aetiologies for his distress and would reveal any possible contraindications to antiplatelet, anticoagulation or antifibrinolytic therapy. Immediate measures would include supplemental oxygen to maintain oxygen saturation > 90% and, if there are no contraindications, aspirin, heparin, nitrate and beta-adrenergic antagonist therapy should be initiated. Continuous cardiac monitoring and defibrillation capability should be established. Immediate consultation with a cardiologist for potential reperfusion therapy should be requested. Laboratory studies including cardiac biomarkers such as troponin T or troponin I, basic haematological and metabolic panels and portable chest radiograph should be obtained. Cardiac imaging with echocardiography would be useful to evaluate for regional wall motion abnormalities and ventricular function.

Heart failure in the ICU

Given this gentleman's medical history and recent surgical procedure, a number of likely possibilities for his acute respiratory embarrassment exist. A quick assessment of ABCs and increasing his supplemental oxygen concentration would be immediate interventions while performing a more complete history and physical examination. While not an exhaustive list, most likely to be included in the differential diagnosis would be:

- Acute myocardial ischaemia with elevated left ventricular filling pressures and/or ischaemic mitral regurgitation (multiple CAD risk factors)
- Heart failure due to diastolic, systolic dysfunction or both, new-onset dysrhythmia (irregular pulse), relative hypervolaemia due to mobilisation of perioperative resuscitation fluids, sleep-disordered breathing (obesity)
- Exacerbation of chronic obstructive pulmonary disease (smoking history)
- Primary pulmonary disturbance such as pneumonia, atelectasis
- Pulmonary embolus.

Recommended early studies would include a review of recent medications, daily fluid balance and/or weight, 12-lead ECG, chest radiograph, complete blood cell panel, basic electrolyte panel and renal function screen. Based on the results of the above preliminary investigation, one could establish a likely diagnosis and initiate therapy or determine whether further studies are warranted including transthoracic echocardiography, computerised chest tomography, thyroid function panel, cardiac enzymes, etc.

Arrhythmias

Emergency defibrillation is indicated for pulseless ventricular tachycardia. With restoration of sinus rhythm, aspirin, a beta-blocker and oxygen should be given. Morphine may be administered if she has chest pain. Thrombolysis should be initiated if there is no contraindication. Blood sugar, cholesterol and electrolytes should be checked. History should be elicited, and examination may yield valuable information. A repeat 12-lead ECG should be obtained. Expert opinion should be sought from a cardiologist and an electrophysiologist. This patient may benefit from stent placement in her coronary arteries or from cardiac surgery. Long-term therapy with a 'statin' and an angiotensin-converting enzyme (ACE) inhibitor may be indicated. An implantable cardioverter/defibrillator may be warranted.

Pacing

Placing the bed 'head-down' and increasing the fraction of inspired oxygen to 100% are sensible initial interventions. Atropine or isoprenaline (isoproterenol) may be useful in temporarily increasing the heart rate. If severe hypotension persists, epinephrine or even chest compression may be required. Emergency transcutaneous or even transvenous pacing may be life saving. The pacemaker may be 'oversensing'. Placing a magnet over the pacemaker may convert it to a 'VOO' mode, which may result in resumption of pacing. Investigation of permanent pacemaker failure to capture should include an arterial blood gas, electrolytes and temperature. Myocardial ischaemia, acid–base abnormalities, electrolyte abnormalities and hypothermia may result in loss of capture. An electrophysiologist should be consulted to interrogate the pacemaker, which may have a fractured lead. Reprogramming the pacemaker may be necessary.

Cardiac surgery

The most likely diagnoses are cardiac tamponade, bronchospasm, autoPEEP and tension pneumothorax. Hypovolaemia is unlikely in view of the jugular venous distension. Bilateral breath sounds with no increase in plateau pressure would be against pneumothorax. No increase in peak airway pressures would be against bronchospasm. Good breath sounds with no wheezing would also weigh against bronchospasm. Brief disconnection of the tracheal tube from the ventilator tubing would exclude autopeep. An urgent chest radiograph would be useful. Echocardiography might show compression of a heart chamber such as the left atrium. But the diagnosis is based on clinical suspicion. If tamponade is suspected, the patient should be taken to the operating theatre for surgical exploration. During transport, fluid resuscitation and adrenaline (epinephrine) may prevent haemodynamic collapse.

Pulmonary hypertension

Pulmonary embolism (PE) is a common postoperative complication. All high-risk patients (e.g. orthopaedic patients) should receive thrombosis prophylaxis. The triad of tachycardia, tachypnoea and (increased) temperature may be present. The ECG may show signs of right heart strain, such as S waves in standard lead 1, Q waves in standard lead 3 and inverted T waves in standard lead III. Echocardiography may also show signs of right heart strain. The low oxygen saturation despite supplementary oxygen may reflect shunting of blood through a patent foramen ovale. A large difference between end-tidal CO_2 and $P_a CO_2$ may be present, reflecting an increase in dead space ventilation and a decrease in cardiac output. Tests to support the diagnosis include a ventilation/perfusion scan, high-resolution CT scan with contrast and pulmonary angiography. Pulmonary angiography is the gold standard, but is rarely used because it is most invasive. The first two tests are preferred; however, the radiation dose associated with the CT scan is substantially higher and intravenous dye is nephrotoxic. Prior to administering intravenous contrast agent for the CT scan, intravenous fluids and bicarbonate (e.g. 150 mL of 8.4% bicarbonate in 1 L of 5% dextrose) may decrease the likelihood of contrast-induced nephropathy. For patients with known renal dysfunction, N-acetylcysteine may also help to reduce the risk of acute renal failure. Anticoagulation with heparin and oxygen should usually be started whenever PE is suspected. Long-term anticoagulation with warfarin is likely to be needed.

Respiratory failure

Analysis of the arterial blood gas reveals the presence of respiratory acidosis and a low ratio of $P_a O_2 / F_i O_2$ (90 mmHg/ 0.6 = 150 mmHg). Normally, this ratio is > 300 mmHg. Although the respiratory acidosis may be explained by opioid-induced respiratory depression, the markedly decreased $P_a O_2 / F_i O_2$ ratio may not be. Further investigation should be initiated for causes of V/Q mismatch. In the clinical setting, pulmonary embolus is an important consideration. Other possibilities include atelectasis, aspiration pneumonia, retained secretions, pulmonary oedema, bronchospasm, ARDS, pneumothorax and fat embolism. Clinical examination is imperative and may suggest such diagnoses as pneumothorax, bronchospasm and pulmonary oedema. Chest radiograph, V/Q scan, echocardiography and CT scan may all yield valuable information in this setting.

Asthma

This patient is about to have a cardiorespiratory respiratory arrest. Emergency intervention is indicated. The decreased wheezing probably represents decreased air movement, and her change in mental status is probably secondary to increasing arterial CO_2. The slow heart rate is sinister and suggests hypoxaemia and imminent cardiac arrest. Check that the patient still has a pulse! Call for help and the cardiac arrest equipment. Administer 100% oxygen with assisted ventilation if possible. Administer fluids and subcutaneous adrenaline (epinephrine) (0.3 mg). If the patient stops breathing and an expert in airway management is not yet present, consider inserting a laryngeal mask airway to facilitate controlled ventilation as a temporising measure.

Chronic obstructive pulmonary disease

It is likely that the combined use of systemic steroids and non-depolarising muscle relaxants have caused a steroid myopathy. To assess the possibility of a steroid myopathy, creatinine kinase and urine myoglobin should be checked. Electromyography, muscle biopsy and nerve conduction studies may yield valuable information. Systemic steroids should be quickly tapered and discontinued. The patient's family should be informed that acute steroid myopathies are associated with failure to wean and protracted ICU stays.

Weakness may persist for months. The use of muscle relaxant infusions is seldom indicated.

The ICU chest radiograph

Rather ominously, the pCXR shows something that looks suspiciously like the feeding tube passing beyond the carina into the right mainstem bronchus and then to a distal airway. Food should not be given through this tube. A capnograph may detect CO_2 at the other end of the tube, providing further evidence of the dangerous misplacement. If there is lingering doubt, a bronchoscope passed through the tracheal tube may be used to clinch the diagnosis. The tube should be withdrawn carefully, with care taken not to displace the tracheal tube. A new feeding tube should be placed, and the same precautions as before should be followed before it is used for feeding.

Renal failure

Diagnoses to consider include post-renal renal failure with lymphadenopathy causing obstruction, gentamicin-induced ATN and prerenal failure. The combination of decreased fluid intake with sepsis suggests that prerenal failure is implicated. There could be more than one factor contributing to the renal dysfunction. The FENA is 0.5% and urea/Cr is 74. The urine Na is only 14. These laboratory tests suggest that the tubules are still functional and able to concentrate urine. Prerenal renal failure is probably the predominant diagnosis. The fact that this patient has been treated with a known nephrotoxic drug should not exclude other possible aetiologies from the differential diagnosis. Apart from fluid administration, consideration should be given to changing the antibiotic or decreasing its dose according to the creatinine clearance.

Gastrointestinal bleeding

The most likely cause is an upper GI bleed. In the ICU, stress-related erosive syndrome (SRES) is the most common cause of upper GI bleeds. This patient's SRES haemorrhage may be severe in view of the need for a blood transfusion. With his history, myocardial ischaemia and infarction should be excluded. An oesophagogastroduodenoscopy may confirm the diagnosis. Other important causes of upper GI bleeds include variceal bleeding, peptic ulcer disease and anticoagulant medications.

Gastrointestinal motility disorders

The most likely cause of her diarrhoea is C. *difficile*. Cephalosporins, clindamycin and quinolones are the antibiotics most commonly implicated in C. *difficile* colitis. A normal white cell count does not exclude the diagnosis. Other important causes of her diarrhoea include hyperosmolar diarrhoea from enteral feeding and ischaemic colitis. The next steps in managing this patient would be to send stool samples for C. *difficile* toxin assay and to start empirical oral metronidazole 500 mg three times daily. Isolation precautions should be instituted. In particular, thorough hand washing with soap and water is required. Alcohol-based hand-cleansing solutions do not destroy clostridial spores. Ideally, intravenous antibiotics should be discontinued.

Cholecystitis and pancreatitis

The differential diagnosis includes sepsis, bowel ischaemia, hepatitis, ruptured abdominal viscus, ileus, pancreatitis and cholecystitis. Blood and urine cultures, blood gas, lactate, liver and renal function tests, hepatitis studies, C-reactive protein, full blood count, amylase and lipase should be checked. Urine output and bladder pressure should be monitored. Abdominal ultrasound, radiograph and CT scan may help to narrow the diagnosis. Supportive therapy, including fluid resuscitation, is vital. Antimicrobial therapy may be broadened pending the results of the cultures. Specific targeted therapy will depend on the final diagnosis.

Liver failure

Admission to an ICU at a liver transplant centre is important. If transport to another hospital is necessary, prophylactic sedation and tracheal intubation may be appropriate; rapid deterioration is frequent with liver failure. The INR should be followed to detect worsening liver function. Frequent blood glucose checks are mandatory. Electrolytes, blood gases and renal function should be monitored. Lactate level may provide prognostic information. Frequent neurological assessment will alert to progression of encephalopathy, which is associated with increased risk of cerebral oedema and brain herniation. ICP monitoring is an option even for grade II encephalopathy. A central venous line for fluid and monitoring should be placed. A cardiac output monitor and an indwelling arterial line may be needed. Cultures should be obtained early, including blood, urine and sputum. Empiric antimicrobial therapy may be appropriate. Following treatment of life-threatening problems, a detailed collateral history and physical examination may provide vital information. A battery of blood tests (e.g. hepatitis serology, toxicology screen) is usually indicated. Further investigations including ultrasound, CT scan and liver biopsy may be indicated. The King's College Hospital's Criteria for liver transplantation in non-paracetamol-induced liver failure are:

- INR > 6.5 or prothrombin time > 100 s; or any three of:
  - Drug-induced, non-A, non-B hepatitis, halothane hepatitis or indeterminate cause
  - Jaundiced > 7 days before onset of encephalopathy
  - Age < 10 or > 40 years
  - INR > 3.5 or prothrombin time > 50 s
  - Serum bilirubin > 299 μmol/L.

Diabetes mellitus in the ICU

Tight glycaemic control in the ICU is extremely controversial. Early enthusiasm (after biased studies advocating extremely tight control) has waned due to an increased incidence of hypoglycaemia and doubts about benefits. It may be reasonable to maintain tight enough control to prevent blood glucose exceeding the renal threshold for glucose (usually about 10 mmol/L) while avoiding hypoglycaemia.

Endocrine emergencies

1. Thyroid storm, pulmonary embolus, myocardial ischaemia/infarction, and phaeochromocytoma are possible causes.
2. Further studies should include electrocardiogram (ECG), routine chemistries, blood counts, myocardial enzymes, thyroid hormone levels and some form of investigation for pulmonary embolus.

Follow-up question and response
Her TSH is undetectable; T4 and T3 are markedly elevated. ECG shows atrial fibrillation with no evidence of ischaemia. Helical computerised tomography (CT) scan of the chest shows no evidence of pulmonary embolus. What is your diagnosis? What therapy would you initiate?

Her thyroid studies suggest hyperthyroidism with a clinical picture suggesting thyroid storm. Treatment consists of initial symptomatic therapy (beta blockade for heart rate control, temperature management) followed by antithyroid therapy (propylthiouracil or methimazole). If desired, definitive therapy includes thyroidectomy or radioactive iodine therapy.

Clotting and bleeding: a delicate balance

While patients with meningitis may be at risk of bleeding, the pathological process is a severe disseminated intravascular coagulopathy. In such circumstances, treatment with platelets and plasma may provide more fuel for intravascular coagulation. Activated protein C has been shown in the PROWESS study to decrease mortality in severe sepsis and may be especially indicated for bacterial meningitis. Recombinant tissue factor pathway inhibitor and recombinant antithrombin have also been administered, but without proven benefit. Some clinicians would consider administering heparin in this setting. There is controversy surrounding all the interventions. The haematologist is probably acting on the best available evidence.

Bleeding in the ICU

After checking for localising neurological signs (e.g. pupil size), analgesia may be administered to treat the hypertension and the tachycardia. A convection warmer may be used to warm the patient, and a buffer such as bicarbonate may be useful to correct the acidaemia. Like most proteins and enzymes, the coagulation proteins work best under normal physiological conditions. Coagulation tests including platelet count should be sent off. If the INR is normal and the PTT is prolonged, small increments of protamine or a slow infusion may reverse residual heparin. Aprotinin, tranexamic acid or epsilon aminocaproic acid may be administered to decrease clot lysis. DDAVP may improve platelet function. Platelet transfusion may be helpful if there is thrombocytopenia or platelet dysfunction. However, it should be borne in mind that platelet transfusions may be associated with increased mortality. If both the INR and the PTT are prolonged, FFP and cryoprecipitate transfusions may be indicated. Surgical bleeding is always a possibility and re-exploration should be considered. If bleeding persists, rFVIIa may be considered to promote clotting.

Thrombosis in the ICU

The rapid decrease in platelet count coupled with a thrombotic event (stroke) in the context of heparin therapy is highly suggestive of type II HIT. This patient was probably exposed to heparin during the admission 6 weeks ago and developed antibodies then. This explains the rapid onset (< 5 days) of HIT during this current admission. Heparin must be stopped. Argatroban should be started for therapeutic anticoagulation. Renal dysfunction weighs against hirudin or bivalirudin. Only when therapeutic anticoagulation has been established with argatroban and the platelet count has recovered (> 150 × 10⁹/L) should warfarin be started. If warfarin is administered without therapeutic anticoagulation, further thrombosis may be precipitated. Blood should be sent for ELISA testing and serotonin release assay to confirm the presence of antibodies to the heparin–platelet factor 4 complex.

Prevention and treatment of infections

Management of intra-abdominal sepsis:

Antibiotics: Which agents?

Polymicrobial infection is likely to be present. Antibiotics active against organisms of bowel flora, including *E. coli* and anaerobes including *Bacteroides fragilis* should be administered. In this case, cefuroxime, gentamicin and metronidazole were given.

Correct dose and route of administration?

The intravenous route was chosen as the patient was starved for possible surgery. Renal function and liver function of the patient should be taken into account, as dose alteration of agents may be required. In this case, standard doses of cefuroxime (1.5 g 8-hourly) and metronidazole (500 mg 8-hourly) were given. Gentamicin was administered according to a once-daily dosing protocol.

Further treatment required?

Antibiotics alone are unlikely to cure this infection. There is a large collection of pus, which must be drained. A percutaneous hepatic drain was placed under CT guidance, and 750 mL of foul-smelling pus was drained over the next 12 h.

Sepsis and septic shock

Invasive monitoring was commenced with placement of a central venous catheter and an arterial line. There was a pulsus paradoxus on the arterial line trace and a low central venous pressure (4 mmHg); both of these suggested intravascular volume depletion. Four litres of colloid fluid were administered with brief restoration of blood pressure. Benzyl penicillin treatment was continued. Vasopressors were introduced, initially noradrenaline (norepinephrine) at 0.1 µg/kg/min, then vasopressin 0.04 units/min was added, after which blood pressure increased. A tracheal tube was inserted, and mechanical ventilation was commenced. Activated protein C at a dose of 24 µg/kg/h was administered by intravenous infusion for 96 h. Urine output failed to improve, and haemofiltration was started for treatment of worsening acidosis. Hydrocortisone 50 mg 6-hourly was administered intravenously, while the results of a short synacthen (synthetic adrenocorticotropic hormone) test was awaited. The dose of noradrenaline (norepinephrine) required to maintain blood pressure decreased following administration of hydrocortisone. An insulin infusion was used to achieve tight glucose control. During her prolonged stay in intensive care, she lost several digits but ultimately recovered and was discharged to the ward after 30 days.

Central nervous system infection

Acute disseminated encephalomyelitis (ADEM) is an acute demyelinating disorder of the CNS occurring days to weeks after an infection or vaccination. It occurs in about 1:1000 children, particularly after measles and rubella infection although it occasionally affects adults. As effective vaccination has reduced these diseases, it is less common.

ADEM is not due to viral invasion of CNS tissue, as live virus cannot be detected; rather, it appears to be an immune-mediated disease occurring after either an infection or vaccination, possibly due to anti-myelin autoreactivity. Common symptoms are the development of motor, sensory and brainstem signs; less commonly, fever, seizures and meningism can occur.

Examination of CSF is often abnormal with minor elevation of white cell count and protein. Monoclonal bands can be present. MRI scanning of the brain reveals numerous demyelinating plaques and together with clinical findings is the cornerstone of diagnosis.

Treatment is supportive, with the majority of patients making a recovery. About 10% of patients will be left with mild to moderate neurological impairment, and a few will be severely disabled. Methyl prednisolone, at high doses, has been used in selected cases with promising results.

Clinical tip: smallpox vaccination, when carried out on large populations, had a high incidence of ADEM. It is possible that smallpox vaccination will be reintroduced in the near future, as a result of bioterrorism threats. Clinicians should be aware of this complication.

Pneumonia

Legionnaire's disease. This case has several risk factors for severe *Legionella pneumophila* infection, including smoking and exposure to air-conditioning systems. However, *Streptococcus pneumoniae* infection is common in the community and cannot be excluded. The chest radiograph (Fig. 3) shows extensive left-sided consolidation. Investigations would include those suggested in Box 2. Specifically, as mechanical ventilation has commenced, non-directed bronchial washings can be collected and cultured for common respiratory pathogens including *L. pneumophila*. In addition, the *L. pneumophila* urinary antigen ELISA can be requested. This test is highly specific (> 95%) and sensitive (80%) and proved to be positive in the case discussed. Empirical antibiotic therapy was commenced with intravenous cefuroxime and erythromycin. Following results supporting the diagnosis of Legionnaire's disease, cefuroxime therapy was ceased. Macrolides such as erythromycin are the mainstay of treatment for Legionnaire's disease, but rifampicin is also thought to be highly active in combination.

Infections associated with prosthetic material in the ICU

The CT scan shows extensive neck inflammation and a probable abscess owing to infection of the internal jugular central cannula. Vancomycin was commenced. Blood cultures and jugular line tip culture subsequently grew MRSA. A large abscess originating from an infected jugular vein was incised and drained under general anaesthesia. Vancomycin was continued for a total of 4 weeks with good resolution and no recurrence of symptoms.

The immunocompromised patient in critical care

Immediately wash the area with plenty of water and soap. Refer to your local hospital policy – make sure you are aware of this when starting a job. Assess the risk:

- Does the patient have risk factors for blood-borne virus infection, e.g. intravenous drug use, high-risk sexual behaviour?
- What kind of injury was it? Deep injection with a needle attached to syringe full of blood is high risk, whereas a splash of body fluid onto a mucosal membrane is lower risk.
- Contact the delegated physician or a senior colleague who has access to post-exposure antiretroviral medication.
- Blood samples should be taken from the recipient of the injury and the donor (if that is possible) for virus antibody testing as soon as possible.

If risk is sufficiently high, then post-exposure prophylaxis (PEP) should be administered as soon as possible while awaiting the results of HIV antibody tests. If the donor is found to be HIV positive, then PEP is administered for 1 month. A typical regimen would be zidovudine, lamivudine and nelfinavir.

Tropical medicine
Case 1: Subsequently, Lassa fever is confirmed on serology. Viral haemorrhagic fevers (VHFs) are some of the most lethal viral infections seen in the world and include Lassa, Ebola, Marburg and Congo-Crimean haemorrhagic fevers. The epidemiology of Ebola and Marburg fever is unknown, but Lassa is acquired from contact with mouse urine in west Africa, and Congo-Crimean haemorrhagic fever from tick bites in Asia and southern Africa. These diseases have a high mortality, from approximately 20% for Lassa to over 80% in cases of Ebola, and are associated with fever, massive bleeding and multiorgan failure. Transmission to other patients and health care workers occurs, especially in resource-poor settings, and isolation and strict barrier nursing should be commenced. Where available, admission of the patient to dangerous pathogen isolation facilities is preferred, and public health services should be informed of a patient with a suspected VHF.

Case 2: A clinical diagnosis of Rickettsial disease is made, with differentials including typhoid fever, malaria, dengue fever and meningococcal sepsis. She gradually improves over the next 7 days with supportive therapy and commencement of ceftriaxone and doxycycline. Gangrenous extremities complicate her recovery. Serology confirms infection with *Rickettsia typhi* (murine typhus), for which the treatment of choice is doxycycline. Rickettsial diseases are prevalent in many countries around the world. They are usually transmitted by an insect vector, often ticks, fleas or lice, and cause febrile diseases associated with spotted skin rashes and eschars (black scab at site of insect bite). Rickettsiae are bacterial infections that respond to treatment with doxycyline.

Clever bugs and defunct drugs
The outbreak was ultimately brought under control after the implementation of draconian strategies. An outbreak committee was called, resulting in the following measures being implemented: cases were cohorted, the ICU was closed to new routine admissions, staff were required to wear gowns and gloves at all times, hand hygiene measures with alcohol were reinforced, intensive cleaning was carried out repeatedly, staff were not rotated around the unit, equipment and consumables were replaced, screening of inpatients took place, and the infection control team visited the unit frequently to reinforce adherence.

The costs to the hospital in financial terms were very high. Direct mortality could not be attributed directly to the outbreak, but there was difficulty in finding beds for patients given the closure to new admissions, and routine surgical cases were cancelled.

Clinical lesson: Infection control precautions should be at a premium at all times. Following the identification of a new infection with the potential to cause an outbreak, appropriate control measures should be adopted promptly and with the full cooperation of the involved parties. Hospital epidemiology and infection control teams should be involved early.

Inflammation
Fever is a common clinical finding in ICU patients. Traditionally, fever has been assumed to be harmful, with treatment aimed at alleviating some of its deleterious effects. The question of whether to treat fever is significant, as the treatments have their own side-effects and carry an estimated cost between $10 000 and $29 000 per year. Fever is defined as an increase in body temperature that is secondary to an upward shift in the hypothalamic set point. This increase is mediated by pyrogens, which endogenously are the cytokines IL-1, TNFα and IL-6, and exogenously are the bacterial products endotoxin and toxic shock syndrome toxin. IL-1 and TNFα induce the synthesis of IL-6, which induces COX-2 activity in the organum vasculosum of the laminae terminalis (OVLT) and the hypothalamic endothelium, producing large amounts of prostaglandin E2 (PGE2). Increased PGE2 leads to increased cyclic adenosine monophosphate (cAMP) production in the preoptic nucleus of the anterior hypothalamus and an elevated thermoregulatory set point. Both paracetamol (acetaminophen) and non-steroidal anti-inflammatory drugs (NSAIDs) inhibit neural COX-2 and thus reduce hypothalamic production of PGE2 and subsequent fever. However, these medicines have side-effects that may be detrimental in severely ill patients, including hepatic and renal dysfunction and decreased gastrointestinal mucosal protection. Non-pharmacological methods of reducing fever include external cooling, which may paradoxically cause decreased heat loss by causing peripheral vasoconstriction.

With regard to clinical evidence, there are no studies to substantiate that elevated core temperature in adults, which rarely exceeds 41°C, is harmful. However, several animal studies have actually demonstrated increased survival with fever. This suggestion of fever having a beneficial effect was supported by a retrospective case series of 612 patients with Gram-negative bacteraemia, which showed that failure to mount a febrile response within the first 24 h was associated with increased mortality. Moreover, a randomised controlled trial of 455 patients with sepsis found no significant difference in 30-day mortality when comparing ibuprofen with placebo. There are also data showing that fever may reduce the production of pro-inflammatory cytokines via suppression of nuclear factor (NF)-κβ. Hence, the current evidence actually supports the concept that fever is a beneficial adaptive response.

Burns
Check the tracheal tube position, and adequacy of ventilation and oxygenation. Arterial blood gas should be obtained along with a carboxyhaemoglobin level. Ventilator F_iO_2 should initially be 1.0. Secure reliable intravenous access through unburned skin and confirm haemodynamic stability. Perform a head-to-toe evaluation to assess the burn's extent and severity, and look for evidence of occult injury. Fluid resuscitation should be guided by a formula and adjusted according to clinical parameters, such as urine output. The burn wounds should be dressed with an appropriate topical agent, such as mupiricin. Large burns (> 20% surface area) or special burns (children, elderly, face, hands, genitalia) should be referred to a specialist burns centre.

Obstetric critical care
Blood pressure > 140/90 or an increase of 30 torr systolic or 15 torr diastolic over baseline in a pregnant patient is

consistent with pregnancy-induced hypertension. Pre-eclampsia also includes features of proteinuria, generalised oedema or both. A careful history and physical examination to evaluate for headache, visual changes, oedema, epigastric pain, along with frequent blood pressure measurements is warranted. Initial laboratory tests should include a complete blood count, platelet count, prothrombin time (PT)/partial thromboplastin time (PTT), renal and hepatic function panels, urinalysis and 24-h protein assessment.

Maternal complications of pre-eclampsia include DIC, convulsions, pulmonary oedema, renal failure, hepatic swelling and/or rupture and intracranial haemorrhage. The major goals of therapy are to prevent convulsions with magnesium sulphate, improve systemic and placental circulation by restoring intravascular volume, minimise the risk of intracranial haemorrhage by controlling blood pressure. In patients who can be relatively well controlled, the pregnancy is allowed to continue until the fetus achieves sufficient size and maturity for survival. In severe pre-eclampsia, eclampsia and the HELLP syndrome, fetal mortality and maternal morbidity is high. The mother should be stabilised quickly for immediate delivery of the fetus and placenta.

Toxicity: poisonings and overdoses

The likely diagnosis is organophosphate insecticide (parathion and malathion) poisoning. These substances bind covalently to cholinesterase, resulting in unremitting muscarinic and nicotinic stimulation. With cholinergic weakness, the patient is at risk of respiratory arrest. A tracheal tube should be positioned. Succinyl choline should be avoided as this can result in prolonged paralysis. Both ventilatory and circulatory support may be required. Atropine and pralidoxime should be administered. One milligram of atropine may be given initially. This may be followed by 2 mg every 15 min until the bradycardia resolves, the pupils dilate, the sweating stops and the secretions dry. Atropine (up to 1500 mg over 24 h!) should be administered until the organophosphate has been metabolised. Pralidoxime 1–2 g intravenously in normal saline reactivates cholinesterase and may be repeated every 6–12 h. Benzodiazepines may be useful to prevent or treat seizures. Hyperglycaemia may occur and should be treated. Nerve gases such as Sarin, which was used by terrorists on the Tokyo subway, are also powerful anticholinesterases. The presentation and treatment are similar to organophosphates.

Trauma

The immediate goals are to ensure that the endotracheal tube is properly placed, and that oxygenation and ventilation are adequate. Tissue perfusion must be assessed. Neurogenic shock is a possibility, but bleeding from his pelvic fracture or missed solid organ injury are more likely sources of hypotension. Invasive monitoring might be helpful. A complete neurological examination is essential to confirm the level of spinal cord injury. Short-acting sedatives may facilitate this.

This patient is at high risk of ventilator-associated pneumonia, DVT and decubitus skin ulceration. Early skeletal stabilisation to facilitate ventilator weaning and mobilisation with physical therapy will help to prevent these complications. Mechanical DVT prophylaxis should be instituted immediately, and pharmacological prophylaxis should be used as soon as bleeding complication risk is minimal. Nutritional support should be started within 48 h if no contraindication exists.

Index

Note: page numbers in *italics* refer to figures and tables

A

ABC (airway, breathing, circulation) 124
advanced cardiac life support team 169
trauma 172–173
Abdominal compartment syndrome 161
Abruptio placentae 162
N-Acetylcysteine 164
Aciclovir 145
Acid burns 161
Acidaemia 185
Acid–base management 44–45, 185
cardiac surgery 93
Stewart approach 45
Acinetobacter baumanii 155, 191
Activated charcoal 164
Activated protein C 131, 133, 189
meningococcal sepsis 190
recombinant human 141
Acute coronary syndrome 84
anatomy 84–85
management 85
Acute disseminated encephalomyelitis (ADEM) 190
Acute fatty liver of pregnancy (AFLP) 163
Acute interstitial nephritis 110, 111
Acute lung injury 143
transfusion-related 61
Acute renal failure *see* renal failure, acute (ARF)
Acute respiratory distress syndrome (ARDS) 33, 46, 100–101, 186
excessive fluid administration 58
outcomes 8
pancreatitis 117
Rickettsial disease 191
ventilation 83
Acute tubular necrosis (ATN) 58, 110–111, 186
gentamicin-induced 188
Adrenal function 122
Adrenal insufficiency 127
Adrenaline 2
asthma respiratory arrest 188
Adrenergic blockade 127
Adrenocorticotropic hormone (ACTH) 122, 127
Advanced cardiac life support 168–169
Aedes mosquito 152, 153
Afterload 40, 96
Agitation 72, 73, 77
Air embolism, vascular access 25
Air space, pressure 32, 33
Aircraft, fixed-wing 10
Airway 22–23, 184
advanced cardiac life support 168
anticipation of problem 22
assessment 22
compliance 100, 102
crisis management 22
dead space 100

patient transportation 11
see also endotracheal tube; lungs
Albumin 53
evidence-based care 9
fluid therapy 59
hypervolaemia 58
Albuterol 102–103, 105
Alcohol
abuse and magnesium disturbances 56
withdrawal 73, 186
Aldosterone 54
Alkali burns 161
Ambulance 10
Amniotic fluid embolism 163
Amphetamine poisoning 164
Analgesia 74–75, 186
non-opiate 186
trauma patients 173
Anaphylaxis 41
Androgens 123
Angina, unstable 84
Angiotensin-converting enzyme (ACE) inhibitors 93, 187
Anion gap (AG) 45
Anopheles mosquito 152
Anterior spinal artery syndrome 68
Anthrax 166, 167
Antibiotics 3, 139
acute tubular necrosis 110, 188
bacterial meningitis 144
benzyl penicillin 143, 151, 190
chickenpox 151
colitis 115, 188
community-acquired pneumonia 146
COPD 105
evidence-based care 8
hospital-acquired pneumonia 146–147
immunocompromised patients 151
intra-abdominal sepsis 189–190
ketotic coma 124
Legionnaire's disease 190
myxoedema coma 127
pancreatitis 117
prophylactic 96
prosthetic material-association infections 147, 148, 190
resistance 154–155, 191
selective decontamination of digestive tract 138
septic shock 142
tuberculosis 145
Antibody deficiency 150
Anti-clotting mechanisms 130, 131
Anticoagulants 131, 132, 134–135
gastrointestinal bleeding 112
Anticoagulation 34
strategies 134–135
Antidiuretic hormone (ADH) 54
Antigen-presenting cells (APCs) 158
Antiplatelet agents 135
see also aspirin
Antithrombin 131, 189
Antithyroid therapy 126, 189
Alpha-1 antitrypsin deficiency 104
Anxiety 72

Aprotinin 133, 189
Argatroban 135, 189
Arrhythmias 88–89, 168, 187
diagnosis 88
magnesium disturbances 56
Artemisinin compounds 153
Arterial lines 25
Aspirin 96, 132, 135, 187
poisoning 165
Asthma 102–103, 188
acid–base management 45, 185
bronchoscopy 27
mechanical ventilation 33, 184
obstructive shock 41
permissive hypercapnia 33
severe attack management 102–103
status asthmaticus 69, 186
Atelectasis 32–33, 139, 187
Atrial fibrillation 89
Atrial flutter 89
Atrioventricular node 88
Atropine 192
Auditory evoked potentials 64, 65
Automated external defibrillator (AED) 168
Automaticity 88
AutoPEEP 187
Autoregulation 40, 41
Avian influenza A 146, 147

B

Bacillus anthracis 166, 167
Bacteria
drug resistance 154–155, 191
see also infection; meningitis, bacterial; *named organisms*
Bag–mask ventilation 168
Barotrauma 32
Bedsores 173, 192
Benzodiazepines 77, 103
alcohol withdrawal 73
organophosphate poisoning 192
poisoning 164
withdrawal 73
Benzyl penicillin 143, 151, 190
Beta-adrenergic antagonists 85, 187
thyroid storm 126
Beta-agonists 102, 105
Bicarbonate, ketotic coma 124
Biliary colic 97
Bilirubin, unconjugated 97
Biofilm formation 148
Biological agent attacks 166
Bioterrorism 166–167
Bivalirudin 135, 189
Bleeding 130–131, 132–133, 189
causes 132–133
congenital 132
gastrointestinal 112–113, 188
haemorrhagic shock 92
intracranial in pre-eclampsia 163, 191, 192
peripartum 162
pharmacological treatment 133
surgical 133
Blood flow, shunt 100

Blood pressure
monitoring 18, 19, 19, 64, 184
postural change 83
see also hypertension; hypotension
Blood transfusions 3, 60–61, 185
incompatibility 61
risks 60, 61
see also transfusion-related acute lung injury (TRALI)
Blood viscosity, pregnancy 162
Blood volume, pregnancy 162
Blood/blood components 60–61
Blue bloater 104
Boston formula 45
Botulinum toxin 166
Bowel obstruction 114
Bowel sounds 53
Bradyarrhythmias 89
Bradycardia 89
Brain
damage 171
temporal lobe necrosis 144–145
Brain death 79
determination 78
Brain injury 66–67
acute head injury 47
traumatic 170, 171
treatment 66–67
Brainstem infarct 101
Breathing
rescue 168
see also ABC (airway, breathing, circulation)
Bronchial anatomy 26
Bronchial/bronchoalveolar lavage (BAL) 26, 27, 147, 190
Bronchitis, chronic 104
Bronchodilators 102
Bronchoscopy 26–27, 184
Bronchospasm 27, 187
Burns 160–161, 191

C

Caecal volvulus 114
Calcium 55
emergency management of derangement 57
Calibration, traceable 18
Candida
infections 139
sepsis 140
Capillaries, leaky 58, 59
Carbon dioxide 46–47
end-tidal 169
narcosis 102
ventilation–perfusion ratio 100
Carbon dioxide partial pressure (P_aCO_2) 2, 32, 44
acid–base balance 45
Carbon monoxide toxicity 160–161
Cardiac arrest
cardiac life support 168
hyperkalaemic 69
pre-arrest period 169
Cardiac biomarkers 85, 187
Cardiac catheterisation 2
Cardiac failure 37, 185

Cardiac index 41, 185
Cardiac life support, advanced 168–169
Cardiac output 40, 41, 43, 185
  pregnancy 162
Cardiac pacemakers 2
Cardiac pacing 90–91, 187
Cardiac shunting 97, 100
Cardiac surgery 92–93, 187
Cardiac tamponade 187
Cardiogenic shock 41, 92
Cardiopulmonary bypass 49
  complications 92
Cardiopulmonary resuscitation 168–169
Cardiovascular system
  function tests 82
  monitoring 82–83, 118–119, 186
  proxies for function 82
Catheters
  chest radiographs 106, 107
  see also central venous catheter; pulmonary artery catheter
Causation 16
CD4 cells 158
Cellular immunity, impaired 150
Central nervous system (CNS)
  infection 144–145, 190
  injury 66–67, 186
  severe disorders 171
Central nervous system (CNS)-mediated disability 170
Central venous catheter 107
  burns 160
  infection 148
Centrifugal rotary pump 36, 37
Cerebral abscess 145
Cerebral blood flow 66
Cerebral perfusion pressure (CPP) 28, 66, 67, 186
  liver failure 119
  monitoring 64
Cerebral vascular occlusion 125
Cerebral vascular resistance (CVR) 66
Cerebral ventricles 28
Cerebrospinal fluid 28–29, 184
  bacterial meningitis diagnosis 144
  leaks 29
Cervical spinal cord injury 173, 192
Chemical attacks 166
Chemical burns 161
Chemotherapeutic agents 132, 150
Chest compressions 168–169
Chest pain 84, 85
Chest radiographs, portable 106–107, 188
Chest wall impedance 32
Chickenpox 151
Child–Turcotte–Pugh scoring system 118, 119
Cholecystectomy 116, 117
Cholecystitis 116, 188
Cholelithiasis 97
Christmas disease 132
Chronic obstructive pulmonary disease (COPD) 59, 104–105, 186, 188
  epidemiology 104
  exacerbation 187
  management 104–105
  obstructive shock 41
  pathophysiology 104

ventilation 101, 105
Circulation 40–41, 185
  fetal 96–97
  neonatal 97
  physiology 40, 41
Circulatory support, mechanical 36–37, 185
Clinical excellence 16–17, 184
Clopidogrel 135
Clostridium difficile 115, 188
Clotting 130–131
Clotting agents 130–131
Clotting factors 132
  recombinant 133, 189
Coagulopathy 131
  acquired 132–133
Cocaine poisoning 164–165
Codes of practice
  brain death determination 78
  see also protocols
Colitis 115
Colloids 186, 190
Colonic pseudo-obstruction 114–115
Colonoscopy 112
Coma
  diabetic 124–125
  ketotic 124–125
  myxoedema 126–127
  persistent 170
Compensatory anti-inflammatory response syndrome (CARS) 140, 159
Computerised tomography (CT)
  central nervous system injury 66
  neurological assessment 64
  pulmonary hypertension 94, 95, 187
  seizures 70
Confusion 72
Congenital heart disease 96–97
Congestive heart failure 86
Constipation 115
Continuous positive airway pressure (CPAP) 32, 101
  COPD 105
Continuous renal replacement therapy (CRRT) 34
Continuous veno-venous haemodialysis (CVVHD) 34, 35, 185
Contractility 40
Convulsions
  pre-eclampsia 163, 191–192
  see also seizures
Coronary artery bypass surgery 93, 187
Coronary artery disease 84, 86
Coronary care units 2
Coronary perfusion pressure 85
Corticosteroids
  gastrointestinal bleeding 112
  spinal cord injury 67
  see also steroids
Corticotrophin-releasing hormone 122
Cortisol 122
Cortisol-binding globulin (CBG) 122
COX-2 191
C-reactive protein 143
Creatine phosphokinase 85
Critical oxygen delivery 42
Cryoprecipitate 61

Crystalloids 186
CURB-65 score 146
Cycle of therapy 12, 13
Cytochrome P450 (CYP) 12–13
Cytokines 158
  anti-inflammatory 158
  proinflammatory 140, 191

D

Daptomycin 155
Dead space 100
Decision-making 171
Decubitus ulcers 67, 173, 192
Deep vein cannulation 25
Deep vein thrombosis 173
  prophylaxis 67
  trauma patient 192
Defibrillation
  advanced cardiac life support 168
  emergency 187
Dehydration 58
Dehydroepiandrosterone (DHEA) 122
Delirium 72, 173, 186
  management/prevention 73
Delirium tremens 73
Dementia 72
Dengue 152–153
Dengue haemorrhagic fever 152–153
Desmopressin (DDAVP) 132, 133
Dexamethasone, evidence-based care 9
Diabetes insipidus 79
Diabetes mellitus 86, 124–125, 189
  complications 125
Diabetic ketoacidosis 17, 124–125, 126, 184
Diagnostic tests, potential errors 16
Dialysis 2
  peritoneal 34
  see also haemodialysis
Dialysis disequilibrium syndrome 35, 185
Diarrhoea, enteral feeding 115
Diastolic augmentation 85
Diastolic dysfunction 92
Diazepam 77
Diets
  organ-specific 53
  see also nutrition
Dilutional acidosis 45
Disability 171, 173
Disseminated intravascular coagulation (DIC) 132–133
  meningococcal sepsis 143
  placental abruption 162
  pre-eclampsia 191
  viral haemorrhagic fever 153
Distributive shock 41, 185
Diuretics 54, 55
  fluid overload 58
Drug interactions 12–13, 184
Drug resistance 154–155, 191
  malaria 153
Ductus arteriosus, patent 97
Dysphagia 67
Dyspnoea 102

E

Eaton–Lambert syndrome 69
Echocardiography 82, 83, 186

cardiac surgery management 93
pulmonary hypertension 95, 187
transoesophageal 134, 186
transthoracic 82, 83
Eclampsia 192
Electrical burns 161
Electrocardiogram (ECG)
  gastrointestinal bleeding 112
  hyperkalaemia changes 55
  ischaemic heart disease 85
  magnesium disturbances 56
  pulmonary hypertension 94, 187
  sinus tachycardia 187
Electroencephalogram (EEG) 64, 65
  seizures 70
Electrolytes
  abnormalities 54–57, 185
  cardiac surgery management 93
Emphysema 104, 105
  surgical 151
Encephalitis, viral 144–145
Encephalomyelitis, acute disseminated 190
Encephalopathy
  hepatic 118, 119
  hypoxic–ischaemic 170
  Wernicke's 73
Endocrine emergencies 126–127, 189
Endocrine function 122–123
End-of-life care 171
Endotracheal tube 26
  advanced cardiac life support 168
  cervical spinal cord injury 192
  cuffed 22
  infection 33
  migration 27, 184
  patient transportation 11
  removal 33
Energy
  provision 53
  requirements 52
Enteral feeding 52
  diarrhoea 115
  pancreatitis 117
  trauma patients 173
Enterobacteriaceae 147
Enterococci 155
Epidural analgesia 74–75
Epileptic seizures 70
Epinephrine see adrenaline
Epsilon aminocaproic acid 133, 189
Errors
  checking 16
  systems approach 17
  trapping 17
Escharotomy 161
Escherichia coli 150
  sepsis 140
Ethics 170–171
Evaporative loss 48
Evidence-based intensive care 8–9, 184
Extracellular fluid (ECF) 54
  pregnancy 162
Extubation 33

F

Face mask 22
Facilities 4

Factor VII 119
Factor VIII 132
Factor IX deficiency 132
False alarms 19
Family 5
  care 171
  consensus 171
  limitation/withdrawal of
      treatment 170
  meetings 170–171
  organ donation 78–79
  relationship with team 170–171
Feeding 3
Feeding tube 106
  misplacement 107, 188
FENA (fractional excretion of
      sodium) equation 110–111
Fever 48–49, 159, 191
  transfusion-induced 60
Fibreoptic bronchoscopy 26–27,
      184
  complications 27
  landmarks 26, 27
  technique 26–27
Fluid balance 54
  diabetes mellitus 125
Fluid overload, diagnosis 58
Fluid restriction 58
Fluid resuscitation 41, 185
  burns 160, 191
  diabetic ketoacidosis 126
  septic shock 142, 190
Fluid status, postural change in
      blood pressure 83
Fluid therapy 58–59, 186
  asthma respiratory arrest 188
  diabetic ketoacidosis 126
  excess 58
  hyperosmolar states 125
  ketotic coma 124
  myxoedema coma 127
  pancreatitis 117
Foramen ovale, patent 97, 134
Frank–Starling curve 40
Fresh frozen plasma 61

G

Gallbladder disease 116
Gastrointestinal tract
  bleeding 112–113, 188
  bowel sounds 53
  gut irrigation 164
  motility disorders 114–115, 188
  selective contamination 138–139
Gastroparesis 67
Ginkgo biloba 132
Glasgow Coma Scale 64, 66, 67,
      186
  traumatic brain injury 170
Glomerular filtration rate,
      pregnancy 162
Glomerulonephritis 110
Glucocorticoids 122, 127
Glucose control 124, 125, 189
Glycogen body stores 52
Granulocytopenia 150
Growth hormone (GH) 122–123
Guidelines 8–9
Guidewire removal 25, 184
Guillain–Barré syndrome 68–69
  pain management 74
Gut irrigation 164

H

Haemodialysis
  continuous veno-venous 34, 35,
      185
  hyperphosphataemia 56
  intermittent 34
Haemodynamic monitoring 59
Haemodynamic stability, patient
      transportation 10–11
Haemofiltration, high-volume 34
Haemoglobin 42, 43, 60
Haemolytic uraemic syndrome
      (HUS) 163
Haemophilia A 132
Haemophilus influenzae 144, 150
Haemophilus meningitis 144
Haemorrhagic shock 92
Hand hygiene 138, 154
Handwashing 3
Head injury, acute 47
Headache, post-lumbar puncture
      29
Hearing loss, sensorineural 144
Heart attack, intravascular
      clotting 131
Heart block 89
  transcutaneous pacing 91
Heart disease
  congenital 96–97
  cyanotic 97
  ischaemic 84–85, 186–187
  valvular 96, 97
Heart failure 86–87, 187
  assessment 86
  clinical syndrome 86
  diastolic 86
  factors 87
  management 87
  right 92
  systolic 86
Heart muscle
  contractility 40
  see also myocardial entries
Heart rate monitoring 19, 184
Heart valves, prosthetic 96
Heat loss 48
Helicobacter pylori 112
Helicopter 10
HELLP syndrome 163, 192
Helper T cells 158
Henderson–Hasselbalch (HH)
      equation 44, 45
Heparin 132, 135, 189
  anticoagulation 34
  bacterial meningitis 189
  disseminated intravascular
      coagulation 133
  pulmonary embolus 173
Heparin-induced thrombocytopenia
      (HIT) 135, 189
Hepatic drain 190
Hepatic encephalopathy 118, 119
Hepatic failure, fulminant 118
Hepatorenal syndrome 119
Herpes simplex virus (HSV)
      encephalitis 144
High-volume haemofiltration
      (HVHF) 34
Histamine-2 receptor blockers 112
History of intensive care 2–3
HIV infection 150–151
  post-exposure prophylaxis 190

tropical areas 152
Human leucocyte antigens
      (HLA) 60, 61
Humoral immunity deficiency 150
Hydrocephalus 28, 144
Hypercalcaemia 55, 56
  hyperphosphataemia
      combination 56
Hypercapnia 100
  hazards 46, 47
  mild 46
  permissive 33
  therapeutic 47
Hypercarbia 53, 185
Hyperglycaemia 123, 124, 125
  sepsis 141
Hyperkalaemia 55
  suxamethonium-induced 69
Hypernatraemia 54
Hyperosmolar non-ketotic coma
      (HONK) 126
Hyperosmolar states 125
Hyperparathyroidism 55
Hyperphosphataemia 56
Hypertension
  pre-eclampsia 163, 191–192
  see also pulmonary hypertension
Hyperthermia 49
Hyperthyroidism 189
Hyperventilation 46
Hyperviscosity 125
Hypervolaemia, total body 58
Hypocalcaemia 55, 185
  magnesium disturbances 56
Hypocapnia, dangers 46–47
Hypokalaemia 35, 54–55, 185
Hyponatraemia 54
Hypoparathyroidism 55, 185
Hypophosphataemia 56
Hypotension
  management 85
  organ donation 79
Hypothalamus–pituitary–adrenal
      axis 122
Hypothermia 49
Hypothyroidism
  myxoedema coma 126
  respiratory failure 101
Hypoventilation 100
Hypovolaemia, intravascular
      58–59
Hypovolaemic shock 11
Hypoxaemia 100
Hypoxia 43, 159
Hypoxic–ischaemic
      encephalopathy 170

I

Ileus 115
Immune cells 158
Immunocompromised patient
      150–151, 190
Immunonutrition 53
Impaired glucose tolerance 125
Implantable cardioverter/
      defibrillator 187
Infection
  bacterial drug resistance 154–155,
      191
  cardiac surgery management 93
  CNS 144–145, 190
  early recognition 124

endotracheal tube 33
hospital-acquired 138, 146–147,
      190
  intracranial 145
  intravascular cannulae 148
  liver failure 119
  peritoneal 34
  prevention 138–139, 190
  prosthetic materials 148–149,
      190
  risk with platelet transfusion 61
  treatment 138–139, 189
  urinary catheter-associated
      148–149
  ventilation 32
  see also HIV infection; named
      organisms; viral entries
Infection control 3
  bronchoscopy 27
  measures 155, 191
Inferior vena cava filters 135
Inflammation 58, 158–159, 191
  activation 158–159
Inflammatory response 158
  balance 159
Inhalation injury 160
Insulin resistance 123, 124, 141
Insulin therapy 125
  intensive 141
  ketotic coma 124
  meningococcal sepsis 190
Intensive care unit 4, 5
Intensivist team
  consensus 171
  responsibilities 170
  trauma patients 173
  see also staff
Intermittent haemodialysis
      (IHD) 34
International normalised ratio
      (INR) 119, 132
Intestinal decompression 115
Intra-abdominal pressure,
      pregnancy 162
Intra-aortic balloon pump 37
Intracranial haemorrhage,
      pre-eclampsia 163, 191, 192
Intracranial infection 145
Intracranial pressure (ICP) 66
  low 29
  monitoring 119
  monitors 64, 65
  raised 28–29, 40
    hypercapnia 46
    lumbar puncture
      contraindication 144
    reduction 186
Intraparenchymal transducers 29
Intravascular cannulae, associated
      infections 148
Intravascular volume depletion 58
Intravenous access, patient
      transportation 11
Intraventricular catheters 29
Intubation 103
  patient transportation 11
Intussusception 114

J

Jejunostomy, feeding 52
Jugular vein abscess 149, 190
Jugular venous oximetry 64

K

Ketamine 103
Ketotic coma 124–125
Klebsiella pneumoniae 150

L

Lactic acid 43
Lactic acidosis 102, 143
Laplace's law *33, 40, 41, 96*
Large bowel obstruction 114
Laryngeal mask airway 22, 23, 188
Laryngospasm 27
Lassa fever 190–191
Left ventricular assist device
    (LVAD) 36, 185
Left ventricular dysfunction 86, 96
Left ventricular heart failure 86, 87
Left ventricular hypertrophy 40
Left-to-right shunts 97
Legionnaire's disease 146, 190
Leucocytes 158
    reduction 61
Leukaemia 150
Life support, advanced cardiac
    168–169
Linezolid 155
Liotta heart 36
Lipogenesis, hepatic 185
Lipopolysaccharide 159
Liver
    deranged function 143
    lipogenesis 185
    transplantation 119, 188–189
Liver failure 118–119, 188–189
    coagulopathy 132
    paracetamol poisoning 164
Lorazepam 77
Lumbar puncture 29, 184
Lundberg A waves 28, 29
Lungs
    acute injury 61, 143
    asthma 102
    collapse 32–33
    compliance 100, 102
    hyperinflated 102, 105
    injury 46
    overdistension 32
    transfusion-related injury 61,
        100–101
Lymphoma 150

M

Magnesium 56
    emergency management of
        derangement *57*
Magnesium sulphate 163
Magnetic resonance imaging
    (MRI) 64
    epidural haematoma 75
    seizures 70
Major incident protocol 167
Malaria 152, 153
Malathion 192
Malignancy 55
Malnutrition 173
Mean arterial pressure (MAP) 40,
    54, 66
    monitoring 64
    raising 186

Mechanical circulatory support
    36–37, 185
Mechanical ventilation 32–33, 184
    asthma 33, 103, 184
    hyperventilation 47, 185
    obstructive shock 41
    pneumonia 47, 185
Medtronic Biomedicus pump 36
Memory of intensive care 77
Meningitis
    bacterial 131, 144, 189
    tuberculous 29, 145, 184
Meningococcal sepsis 143, 190
Mental state, altered 72–73, 186
Meperidine *see* pethidine
Mesenteric vasculopathy 112
Metabolic acidosis 43
Metabolic carts 52
Metabolic needs 52
Metabolic rate, shivering 49, 185
Methadone 73
    analgesia 75
    drug interactions 13, 184
Methicillin-resistant *Staphylococcus
    aureus* (MRSA) 138, 147, 154
    new drugs 155
Methimazole 126, 189
Microcirculation 82–83
Midazolam 77, 103
Middle cerebral artery *65*
Mitral valve, systolic anterior motion
    of the leaflet 92
Models 17
Monitoring 18–19, 184
    accuracy 18–19
    adverse effects 18–19
    burns 160, 191
    cardiovascular system 82–83,
        118–119, 186
    false alarms 19
    haemodynamic 59
    intracranial pressure 29, 66, 119
    liver failure 118–119
    neurological 64, 119, 186
    nutritional 53, 118
    oxygen delivery 43
    precision 18–19
    renal system 119
    respiratory system 119
    transportation 11
Monro–Kellie doctrine 28, 66
Morphine 75, 187
Mosquitoes 152, 153
Multiorgan dysfunction
    medical commendations 171
    meningococcal sepsis 143
    prognosis 170
    weakness 68
Multiorgan dysfunction syndrome
    (MODS) 159
Multiple endocrine neoplasia
    (MEN) type II 127
Multiple myeloma 151
Murine typhus 191
Muscle relaxants, non-depolarising
    103
Myasthenia gravis 69
Mycobacterium tuberculosis 145
    see also meningitis, tuberculous
Myocardial contractility 40
Myocardial infarction (MI) 43, 84
    complications *84*
    gastrointestinal bleeding 112, 188

Myocardial ischaemia, acute 186–187
Myocardial oxygen demand 84
Myocardial stunning 92
Myopathy of intensive care 68, 69,
    168
    steroid 188
Myxoedema coma 126–127

N

N-acetylcysteine 164
Naloxone 165
Nasojejunal tube 52
Necrotising myopathy of intensive
    care 168
Needle cricothyroidotomy 23
Neisseria meningitidis 144, 150
Nerve gas 192
    chemical attacks 166
Neurogenic shock 67
Neurological injuries, seizures 70
Neurological system
    assessment 64–65, 186
    function preservation 71
    monitoring 119
Neuromuscular blocking agents 69,
    168
    sedation 76
Neuropathic pain 75
Nitrates 85, 187
Nitric oxide 95
Non-depolarising muscle relaxants
    103
Non-positive pressure ventilation
    (NIPPV) 101
Non-ST elevation myocardial
    infarction (NSTEMI) 84
    management 85
Non-steroidal anti-inflammatory
    drugs (NSAIDs) 112
Noradrenaline 2, 190
Norepinephrine *see* noradrenaline
Nuclear factor (NF)-κB 191
Nutrition 3, 52–53, 185
    monitoring 118
    trauma patients 173, 192
    see also enteral feeding; total
        parenteral nutrition (TPN)
Nutritional assessment 53

O

Obstetric critical care 162–163,
    191–192
Obstructive shock 41, 102
Oesophagogastroduodenoscopy
    112, 188
Ogilvie's syndrome 114–115
Ondine's curse *101*
Opiates 75, 85
    respiratory depression 101, 188
Opioids
    intoxication 165
    withdrawal 72–73, 165
Organ donation 78–79
    offering option to family 78–79
    process 78
    recipients 79
    responsibilities 78
Organ dysfunction 43
Organ perfusion 59
Organ transplantation, weakness 68
Organophosphates

chemical attacks 166
    poisoning *165*, 192
Orotracheal tube, armoured 23, 184
Otitis media 145
Overdoses 164–165
Oxycodone 75
Oxygen
    arterial saturation 43
    delivery 42–43, 185
    partial pressure 32
    supplemental 168
    venous saturation 43, 185
    ventilation–perfusion ratio 100
Oxygen consumption
    pregnancy 162
    valvular heart disease 96
Oxygen electrodes 2
Oxygen extraction ratio (OER) 42
Oxygenation 22, 23
Oxyhaemoglobin dissociation
    curve 46

P

Pacemakers
    biventricular 91, 187
    capture 91
    leads 25
    oversensing 90, 187
    permanent 90, 93, 96
    temporary 90–91
Pacing 90–91, 187
    biventricular 90, *91*
    epicardial 90, *91*
    modes 90
    sense 90, 91
    transcutaneous 91, 187
    transvenous 91, 187
Packed red blood cells 60
Pain
    assessment 74
    burn victims 161
    management 74, 161
    monitoring 64
    relief 74–75
    see also analgesia
Pancreatic necrosis, infected 117
Pancreatitis 116–117, 188
Papilloedema 28, *29*
Paracetamol 74
    poisoning 164
Paranasal sinuses, chronic
    infection 145
Parathion 192
Parathyroid hormone 55
Parkinson's disease 74
Patient
    care 171
    limitation/withdrawal of treatment
        170
    outcomes 5
Patient-controlled analgesia (PCA) 75
Peak expiratory flow rate 103
Penicillin 3
Peptic ulcer disease 112
Peripartum haemorrhage 162
Peritoneal dialysis 34
Pethidine 165
Petrol burns 161
pH
    gastric intramucosal 82
    regulation 44
Phaeochromocytoma 127

Phenol burns 161
Phosphates 56, 57
Physiological stability maintenance for organ donation 79
Pink puffer 104
Placenta praevia 162
Plague 166
Plasmodium 152, 153
Platelets 60–61
  contamination 61
  transfusion 60–61, 189
Pneumocystis jiroveci pneumonia (PCP) 101, 151
Pneumonia 41, 46, 185, 187
  biventricular pacemaker 91, 187
  community-acquired 146, 147, 190
  hospital-acquired 146–147, 190
  mechanical ventilation 47, 185
  PCP 101, 151
  ventilator-associated 33, 147, 173, 192
  viral vectors 147
Pneumothorax 92, 93, 107, 187
Poisoning 164–165
  exposure reduction 164
Poliomyelitis epidemic 2
Polyneuropathy, critical illness 68, 69
Positive end-expiratory pressure (PEEP) 32
  COPD 105
  intrinsic 102, 103
  loss 27
Post-antibiotic era 154
Post-exposure prophylaxis (PEP) 190
Potassium 35, 54–55, 185
  diabetes mellitus 124, 125
  emergency management of derangement 57
  ketotic coma 124
Pralidoxime 192
Pre-eclampsia 163, 191 192
Pregnancy, physiological changes 162
Preload 40
Pressure control ventilation 32
Pressure–volume loops 96
Prognosis assessment 170
Prolactin 123
Propofol 77
Propylthiouracil 126, 189
Prostacyclin, inhaled 95
Prostaglandin E2 (PGE2) 191
Prosthetic materials, associated infections 148–149, 190
Protocols 8–9
  major incident 167
Proton pump inhibitors 112
Pseudomonas aeruginosa 147
  resistance 154
Puerperal sepsis 3
Pulmonary artery
  catheterisation 82, 83
  occlusion pressure 83
  pulmonary hypertension 94
Pulmonary artery catheter 25, 82, 83
  chest radiograph 106, 107
  complications 25
  evidence-based care 9
  pacing 91
Pulmonary embolus 130, 131, 134, 187, 188

trauma patients 173
Pulmonary hypertension 94–95, 187
Pulmonary oedema
  opioid withdrawal 165
  pre-eclampsia 191
  tocolytic-induced 162
Pulmonary vascular resistance 46
Pulsatile blood pump 36, 37
Pulse check 168
Pulse oximetry, burns 160
Pulsus paradoxus 59

Q
QRS complex 88

R
R on T phenomenon 90
Radiation exposure 166–167
Ramsay scale 76
Rapid-sequence induction (RSI) 23
Recoil pressure 33
Red cell transfusion 60
Refeeding 52
Reid index 104
Renal failure 110–111, 188
Renal failure, acute (ARF) 34–35
  aetiology 111
  causes 110–111
  definition 110
  pre-eclampsia 163, 191
  treatment 111
Renal impairment 143
Renal protection 111
Renal replacement therapy 2, 34–35, 185
  acute tubular necrosis 186
  complications 35
  discontinuation 35
Renal system monitoring 119
Respiratory acidosis 46, 188
Respiratory arrest, cardiorespiratory 188
Respiratory depression 101, 188
Respiratory failure 32, 100–101, 188
  asthma 102
  community-acquired pneumonia 146
  trauma 173
  see also acute respiratory distress syndrome (ARDS)
Respiratory quotient 53, 185
Respiratory system monitoring 119
Rest, non-pharmacological methods 77
Restrictive shock 41
Rewarming 49, 185
Rickettsial disease 191
Right atrial enlargement 94
Right heart failure 92
Right-to-left shunts 97
Right ventricular heart failure 86, 87
Right ventricular hypertrophy 94

S
Safety in transportation 10
Salicylates
  poisoning 165
  see also aspirin
Saline 59

Sarin 166, 192
Scientific induction 17
Scientific theory 17
Sedation 76–77, 186
  assessment 76
  drugs 77
  goals 76–77
  management 76–77
  monitoring 64
  tracheal intubation 103
  trauma patients 173
Seizures 64, 70–71, 186
  alcohol withdrawal 73
  cocaine poisoning 164, 165
  opioid withdrawal 165
  pre-eclampsia 163, 191–192
Selective decontamination of digestive tract 138–139
Sepsis 41, 58, 140–143
  bleeding 132, 133
  community-acquired pneumonia 146
  complications 140, 141
  medical recommendations 171
  prognosis 170
  treatment 142
Septic shock 140–143
  treatment 142
Severe acute respiratory syndrome (SARS) 146, 147, 150
Sharps injuries 151, 190
Shivering 49, 185
Shock 41, 102, 185
  dengue syndrome 152–153
  heart surgery 92
  neurogenic 192
  septic 140–143
  spinal 67
  treatment 142
Shock liver 118
Shunt 97, 100
Shunt surgery 112
Sick sinus syndrome 89
Sigmoid volvulus 114
Sinoatrial node 88
Sinus tachycardia 89, 187
Sleep apnoea, central 101
Slow low-efficiency daily dialysis (SLEDD) 34
Small bowel obstruction 114, 115, 188
Smallpox 166, 167
  vaccination 190
Smoking 104
Sodium 54
  correction with glucose level 125
  emergency management of derangement 57
Somatosensory evoked potentials 170
Somatotropic axis 122–123
Spinal cord injury 67
Spinal immobilisation 67
  patient transportation 11
Spinal shock 67
Spiral impeller 36, 37
Splenectomy 150, 151
Sputum, microbiological examination 147
ST elevation myocardial infarction (STEMI) 84
  diagnosis/management 85
Staff 8

outcomes 5
  synergy between 17
  team 170, 171
  trauma patients 173
Staphylococcus aureus
  sepsis 140
  vancomycin-resistant 155
  see also methicillin-resistant Staphylococcus aureus (MRSA)
Starvation 52, 185
  recovery 52
Statins 187
Status asthmaticus 69, 103, 186
Status epilepticus 70–71, 168
  management algorithm 71
Steroids
  asthma 102, 103
  bacterial meningitis 144
  COPD 105
  myopathy 188
  tuberculosis 145
  see also corticosteroids
Streptococcus pneumoniae 144, 146, 150, 151
  sepsis 140
Streptokinase 135
Stress 122
  hyperglycaemia 123
Stress ulcers 67
Stress-related erosive syndrome (SRES) 112, 188
Stroke 43, 69
  intravascular clotting 131
  ischaemic 47
  respiratory failure 101
Stroke volume 40, 96
  pregnancy 162
Strong ion difference (SID) 45, 124
Subdural empyema 145
Sulphonamides 3
Supraventricular tachycardia 89
Surfactant 33
Suxamethonium 69
Sweating 48
Synchronised intermittent mandatory ventilation with pressure support (SIMV + PS) 32
Synercid® 155
Systemic inflammatory response syndrome (SIRS) 41, 58, 140
  cardiac surgery complications 92
  transfusion-induced 60
  weakness 68
Systemic vascular resistance, pregnancy 162
Systolic anterior motion of the mitral valve leaflet (SAM) 92

T
T helper cells 158
Tachyarrhythmias 88–89
Tachycardia 89, 187
Tamponade 93
Technical components 2–3
Temperature, interthreshold range 48
Tension pneumothorax 92, 93, 187
Testosterone 123
Tetany 55
Thermal disorders 48–49, 185
Thermoregulation 48, 49

Thiamine 73
Thoracostomy tube 106, *107*
  patient transportation 11
Thrombocytopenia, heparin-induced 135, 189
Thromboembolic disease 173
Thrombophilia 131, 134
Thrombosis 130, 131, 134–135, 189
  prophylaxis 134, 135
  risk factors *134*
  trauma patient 173, 192
Thrombotic thrombocytopenic purpura (TTP) 163
Thyroid function 122
Thyroid storm 126, 189
Thyroidectomy 57, 185
Thyroid-stimulating hormone (TSH) 122, 126
Thyrotrophin-releasing hormone (TRH) 122
Thyroxine (T4) 122
  myxoedema coma 126, 127
Tissue factor pathway inhibitor 133, 189
Tissue hypoxia 43
Tissue plasminogen activator 135
Tocolytic therapy, pulmonary oedema 162
Toll-like receptors 158–159
Tongue microcirculation 83
Total body water (TBW) 54
Total parenteral nutrition (TPN) 52, 173
Toxicity 164–165
Tracheal extubation 33
Tracheal intubation 103
  patient transportation 11
Tracheostomy

COPD 105
  dislodged 22, 23
Tracheostomy tubes 26
Tramadol 75
Tranexamic acid 133, 189
Transcranial Doppler ultrasonography (TCD) 64
Transfusion-induced immunomodulation (TRIM) 60
Transfusion-related acute lung injury (TRALI) 61, 100–101, 186
Transjugular intrahepatic portosystemic shunt (TIPS) 112
Transoesophageal echocardiography (TOE) 134, 186
Transportation 10–11, 184
Transthoracic echocardiography (TTE) 82, 83
Trauma 172–173, 191
  evaluation 172–173
  multidisciplinary approach 173
Traumatic brain injury 170, 171
Treatment limiting/withdrawal 170–171
Triiodothyronine (T3) 122
  myxoedema coma 126, 127
Tropical medicine 152–153, 191
Troponins 85, 187
  gastrointestinal bleeding 112
Trousseau's sign 55
Tuberculosis
  treatment 145
  see also meningitis, tuberculous
Tubes
  chest radiographs 106, *107*
  orotracheal armoured 23, 184

tracheal/tracheostomy 26
see also endotracheal tube; feeding tube
Typhus 191

U

Ultrasound
  transcranial Doppler 64
  vascular access 24–25
Urinary catheters, infections 148–149
Urinary tract infection 148–149
Urine output 59

V

Vancomycin-resistant enterococci (VRE) 138, 154, 155
Variola major 166, *167*
Vascular access 24–25, 184
  complications 25
Vascular puncture, complications 25
Vasoplegia *92*, 93
Vasopressin 141, 190
Vasopressor therapy 142, 190
Vecuronium 103
Ventilation 2
  assisted 101
  control 100
  COPD 101, 105
  plateau pressures 32
  small volume 32
  terminology 32
  during transportation 10–11
  see also mechanical ventilation
Ventilation–perfusion mismatch 100, 188

Ventilation–perfusion ratio 100
Ventilation–perfusion scan *100*
  pulmonary hypertension 187
Ventilator problems 32–33
Ventilatory monitoring 2
Ventricular fibrillation 89
  cardiac arrest 168
  see also left ventricular *entries*; right ventricular *entries*
Ventricular hypertrophy 96
Ventricular tachycardia 89
Ventriculostomy catheters 64, *65*
Viral encephalitis 144–145
Viral haemorrhagic fever 153, 190–191
Virchow's triad 134
  trauma patients 173
Vitamin B12 73
Vitamin D 55
Volutrauma 32
Volvulus 114
Von Willebrand factor (vWF) 132, 133
Von Willebrand's disease 132

W

Warfarin 132, 134–135, 189
Weakness 68–69, 186
Wernicke's encephalopathy 73
Withdrawal of treatment 170–171
World Health Organization (WHO) pain ladder 74
Wound care, burns 161

Y

Yersinia pestis 166

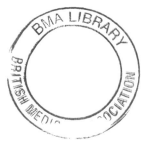